Fundamentals of Pain Medicine

Jiangguo Cheng • Richard W. Rosenquist
Editors

Fundamentals of Pain Medicine

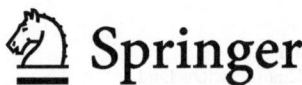
Springer

Editors
Jianguo Cheng, MD, PhD
Professor of Anesthesiology
President-elect, American Academy of Pain Medicine
Director, Cleveland Clinic Multidisciplinary Pain Medicine Fellowship Program
Departments of Pain Management and Neurosciences
Cleveland Clinic Anesthesiology Institute and Lerner Research Institute
Cleveland, OH, USA

Richard W. Rosenquist, MD
Chairman, Department Pain Management
Cleveland Clinic
Cleveland, OH, USA

ISBN 978-3-319-64920-7 ISBN 978-3-319-64922-1 (eBook)
https://doi.org/10.1007/978-3-319-64922-1

Library of Congress Control Number: 2017958545

Printed on acid-free paper

This Springer imprint is published by Springer Nature
The registered company is Springer International Publishing AG
The registered company address is: Gewerbestrasse 11, 6330 Cham, Switzerland

Contents

Contributors

Salahadin Abdi, MD, PhD Department of Pain Medicine, The University of Texas MD Anderson Cancer Center, Houston, TX, USA

Magdalena Anitescu, MD, PhD Department of Anesthesia and Critical Care, University of Chicago Medicine, Chicago, IL, USA

Alexander Bautista, MD Anesthesiology and Pain Medicine, University of Oklahoma Health Sciences Center, Oklahoma City, OK, USA

Rodrigo Benavides, MD Alan Edwards Pain Management Unit, McGill Anesthesia Department, McGill University Health Centre, Montreal, QC, Canada

Robert Bolash, MD Department of Pain Management, Cleveland Clinic, Cleveland, OH, USA

Daniel C. Callahan, MD Department of Pain Management, Cleveland Clinic, Cleveland, OH, USA

Kenneth D. Candido, MD Department of Anesthesiology, Advocate Illinois Masonic Medical Center, University of Illinois College of Medicine, Chicago, IL, USA

Martin J. Carney, BS Tulane University School of Medicine, New Orleans, LA, USA

Siu Fung Chan, MD Department of Anesthesiology, University Hospitals Case Medical Center, Cleveland, OH, USA

Jennifer L. Chang, MD Department of Anesthesiology and Pain Medicine, University of Florida Health, Gainesville, FL, USA

Lucy Chen, MD Associate Professor, Harvard Medical School, MGH Center for Translational Pain Research, MGH Center for Pain Medicine, MGH Center for Pain Medicine, Department of Anesthesia, Critical Care and Pain Medicine, Massachusetts General Hospital, Harvard Medical School, Boston, MA, USA

Jianguo Cheng, MD, PhD Departments of Pain Management and Neurosciences, Cleveland Clinic Anesthesiology Institute and Lerner Research Institute, Cleveland, OH, USA

Steven P. Cohen, MD Anesthesiology, Neurology, and Physical Medicine & Rehabilitation, Johns Hopkins School of Medicine and Walter Reed National Military Medical Center, Baltimore, MD, USA

Edward Covington, MD Center for Neurological Restoration, Cleveland Clinic, Cleveland, OH, USA

Sara Davin, PsyD, MPH Center for Neurological Restoration, Cleveland Clinic, Cleveland, OH, USA

Mellar P. Davis, MD Taussig Cancer Institute, Cleveland Clinic, Cleveland, OH, USA

Jagan Devarajan, MD Department of Anesthesiology, Cleveland Clinic Medina Hospital, Westlake, OH, USA

Justin T. Drummond, MD Comprehensive Pain Management Specialists, Cleveland Clinic Akron General, Akron, OH, USA

Wael Ali Sakr Esa, MD, PhD General Anesthesia and Pain Management, Cleveland Clinic, Cleveland, OH, USA

Ehab Farag, MD, FRCA Cleveland Clinic Lerner College of Medicine, Departments of General Anesthesia and Outcomes Research, Cleveland Clinic, Cleveland, OH, USA

Salim M. Hayek, MD, PhD Department of Anesthesiology, University Hospitals Case Medical Center, Cleveland, OH, USA

Douglas Henry, MD Department of Developmental and Rehabilitative Pediatrics, Cleveland Clinic Children's, Cleveland, OH, USA

Michael Stanton-Hicks, MD Department of Pain Management, Cleveland Clinic, Cleveland, OH, USA

Robert W. Hurley, MD, PhD Department of Anesthesiology and Public Health Sciences, Wake Forest School of Medicine, Winston-Salem, NC, USA

Michael B. Jacobs, MD, MPH Physical Medicine & Rehabilitation, Walter Reed National Military Medical Center, Bethesda, MD, USA

Mark R. Jones, MD Brigham and Women's Hospital/Harvard Medical School, Department of Surgery, Boston, MA, USA

Leonardo Kapural, MD, PhD Carolinas Pain Institute, Winston-Salem, NC, USA

Wake Forest University, School of Medicine, Winston-Salem, NC, USA

Alan David Kaye, MD, PhD, DABA, DABPM, DABIPP Department of Anesthesiology, Hospital Director of Anesthesia, Department of Pharmacology, LSU School of Medicine T6M5, Tulane School of Medicine, New Orleans, LA, USA

Meredith Konya, MD Musculoskeletal Physical Medicine and Rehabilitation, Cleveland Clinic, Cleveland, OH, USA

Jennifer S. Kriegler, MD Department of Neurology, Center for Neurological Restoration, Headache and Facial Pain, Cleveland Clinic, Cleveland, OH, USA

Bryan S. Lee, MD Department of Neurological Surgery, Cleveland Clinic, Cleveland, OH, USA

Andre G. Machado, MD, PhD Department of Neurological Surgery, Center for Neurological Restoration, Cleveland Clinic, Cleveland, OH, USA

Department of Neurosciences, Lerner Research Institute, Cleveland Clinic, Cleveland, OH, USA

Beth H. Minzter, MD, MS Department of Pain Management, Cleveland Clinic, Cleveland, OH, USA

Brian R. Monroe, MD Lewis Katz School of Medicine, Department of Anesthesiology and Pain Medicine Geisinger Health System, Danville, PA

Sean J. Nagel, MD Department of Neurological Surgery, Center for Neurological Restoration, Cleveland Clinic, Cleveland, OH, USA

Samer Narouze, MD, PhD Department of Anesthesiology, Ohio University, Athens, OH, USA

Department of Neurological Surgery, Ohio State University, Columbus, OH, USA

Timothy J. Ness, MD, PhD Department of Anesthesiology and Perioperative Medicine, University of Alabama at Birmingham Hospital, Birmingham, AL, USA

Kent H. Nouri, MD Department of Pain Medicine, The University of Texas MD Anderson Cancer Center, Houston, TX, USA

Chirag A. Patel, MD Taussig Cancer Institute, Cleveland Clinic, Cleveland, OH, USA

Carlos A. Pino, MD Department of Anesthesiology, University of Vermont College of Medicine, Burlington, VT, USA

Kiran Rajneesh, MD Department of Pain Management, Cleveland Clinic, Cleveland, OH, USA

Michael Ritchey, MD Department of General Anesthesia, Cleveland Clinic, Cleveland, OH, USA

Richard W. Rosenquist, MD Department Pain Management, Cleveland Clinic, Cleveland, OH, USA

Michael P. Schaefer, MD Musculoskeletal Physical Medicine and Rehabilitation, Cleveland Clinic, Cleveland, OH, USA

Associate Professor of Medicine, Cleveland Clinic Lerner College of Medicine, Case Western Reserve University, Cleveland, OH, USA

Judith Scheman, PhD Digestive Disease and Surgery Institute, Cleveland Clinic, Cleveland, OH, USA

Jay P. Shah, MD Rehabilitation Medicine Department, Clinical Center, National Institutes of Health, Bethesda, MD, USA

Loran Mounir Soliman, MD General Anesthesia and Critical Care & Comprehensive Pain Management, Cleveland Clinic, Cleveland, OH, USA

Stewart J. Tepper, MD Department of Neurology, Dartmouth-Hitchcock Medical Center, Lebanon, NH, USA

Nikki Thaker, BS Rehabilitation Medicine Department, Clinical Center, National Institutes of Health, Bethesda, MD, USA

Chiedozie Udeh, MBBS, MHEcon Center for Critical Care Medicine, Anesthesiology Institute, Cleveland Clinic, Cleveland, OH, USA

Mercy A. Udoji, MD Department of Anesthesiology and Perioperative Medicine, University of Alabama at Birmingham, Birmingham, AL, USA

Elias Veizi, MD, PhD Department of Anesthesiology, University Hospitals Case Medical Center, Cleveland, OH, USA

Brinder Vij, MD, FACP, FAHS Neurology & Rehabilitation Medicine, University of Cincinnati Medical Center, Cincinnati, OH, USA

Austin L. Weiss, MD Wake Forrest School of Medicine, Department of Anesthesiology, Winston-Salem, NC, USA

Maria Yared, MD Anesthesiology Institute, Cleveland Clinic, Cleveland, OH, USA

Ying (Amy) Ye, MD, MPH Department of Neurology, Center for Neurological Restoration, Headache and Facial Pain, Clevelanad Clinic, Cleveland, OH, USA

Sherif Zaky, MD, PhD Pain Management & Anesthesiology, Firelands Physicians Group, Sandusky, OH, USA

Part I

Diagnosis of Pain States

1 Overview of Pain States

Jianguo Cheng

Key Concepts

- Pain medicine is a subspecialty of medicine dedicated to the relief and/or control of pain in patients with various painful conditions/states. It is rapidly expanding and has become a true multidisciplinary specialty to meet the enormous needs of patients. The complexity of pain conditions often requires multimodal, multidisciplinary approaches to prevention, management, and rehabilitation.
- Therapeutic strategies depend on proper clinical assessment and, to some extent, mechanistic understanding of each pain condition in each patient. Adequate and effective clinical assessment with appropriate methodology (history, physical exam, and diagnostic imaging and diagnostic procedures) holds the key to clinical understanding of pain conditions. Relevant anatomy, cellular and molecular pathophysiology, and pharmacology are fundamental elements in the mechanistic understanding of pain states.
- Effective treatment of pain may involve mechanistic therapy, evidence-based therapy, and personalized therapy. In many cases, mechanistic and evidence-based therapy may not be readily available. Each patient is unique in their pain presentation and response to therapy. Therefore, physicians need to weigh the risk and benefits of available treatment options and tailor therapeutic strategies to fit the individual needs of each patient.

Defining Pain

"Pain is an unpleasant sensory and emotional experience associated with actual or potential tissue damage or described in terms of damage." Pain sensation is essential to the survival, well-being, learning, and adaptation of human beings. The ability to detect noxious stimuli is a key function of the nervous system through which humans interact with the ever-changing environment to anticipate, plan, react, and adapt. However, pain may become pathological when it is no longer useful as an acute warning system and instead becomes chronic and debilitating. The mechanisms of transition from acute to chronic pain, from physiological to pathological pain, and from protective to harmful pain are poorly understood. However, peripheral and central sensitizations seem to be critical elements in the development of pathological pain. Alterations of the pain pathway lead to hypersensitivity, hyperalgesia (exaggerated pain to

J. Cheng, MD, PhD (✉)
Departments of Pain Management and Neurosciences, Cleveland Clinic Anesthesiology Institute and Lerner Research Institute, Cleveland, OH, USA
e-mail: CHENGJ@ccf.org

J. Cheng, R.W. Rosenquist (eds.), *Fundamentals of Pain Medicine*,
https://doi.org/10.1007/978-3-319-64922-1_1

painful stimuli), and allodynia (pain response to non-painful stimuli). For instance, individuals who suffer from arthritis, postherpetic neuralgia, or bone cancer often experience intense and unremitting pain that is not only physiologically and psychologically debilitating but may also hamper recovery. Chronic pain may even persist long after an acute injury, such as trauma or surgery. The elucidation of molecules and cell types and the interactions that are involved in normal (acute) pain sensation are key to understanding the mechanisms underlying the transition from physiological to pathological pain states.

Classification of Pain States

Pain is the most common presenting symptom in medicine. It can occur in any part of the body, from the head to the toes, and affect any system. It can be acute or chronic, episodic or continuous, and occurring regularly or irregularly. It is necessary to classify pain states to provide an understanding of pain disorders, establish standards for diagnosis and description, and allow exchange of standardized information. Although it may be classified in many ways, pain is generally classified as nociceptive, neuropathic, idiopathic, psychogenic, and mixed. The use of specific classifications makes it possible to compare statistical data between professionals within countries and internationally. The International Classification of Diseases, tenth revision (ICD-10), copyrighted by the World Health Organization (WHO) is used worldwide for the purpose of documenting mortality and morbidity. A slightly modified version with clinical modification (ICD-10-CM) was adopted in the USA in 2015. This classification system facilitates statistical comparisons of the occurrence of disease and management outcomes but also serves as a means of defining work and providing standards for billing and payment.

Common Pain States

Acute Pain Acute pain begins suddenly and is usually sharp in quality. It serves as a warning of disease or a threat to the body. Acute pain may be mild and last just a moment, or it may be severe and last for weeks or months. In most cases, acute pain does not last longer than 3–6 months, and it disappears when the underlying cause of pain has been treated or has healed. Typical acute pain states include surgical pain, traumatic pain, labor pain, and ischemic pain.

Chronic Pain Unrelieved acute pain may lead to chronic pain. Chronic pain persists longer than 6 months, often despite the fact that an injury has healed. Physical effects include tense muscles, limited mobility, lack of energy, and changes in sleep and appetite. Emotional effects include depression, anger, anxiety, and fear of reinjury. These effects frequently hinder a person's ability to return to normal work or leisure activities. Typical chronic pain conditions include neuropathic pain, arthritic pain, and fibromyalgia.

Nociceptive Pain Nociceptive pain is caused by activation of nociceptive afferent fibers typically through thermal, mechanical, or chemical stimulation. Based on the location of the nociceptors in body structures, nociceptive pain may also be divided into visceral pain, deep somatic pain, and superficial somatic pain.

Neuropathic Pain Neuropathic pain is caused by damage or disease affecting any part of the somatosensory system. Peripheral neuropathic pain is caused by damage or dysfunction of peripheral nerves. Painful diabetic neuropathy, complex regional pain syndrome type II (causalgia), postherpetic neuralgia, and radicular pain are examples of this type of pain. Neuropathic pain is often described as "burning," "tingling," "electrical," "stabbing," or "pins and needles." Central pain is caused by a primary lesion or dysfunction in the central nervous system and is usually associated with abnormal sensibility to temperature and noxious stimulation. Common examples include poststroke pain, pain related to spinal cord injury, and pain due to multiple sclerosis. Phantom pain (pain felt in a part of the body that has been lost or from which the brain no longer receives signals) may also be considered in this category.

Idiopathic Pain Idiopathic pain is a pain that persists after the trauma or pathology has healed or that arises without any apparent cause. Some argue that such pain is psychogenic.

Psychogenic Pain Psychogenic pain is pain caused, increased, or prolonged by mental, emotional, or behavioral factors. This type of pain is also called *psychalgia* or *somatoform pain*. Sufferers are often stigmatized, because such pain may be considered as "not real." However, specialists believe that it is no less actual or hurtful than pain from any other source.

Mixed Type of Pain The mechanisms of pain are complex, and the classification of pain conditions is often complex as well. Many types of pain can coexist in the same individual, leading to a mixed type of pain. Examples of this type of pain include complex regional pain syndrome (CRPS) and fibromyalgia. In such circumstances, identifying the chief component of the pain may facilitate planning of therapeutic strategies.

- *Complex regional pain syndrome (CRPS)*, formerly called reflex sympathetic dystrophy (RSD) or causalgia, is a chronic systemic disease characterized by severe pain, swelling, and changes in the skin. It often initially affects an arm or a leg and often spreads throughout the body. It is a multifactorial disorder with clinical features of neurogenic inflammation, nociceptive sensitization, vasomotor dysfunction, and maladaptive neuroplasticity, generated by an aberrant response to tissue injury. There are two types of CRPS:
  - Type I, formerly known as RSD, does not have demonstrable nerve lesions. The vast majority of patients diagnosed with CRPS are of this type.
  - Type II, formerly known as *causalgia*, has evidence of specific nerve damage and therefore is a neuropathic pain state. This type tends to be a more painful and difficult to control form of CRPS.
- *Fibromyalgia* is characterized by chronic widespread pain and allodynia (a heightened and painful response to pressure). Pain is considered widespread when it is present in all of the following: the left and right sides of the body and above and below the waist. In addition, axial skeletal pain (cervical spine or anterior chest or thoracic spine or low back) must be present. Its exact cause is unknown but is believed to involve psychological, genetic, neurobiological, and environmental factors that lead to central sensitization. Fibromyalgia symptoms are not restricted to pain. Other symptoms include debilitating fatigue, sleep disturbance, and joint stiffness.

In addition to these common pain states, pain in special patient populations deserves special attention. Distinct assessment and therapeutic skills are required to effectively manage pain in patients with cancer, pain in pediatric patients, pain in geriatric patients, pain in critically ill patients, and pain in those with substance abuse.

Global Strategies of Pain Assessment and Treatment

Therapeutic strategies depend on proper clinical assessment and mechanistic understanding of the pain condition affecting each patient. Adequate and effective clinical assessment with appropriate methodology (history, physical exam, and diagnostic imaging and diagnostic procedures) holds the key to developing a clinical understanding of the pain conditions in question. Relevant anatomy, cellular and molecular pathophysiology, pharmacology, and psychological effects are fundamental elements involved in the mechanistic understanding of a pain state and its treatment.

Effective treatment of pain involves mechanistic therapy, evidence-based therapy, and personalized therapy. Examples of mechanistic therapy include antivirals for herpes zoster, decompression of spinal stenosis for neurogenic claudication and pain, and control of glucose in cases of diabetic neuropathy. Examples of evidence-based therapy include spinal cord stimulation for failed back surgery syndrome, radiofrequency ablation of facet joint innervation for neck and back pain, and pharmacological interventions for neuropathic pain. Mechanistic or evidence-based therapy may not be readily available for many painful conditions and because each patient is unique in their presentation of pain and responses to pain therapy. Therefore, it is extremely important to weigh the risks and benefits of the available treatment options and tailor therapeutic strategies to fit the individual needs of each patient.

Suggested Reading

1. Basbaum AI, Bautista DM, Scherrer G, Julius D. Cellular and molecular mechanisms of pain. Cell. 2009;139(2):267–84.
2. Benzon HT. Taxonomy: definition of pain terms and chronic pain syndromes. Chapter 3. In: Benzon HT, et al., editors. Essentials of pain medicine and regional anesthesia. 2nd ed. Philadelphia: Elsevier; 2005.

2 Pathways of Pain Perception and Modulation

Kiran Rajneesh and Robert Bolash

Key Concepts

- Pain sensation occurs in the periphery via specialized nociceptors with free nerve endings.
- The first sensation of pain is transmitted by myelinated Aδ fibers which carry a well-localized pain signal.
- C fibers are unmyelinated fibers which transmit poorly localized pain to the dorsal horn of the spinal cord.
- First-order neurons synapse with second-order neurons within Rexed lamina I. Second-order neurons then cross midline and ascend to the brainstem via the spinothalamic tracts.
- Second-order neurons synapse with third-order neurons in the thalamus. Third-order neurons project to the cortex.
- These second- and third-order neurons relay to brain and brainstem centers responsible for arousal, emotional experience, and behavior.
- Afferent pain signals are modulated at the level of the dorsal horn, brainstem, and cortex via inhibitory interneurons and inhibitory and excitatory descending pathways.
- Therapeutic targets exist on the afferent neurons, ascending pathways, and descending pathways.
- Acute pain can be adaptive and life-sustaining, while chronic pain often results in comorbid maladaptive behavioral and arousal patho logies.

Introduction

Pain perception is essential to human well-being and survival. The sensation of pain originates through complex signaling pathways which begins in the periphery, ascends in the spinal cord or brainstem (cranial sensory input), and is ultimately interpreted in the cortex of the brain. These ascending pathways are susceptible to injury owing to mechanical, toxic, or pathological aberrations originating at any point along their course.

More complex than a simple one-way circuit, pain is also modulated by descending pathways which serve to mitigate painful inputs throughout the classic pain pathways. An understanding of the pain pathways provides a foundation for discussions of both pathological processes and therapeutic interventions.

K. Rajneesh, MD • R. Bolash, MD (✉)
Department of Pain Management, Cleveland Clinic, 9500 Euclid Ave / C25, Cleveland, 44195 OH, USA
e-mail: robert@bolash.org

J. Cheng, R.W. Rosenquist (eds.), *Fundamentals of Pain Medicine*,
https://doi.org/10.1007/978-3-319-64922-1_2

Peripheral Receptors for Pain

Nociceptors are capable of sensing thermal, mechanical, or chemical insults via specialized receptors or free nerve endings located throughout the body. Nociceptors are the peripherally located terminal ends of specialized pseudounipolar neurons called Aδ and C fibers.

Aδ fibers are medium-diameter fibers that carry well-localized pain signals. Because they are thinly myelinated, Aδ fibers permit relatively rapid transmission of impulses toward the spinal cord and are responsible for the initial sensation of pain. Aδ fibers are further divided into two main subtypes: type I, or high-threshold mechanical nociceptors, that respond to both mechanical and chemical stimuli, and type II nociceptors which have a heat threshold close to 42 °C and are responsible for the transmission of painful thermal insults.

C fibers are small-diameter, unmyelinated fibers that mediate poorly localized pain. Their impulses reach the spinal cord at a tenfold slower rate than Aδ fibers and are responsible for the second pain. The majority of unmyelinated C fibers are polymodal, carrying painful stimuli arising from both chemical and noxious insults.

Ascending Pathways

Aδ and C fibers enter the central nervous system through the dorsal horn of the spinal cord and many synapse at the same level in a histologically defined area of the dorsal horn. Some of the fibers either ascend or descend in a specialized pathway called Lissauer's tract before synapsing with their second-order neuron. Among these laminae, Rexed laminae I, II, and V are the most important in pain signaling with C fibers synapsing in laminae I and II, while Aδ fibers synapse in laminae I and V.

Lamina V receives convergent input from Aδ and Aβ fibers conducting proprioception and fibers arising from the viscera. Because of the diversity of inputs into lamina V, these neurons are termed wide dynamic range (WDR) neurons. Projection neurons within laminae I and V constitute the major output from the dorsal horn to the brain. These neurons are at the origin of multiple ascending pathways, including the spinothalamic and spinoreticulothalamic tracts, which carry pain messages to the thalamus and brainstem, respectively (Fig. 2.1). The former is particularly relevant to the sensory-discriminative aspects of the pain experience, whereas the latter may be more relevant to poorly localized pains. In addition, spinal cord projections to the parabrachial region of the dorsolateral pons of the brainstem provide for a very rapid connection with the amygdala, a region generally considered to process information relevant to the aversive properties of the pain experience.

There is somatotopic organization of the second-order neurons within the spinothalamic tract with medial fibers carrying information about the arms and lateral fibers carrying painful sensation from the legs. This becomes important in pathological conditions such as syringomyelia when the central canal becomes pathologically enlarged and pushes on the anterior commissure. Because of this, second-order neurons of the spinothalamic tract crossing the midline are preferentially affected. Patients complain of pain in "cape-like distribution" affecting both shoulders due to the somatotopic distribution of fibers.

The spinothalamic tracts ascend through the medulla and pons before reaching the ventral posterior nucleus of the thalamus. Along its course to the thalamus, the spinothalamic tracts interact with numerous collaterals. In the medulla, branches of the spinothalamic tract transmit to the reticular formation which modulates alertness when pain is perceived. In the pons, spinothalamic projections transmit to the hypothalamus and amygdala to modulate mood and motivation.

Within the thalamus, the spinothalamic tracts synapse with third-order neurons in the ventral posterior lateral nucleus. These third-order neurons project to the cortex and enable perception of discrete sensations of pain such as the quality and location from which the painful signal originates. Simultaneously, nuclei adjacent to the thalamus receive projections from the spinothalamic tract and mediate some pain behavior such as arousal and emotion.

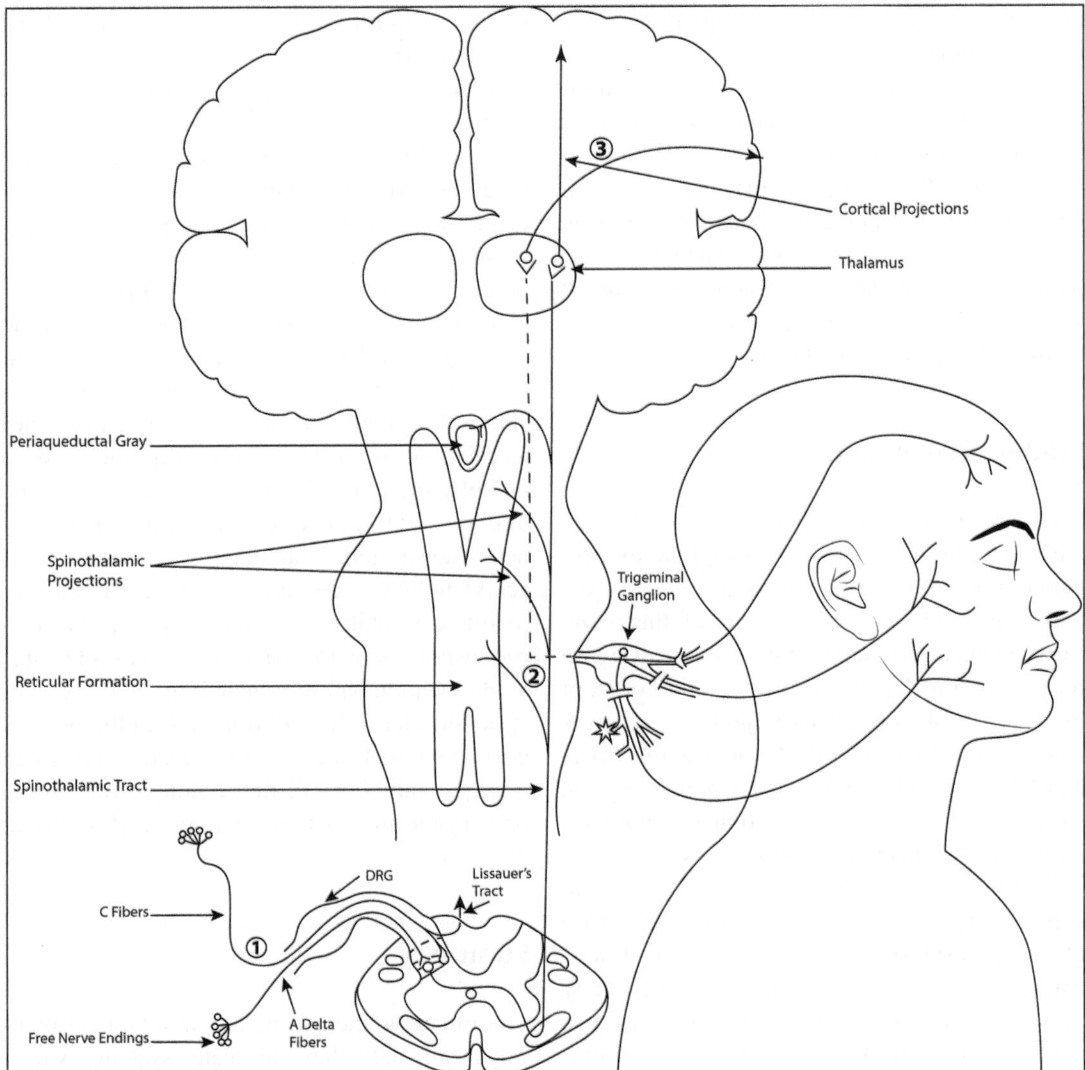

Fig. 2.1 Nociceptive input from the body is sensed at the free nerve endings before traveling (*1*) to the dorsal horn of the spinal cord via A delta and C fibers. Second-order neurons ascend in the spinothalamic and spinoreticulothalamic tracts (*2*) before synapsing in the thalamus and brainstem. Third-order neurons project (*3*) to the cortex. Neurons transmitting facial pain transit through the trigeminal ganglion and synapse in the spinal nucleus of the trigeminal nerve. Second-order neurons run parallel and medial to the spinothalamic tract before synapsing in the thalamus

Pain transmission from the face and sinuses follows a pathway which does not involve the spinal cord. Instead, nociceptive neurons from the face, transit the trigeminal ganglion, and terminate in the spinal nucleus of the trigeminal nerve. Fibers of the second-order neurons in the trigeminal spinal nucleus then ascend through the brainstem and synapse directly in the ventral posterior medial nucleus of the thalamus.

Pain Perception in the Cerebral Cortex

From the thalamus, third-order neurons carry projections to the primary somatosensory cortex in the postcentral gyrus, specifically to Brodmann areas 1–3. Projections from the primary somatosensory cortex then transit to the secondary somatosensory cortex which acts to integrate pain with visual, auditory, and gustatory inputs.

The importance of these thalamic connections is seen in central pain syndromes such as Dejerine-Roussy syndrome. After suffering an ischemic insult to the posterior cerebral artery, thalamic pain may develop. Though arising from a central source within the thalamus, these patients perceive pain throughout the body at locations which are remote from the area affected by the ischemic thalamic insult.

Modulation of Pain

Pain perception is modulated at several discrete areas including the dorsal root ganglion, the spinal cord dorsal horn, the reticular system of the brainstem, and the cortical areas of the brain. These mechanisms serve to increase or decrease the painful impulses before reaching the cortex of the brain. In the dorsal horn, lamina V receives convergent input from both $A\delta$ nociceptive fibers and $A\beta$ sensory fibers which carry proprioception such as touch. It is hypothesized that within lamina V, the gate theory of pain operates.

In 1965, Melzack and Wall described a "gate control theory of pain" whereby sensation of non-painful stimuli, such as touch, diminishes the ability to sense painful input. They theorized that non-painful stimuli "close a gate" to the transmission of noxious stimuli. The theory was subsequently refined with the description of an inhibitory interneuron located within the dorsal horn of the spinal cord. In the presence of mechanical $A\beta$ stimulation, the inhibitory interneuron is activated and thus diminishing transmission through the nociceptive C fibers. Though the gate theory has undergone further clarification since its initial description, this observation has been exploited therapeutically with the development of transcutaneous electrical nerve stimulation (TENS). TENS acts to selectively trigger $A\beta$ sensory fibers, thereby inhibiting the transmission of noxious stimuli at the level of the dorsal horn via an interneuron.

Following the description of the gate theory, further descending pain-modulating pathways were elucidated. The raphe nuclei, rostral ventral medulla, and periaqueductal gray have high concentrations of enkephalins, endorphins, and dynorphins which act to diminish painful input via descending pathways. These pathways arise from the brainstem and impart their effect at the dorsal horn of the spinal cord. Originally thought to function only as inhibitors of pain transmission, descending pathways serve to either amplify or mitigate pain transmission. Most notably, the periaqueductal gray matter of the midbrain utilizes both excitatory and inhibitory neurotransmitters including norepinephrine, acetylcholine, serotonin, and dopamine to facilitate or inhibit nociceptive input. These neurotransmitters work throughout multiple sites along the pain pathway including the distal synaptic terminals, dorsal horn, and midbrain. It is postulated that the use of selective serotonin reuptake inhibitors in the treatment of chronic pain syndromes act through these descending pathways.

Summary

More than simple ascending circuits, pain pathways are redundant intricate systems which undergo modulation at peripheral, spinal cord, brainstem, and cortical sites. Because of connections with behavioral, arousal, and physiological centers, acute pain can enable an organism to survive, while chronic pain can lead to maladaptive behavior. A variety of pathological processes affect both pain signaling and processing at sites both peripherally and centrally. Both pharmacological and surgical treatments have been developed to target these pathological processes, and an understanding of the mechanism of pain transmission serves as the basis for understanding therapeutic strategies.

Suggested Reading

1. Akil H, Richardson DE, Hughes J, Barchas JD. Enkephalin-like material elevated in ventricular cerebrospinal fluid of pain patients after analgetic focal stimulation. Science. 1978;201(4354):463–5.
2. Basbaum AI, Bautista DM, Scherrer G, Julius D. Cellular and molecular mechanisms of pain. Cell. 2009;139(2):267–84.
3. Melzack R, Wall P. Pain mechanisms: a new theory. Science. 1965;150(3699):971–9.
4. Roberts WJ, Foglesong ME. Spinal recordings suggest that wide-dynamic-range neurons mediate sympathetically maintained pain. Pain. 1988;34(3):289–304.
5. Wilkins RH, Brody IA. The thalamic syndrome. Arch Neurol. 1969;20(5):559–62.

3 Mechanisms of Physiologic Pain

Siu Fung Chan, Salim M. Hayek, and Elias Veizi

Key Concepts

- Physiological pain is an adaptive protective mechanism.
- Nociceptors are primary sensory neurons specialized to detect environmental threatening or damaging inputs to initiate a protective response.
- The pain perception is a cascade of events starting with transduction, followed by conduction, transmission, and eventually modulation and perception.
- Endogenous attenuation of the nociceptive pain signal involves segmental inhibition, the endogenous opioid system, and the descending inhibitory system.

Introduction

Nociception and pain perception comprise two different events. *Nociception* is the activation of sensory neuronal pathways upon stimulation by noxious stimuli, while *pain* refers to one's perception of this experience after the brain processes the transmitted signal. Nociception may lead to pain, yet a person may experience pain without activation of the nociceptive pathway. Noxious perception is a complex process that begins in periphery, extends along the neuraxis, and terminates in supraspinal regions responsible for perception, interpretation, and reaction. This process includes nociceptor activation, neural conduction, spinal transmission, and modulation of the stimuli and ultimately spinal and supraspinal responses (Fig. 3.1).

Transduction

Transduction is the process by which potential harmful mechanical, chemical, or thermal stimuli are converted by peripheral nociceptors into action potential within the distal fingerlike nociceptor endings.

Nociceptors

Sherrington first described nociceptors about a century ago. These are sensory neurons with free nerve endings consisting of receptor subtypes that can be excited by mechanical, temperature, and chemical stimuli applied to skin, muscles, joints, bone, viscera, and dura. Yet, they are not excited by innocuous stimuli (e.g., gentle warming or light touch). The intensity of the stimulus determines the initial response. Nociceptors have a high threshold and normally respond only to stimuli of sufficient energy to potentially or actually damage tissue.

S.F. Chan, MD (✉) • S.M. Hayek, MD, PhD
E. Veizi, MD, PhD
Department of Anesthesiology, University Hospitals Case Medical Center, Cleveland, OH, USA
e-mail: SiuFung.Chan@UHHospitals.org

J. Cheng, R.W. Rosenquist (eds.), *Fundamentals of Pain Medicine*,
https://doi.org/10.1007/978-3-319-64922-1_3

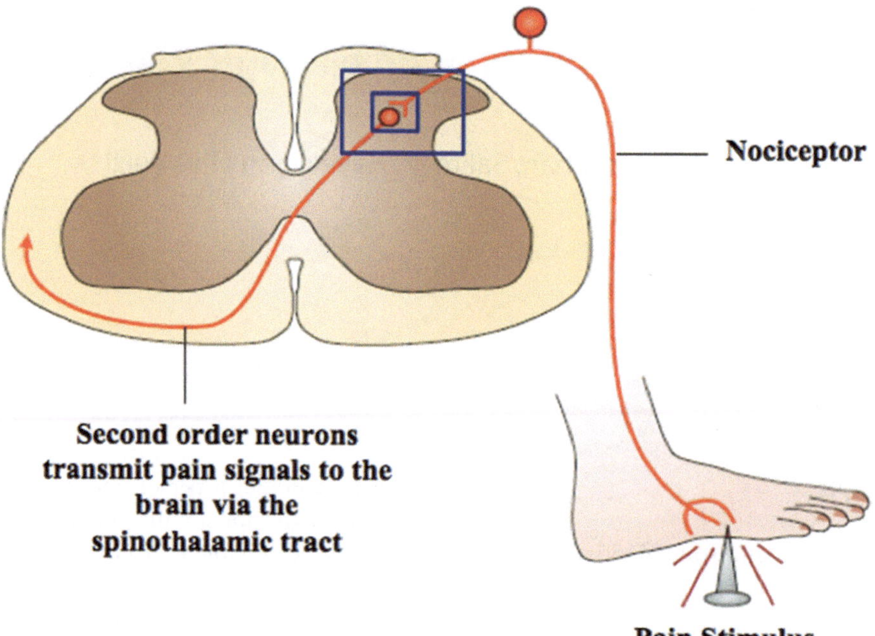

Fig. 3.1 General schematic diagram showing nociception from the site of injury to the spinal cord (CNS). Transmission occurs in the blue boxes, which are discussed in more detail in Fig. 3.3 (With permission from Nature Publishing Group, GLIA: Watkins LR, Maier SF. A novel drug discovery target for clinical pain. *Nat Rev Drug Discov*. 2003;2(12), fig 1)

There are two categories of nociceptors: (a) thinly myelinated (Aδ fibers) and (b) unmyelinated (C fibers). These primary sensory neurons have their cell bodies in dorsal root ganglia [DRG] and give rise to a single axon that bifurcates into a peripheral branch that innervates peripheral target tissue and a central axon that enters the CNS to synapse on nociceptive second-order neurons in the dorsal horn of the spinal cord. As such the unit components of the nociceptor include:

- Peripheral terminal that innervates target tissue and transduces noxious stimuli
- Axon that conducts action potentials from the periphery to the central nervous system
- Cell body in the dorsal root ganglion
- Central terminal where information is transferred to second-order neurons at central synapses.

Following their origin from the neural crest, nociceptors undergo a distinct differentiation pathway that leads to formation of two characteristic subgroups:

(a) "Peptidergic": Express CGRP and substance P. Calcitonin gene-related protein [CGRP] is a 37-amino acid peptide found in peripheral and central terminal of nearly 50% of the C fibers and 35% of Ad fibers. Substance P is an 11-amino acid peptide found in a subset of nociceptive neurons.
(b) "Non-peptidergic": Do not express peptides but express signaling components to respond to glial cell-derived growth factor [GDNF].

Nociceptor Activation

Noxious stimuli are converted into an ion flux. A heterogeneous group of receptors is present on the surface of nociceptors, and they are responsive to various stimuli [polymodal] primarily due to the presence of polycationic channels. Tissue injury mediators activate transducer molecules such as transient receptor potential [TRP] ion channel. TRP channels are a diverse family of ion channels that respond to thermal [TRPV1], traumatic, and chemical [TRPA and TRPM] stimuli. TRPV1/capsaicin receptor is the best-described member of the family. It is a 4 subunit receptor which upon stimulation by H^+ ions, heat, or capsaicin permits an inward flux of Ca^{2+} and Na^+. This inward flux is responsible for generation of action potential by causing membrane depolarization and lowering the activation threshold (Fig. 3.2).

Tissue injury and cellular damage are associated with the release of noxious mediators such as arachidonic acid [AA] from lysed cell membranes as well as intracellular H^+ and K^+ ions. Furthermore, active metabolites of AA such as PGE2 PGG2 bradykinin play a significant role in the activation of peripheral nociceptor. They bind G-protein receptor proteins and activate intracellular signaling cascade such as extracellular-regulated kinase and adenylate cyclase which in turn a) activate ion channels by phosphorylation [e.g., TrpV1 phosphorylation] and b) increase the cell membrane ion channel turnover from internal stores. The net result is activation of Ca^{2+} and Na^+ influx and membrane depolarization. There are different sodium channels expressed in somatosensory neurons. These include tetrodotoxin (TTX)-sensitive channels (Nav 1.1, 1.6, and 1.7) and TTX-insensitive channels (Nav 1.8 and 1.9). Of particular note, Nav 1.7 is largely involved with pain perception, as patients with loss-of-function mutations of this gene cannot detect noxious stimuli. The C nociceptors express both Nav 1.7 and Nav 1.8 sodium channels. These voltage-gated sodium channels are targets of local anesthetic drugs.

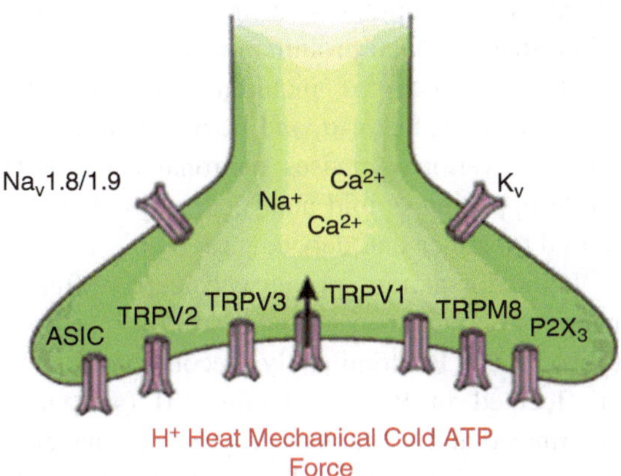

Fig. 3.2 This is an illustration of a close-up area of the circle in Fig. 3.1. A heterogeneous group of receptors on nociceptors respond to various stimuli, leading to an influx and calcium and sodium, generating an action potential. While TRP channels respond to trauma, heat, and chemical stimuli, there are other channels that may be expressed. Na 1.8/1.9, TRPM8, and ASIC channels respond to mechanical, cold/menthol, and protons, respectively. P2X3 channels respond to ATP released from inflamed cells (Adapted from Macmillan Publishers Ltd., Scholz J, Woolf CJ. Can we conquer pain? *Nat Neurosci.* 2002;5:1062–7, fig 2)

Conduction

The action potentials generated by activated nociceptors are conducted through different types of nociceptive fibers: thinly myelinated afferent nociceptors (Aδ nociceptors) and smaller diameter unmyelinated afferent nociceptors (C nociceptors) (Table 3.1). The Aδ fibers mediate the "first" wave of pain (acute, sharp pain), while the C fibers mediate the "second" wave of pain (delayed, diffuse, dull) perceived by the brain. These fibers conduct pain signals through the cell bodies, which are located in the dorsal root ganglia and the trigeminal ganglion for the body and face, respectively, and continue toward the dorsal horn of the spinal cord, where the nociceptive fibers synapse with second-order neurons.

While it is anticipated to think of the nociceptive pathway as a one-way process, in reality it is more complicated. Primary afferent fibers are described as "pseudounipolar," where the nociceptor can send and receive input from either the periphery or central terminals. Both ends serve as targets for endogenous regulatory factors and pharmacotherapy that alter the neuron's threshold to fire in order to regulate pain.

Nociceptive signals are transduced to synapses in the dorsal horn through action potentials mediated mostly through voltage-gated sodium and potassium channels. Voltage-gated calcium channels facilitate neurotransmitter release at the dorsal horn synapse of nociceptor terminals to transmit pain signals. The activation of the various nociceptors

Table 3.1 Classification of primary sensory neurons

Fiber type	Aβ	Aδ	C
Myelination	Myelinated	Thinly myelinated	Unmyelinated
Diameter size	Largest (20–45 μm)	Small (~15 μm)	Very small (~8 μm)
Conduction velocity, m/s	14–30	2.2–8	0.4–2
Activation stimulus	Light touch, movement, and vibration	Brief, intense	High intensity, long duration
Threshold	Low	High	High
Localization	Joints, skin	Skin, deep somatic, viscera	Skin, deep tissues, viscera

and ion channels leads to the propagation of action potentials from peripheral nociceptive endings via myelinated and unmyelinated nerve fibers, in a process termed conduction.

A heterogeneous group of voltage-gated calcium channels are also expressed on nociceptors. All calcium channels are heteromeric proteins, consisting of α1 pore-forming subunits and modulatory subunits α2δ, α2β, or α2γ. In C nociceptors, the α2δ subunit is upregulated in nerve injury and contributes to hypersensitivity and allodynia. This is the target of gabapentin and pregabalin, used to treat neuropathic pain.

Transmission

Transmission refers to the transfer of noxious impulses from primary nociceptors to cells in the spinal cord dorsal horn. Both Aδ and C fibers conduct nociceptive input via first-order neurons, which upon entering the spinal cord travel up or down for one to two vertebral levels in Lissauer's tract before synapsing with second-order neurons in the dorsal horn of the spinal cord. When the signal arrives at the central terminals of nociceptors, depolarization leads to activation of the N-type calcium channel. The influx of calcium leads to the release of the predominant excitatory neurotransmitters at the level of the dorsal horn, glutamate, and substance P (see Fig. 3.3).

Glutamate activates postsynaptic AMPA and kainate subtypes of ionotropic glutamate receptors. Substance P activates postsynaptic NK1 receptors (Table 3.2). The activation of these receptors generates excitatory postsynaptic currents (EPSCs) in the second-order neurons located in the dorsal horn. The summation of subthreshold EPSCs results in action potential firing and transmission of pain signals to higher-order neurons. Transduction of pain is also modulated by neurotransmitters and neuropeptides that influence nerve transmission threshold, thus affecting one's increased or decreased sensitivity of pain perception.

Of note, glutamate and substance P lead to activation of glial cells. Microglia function as macrophages and are homogeneously dispersed in the gray matter of the spinal cord. These are presumed to function as sentinels of injury or infection. Glia found outside of the spinal cord may be involved in pain enhancement. Their expression is upregulated in pain conditions while they produce proinflammatory and neuroexcitatory substances, including interleukin-1β, tumor necrosis factor-α, and IL-6, among others. Glial activation increases neuronal excitability while opposing opioid analgesia and enhancing opioid tolerance and dependence.

In the dorsal horn, primary nociceptor afferent nerve fibers synapse into specific laminae (Table 3.3). Predominantly, second-order cells are located in Rexed's laminae II (substantia gelatinosa) and V (nucleus proprius). Spinal cord neurons within lamina I and II are generally responsive to noxious stimulation, while neurons located in laminae III and IV are responsive to non-noxious stimuli (Aβ fibers). Neurons in lamina V receive both non-noxious and noxious inputs via direct Aδ/Aβ inputs and non-direct C fiber inputs through interneurons in lamina II.

The second-order neurons in lamina V are collectively referred to as wide dynamic range (WDR) neurons as they respond to a wide range of stimulus intensities. It is also the location of where some

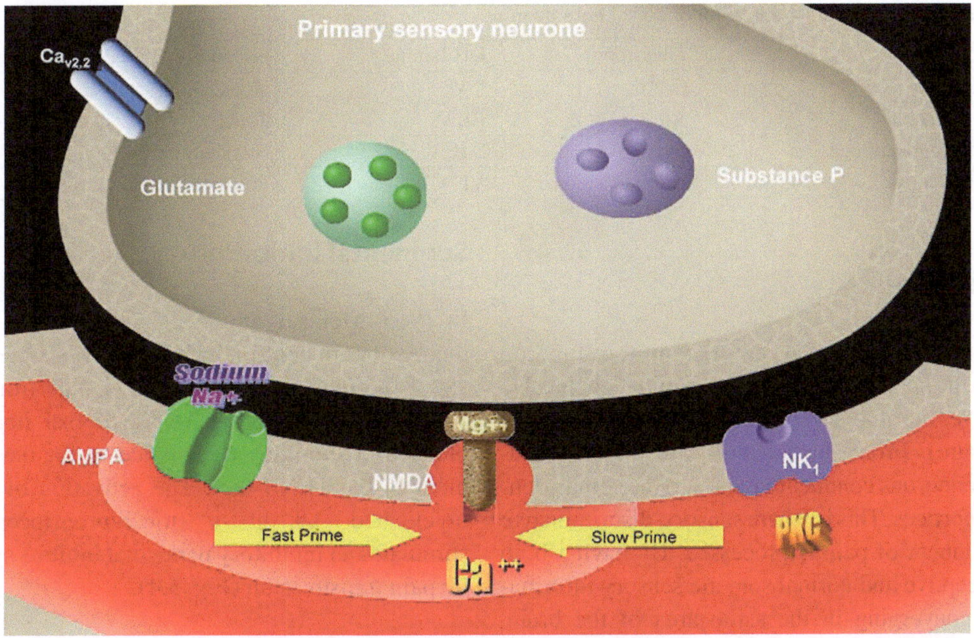

Fig. 3.3 This is a close-up of the area in the smaller square of Fig. 3.1. The release of vesicles containing excitatory neurotransmitters, substance P, and glutamate is Ca dependent (With permission from Springer, Rodger IW. Analgesic targets: today and tomorrow. *InflammoPharmacology* 2009;17(3))

Table 3.2 Receptors associated with dorsal horn noxious signals

Receptor	Type	Ligand	Action	Function
GABA	Ionotropic	Gaba	Inhibitory	K^+ flux inhibition
NK-1	Metabotropic	Substance P	Excitatory	G-protein–coupled rec
AMPA	Ionotropic	Glu	Excitatory	Na^+ flux
Glycine	Ionotropic	Gly	Inhibitory	Cl^- flux
NMDA	Ionotropic	Glu	Excitatory	Ca^{++} flux
ENK	Metabotropic	ENK	Inhibitory	G-protein–coupled rec

visceral inputs occur. The convergence of somatic and visceral inputs explains the phenomenon of referred pain, where pain from an injury to a visceral tissue is referred to a somatic structure (e.g., shoulder discomfort with a heart attack). Second-order neurons conducting nociceptive stimuli cross the spinal midline and ascend via the spinothalamic tract to the thalamus where a synapse occurs with the third-order neurons. This pathway describes how pain information is transmitted as well as how normal thermal stimuli <45°C are transmitted. Thalamic stroke patients may have a dysfunctional thalamus which may be a source of pain without involvement of the spinothalamic pathway. This is referred to as "thalamic pain."

In the facial area, noxious stimuli are transmitted through nerve cells in the trigeminal ganglion and cranial nuclei VII, IX, and X. These travel to the medulla, cross the neural midline, and ascend to the thalamic nerve cells on the contralateral side. Spontaneous firing of the trigeminal nerve ganglion may give rise to "trigeminal neuralgia." This is commonly caused by local trigeminal nerve damage as a result of a mechanical compression by the cerebellar artery.

Table 3.3 Functional classification of dorsal horn neurons

Neuronal Type	Fiber input	DH lamina	Function
Nociceptive	C, Aδ	I, V	Nociception
Low threshold	Aβ	III, V	Touch
Wide dynamic range	C, Aδ, Aβ	I, II, V	Nociception
Proprioceptive	Aα	VI	Proprioception

Perception

The thalamic region receiving pain transmission from the spinal cord and the trigeminal nuclei also receives normal sensory stimuli (i.e., touch and pressure). From the thalamic nuclei, the third-order neurons conduct impulses to the somatosensory cortices. This is where sensory-discriminative component of pain is processed. By having both nociceptive and normal somatic sensory information converging in the same area of the brain, location and intensity of pain can be processed into a localized perception of pain. The cortical representation of the body (described by Penfield's homunculus) may change after limb amputations, causing "phantom pain" as well as non-painful sensations like "telescoping phenomena."

The third-order neurons also project the pain signal to the limbic structures, namely, the anterior cingulate cortex and the insula. Here, the emotional and cognitive components of pain are processed.

Modulation

The concept of modulation refers to pain-suppressive mechanisms within the spinal cord dorsal horn and at the higher levels of brain stem and midbrain. Studies of endogenous inhibition of pain started around the time of World War II when Dr. Beecher noted injured soldiers often experience little or no pain despite sustaining severe battle wounds. There have been studies on the dissociation between body injury and pain, and three mechanisms have been described in literature: segmental inhibition, the endogenous opioid system, and the descending inhibitory nerve system.

Segmental Inhibition

In 1965, Melzack and Wall proposed the "gate theory of pain control," which describes the ability of the transmission of pain signals from the Aδ and C nerve fibers to the dorsal horn be blocked or diminished. This led to the development of the TENS unit. The activation of large myelinated Aβ fibers (touch/proprioception) stimulates an inhibitory nerve that inhibits synaptic pain transmission (Fig. 3.4).

Endogenous Opioid System

Since the 1960s, opioid receptors have been found to be concentrated in the periaqueductal gray matter, lamina II of the dorsal horn of the spinal cord, as well as the ventral medulla. Studies have shown that mammals produce enkephalins, endorphins, and dynorphin, three endogenous compounds that bind to these opioid receptors. Along with the descending inhibitory nerve system, this serves as a pain modulatory system that may partly explain the subjective variability in pain perception among individuals.

Descending Inhibitory System

The periaqueductal gray matter in the upper brain stem, the locus coeruleus, the nucleus raphe magnus, and the nucleus reticularis gigantocellularis in the rostroventral medulla contribute to the descending pain suppression pathway. This inhibits ascending nociceptive information from the nociceptive pain pathway (Fig. 3.5). The axons involved in this pathway descend down the bilateral dorsolateral funiculus and synapses in laminae I, II, and V of the

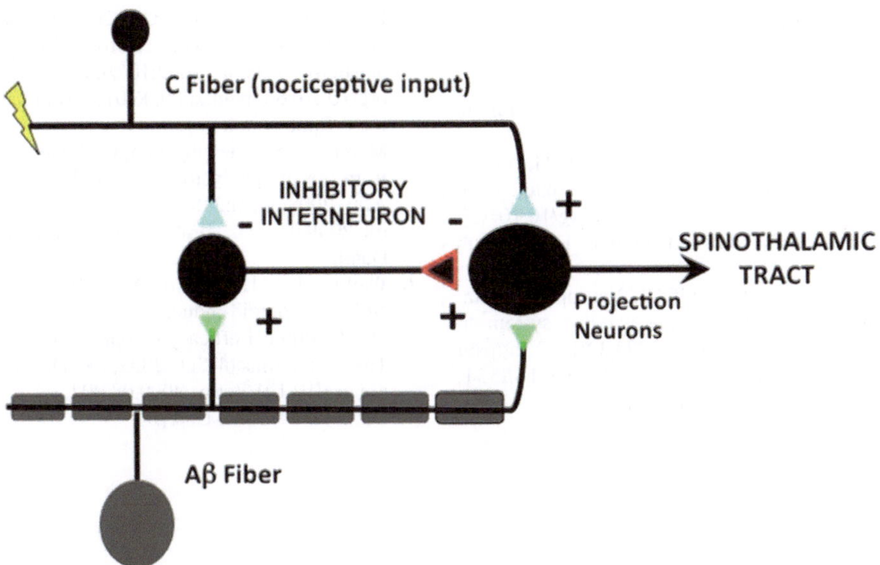

Fig. 3.4 The gate control theory of pain (Melzack and Wall). Nociceptive signals from the peripheral C fibers inhibit the inhibitory interneuron while propagating excitatory signals to the spinothalamic tract. When mechanoreceptors are activated, the inhibition from the C fiber at the inhibitory interneuron is lessened, and the nociceptive signal to the spinothalamic tract is in competition with proprioceptive signals from the mechanoreceptors. + Excitatory synapse, – inhibitory synapse

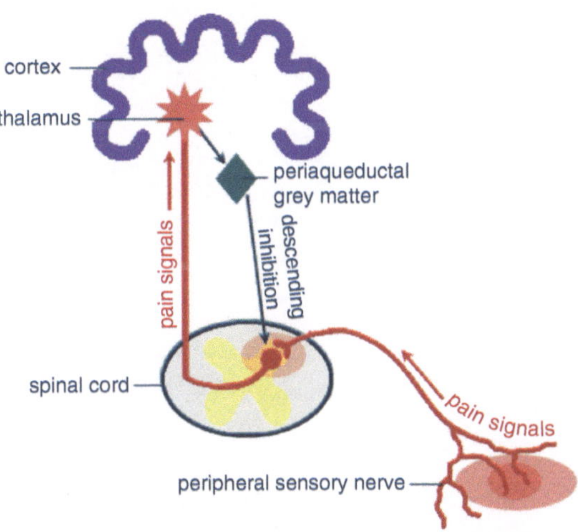

Fig. 3.5 Diagram showing the descending inhibitory pathway. Pain signals from the peripheral sensory nerves are transmitted rostrally via the spinothalamic tract. At the thalamus, descending inhibition is initiated, and the inhibitory signals descend down and synapse in the dorsal horn of the spinal cord (With permission from Elsevier, Livingston A, Chambers P. *Pain management in animals*. 2000. p. 9–19, fig 2.2)

spinal cord. Some of the common inhibitory neurotransmitters are serotonin as well as norepinephrine. Drugs that serve to block reuptake of these neurotransmitters prolong their inhibitory action on the spinal cord neurons involved with pain transmission, leading to pain relief. This explains the use of serotonin-norepinephrine reuptake inhibitors and tricyclic antidepressants for their analgesic properties.

Conclusion

The nociceptive pain pathway is complex, and this chapter provides for a broad overview to simplify for easier understanding. It is important to learn this system well in order to understand targeted pharmacological therapies to alleviate the perception of nociceptive pain as well as to understand pathologies described in later chapters that lead to dysfunction of this nociceptive pain pathway through peripheral and central sensitization.

Suggested Reading

1. Basbaum DJA. Molecular mechanisms of nociception. Nature. 2001;413:203–10. Macmillan Magazines Ltd.
2. Basbaum AI, Bautista DM, Scherrer G, et al. Cellular and molecular mechanisms of pain. Cell. 2009;139(2):267–84. https://doi.org/10.1016/j.cell.2009.09.028. [Published Online First: Epub Date].
3. Costigan M, Scholz J, Woolf CJ. Neuropathic pain: a maladaptive response of the nervous system to damage. Annu Rev Neurosci. 2009;32:1–32. https://doi.org/10.1146/annurev.neuro.051508.135531. [Published Online First: Epub Date].
4. Latremoliere A, Woolf CJ. Central sensitization: a generator of pain hypersensitivity by central neural plasticity. J Pain. 2009;10(9):895–926. https://doi.org/10.1016/j.jpain.2009.06.012. [Published Online First: Epub Date].
5. Marchand S. The physiology of pain mechanisms: from the periphery to the brain. Rheum Dis Clin N Am. 2008;34(2):285–309. https://doi.org/10.1016/j.rdc.2008.04.003. [Published Online First: Epub Date].
6. Watkins LR, Hutchinson MR, Rice KC, et al. The "toll" of opioid-induced glial activation: improving the clinical efficacy of opioids by targeting glia. Trends Pharmacol Sci. 2009;30(11):581–91. https://doi.org/10.1016/j.tips.2009.08.002. [Published Online First: Epub Date].

4 Mechanisms of Pathologic Pain

Jianguo Cheng

Key Concepts

- Pain becomes pathological when it outlives its usefulness as an acute warning system and instead becomes chronic and debilitating.
- The mechanisms of transition from acute to chronic pain, from physiological to pathological pain, and from protective to harmful pain are poorly understood despite intensive research.
- Peripheral sensitization is used to describe a phenomenon, where aberrant regeneration or change of function may occur after a peripheral nerve insult or lesion. Sensory neurons become abnormally sensitive and develop spontaneous pathological activity, unusual excitability, and augmented sensitivity to chemical, thermal, and mechanical stimuli.
- Central sensitization is used to describe a phenomenon where neuroplasticity occurs in the central nervous system. The dorsal horn of the spinal cord serves as an interface in pain processing. Increased volley of afferent input from nociceptors can trigger a prolonged but reversible increase in the excitability and synaptic efficacy of neurons in nociceptive pathways.
- The mechanisms of peripheral and central sensitization are being to be understood at the cellular and molecular levels. The processes of neuroplasticity involve activation of inflammatory cells, such as macrophages (and microglia in the central nervous system), mast cells, platelets, endothelial cells, fibroblast, and other immune cells, and release of inflammatory mediators such as cytokines, chemokines, and a host of other mediators. Interactions of these mediators with specific receptors in the nociceptors or the spinal cord neurons may lead to phosphorylation or changes in expression of ion channels, receptors, transporters, and other effectors through specific signaling pathways. These events ultimately lead to changes in excitability, conductivity, and transmissibility of neurons in the pain processing pathways. Peripheral or central sensitization thus develops.
- In addition to peripheral and central sensitization, other contributing factors may include sprouting of afferent fibers in the spinal cord, changes in descending inhibitory and excitatory pathways, and reorganization of the cortical areas and their interconnections.

J. Cheng, MD, PhD (✉)
Departments of Pain Management and Neurosciences, Cleveland Clinic Anesthesiology Institute and Lerner Research Institute, Cleveland, OH, USA
e-mail: CHENGJ@ccf.org

Definition of Pathologic Pain

Pain becomes pathological when it outlives its usefulness as an acute warning system and instead becomes chronic and debilitating. It is

J. Cheng, R.W. Rosenquist (eds.), *Fundamentals of Pain Medicine*,
https://doi.org/10.1007/978-3-319-64922-1_4

difficult to clearly separate physiological pain and pathological pain in timing, clinical manifestation, and mechanisms. However, pathological pain usually lasts more than 6 months and outlives tissue injury and recovery, has more debilitating effect than protective effect, and may involve more complex changes at the molecular, cellular, and neural network levels.

Current Understanding of Pathologic Pain

Despite intensive research, the mechanisms of transition from acute to chronic pain, from physiological to pathological pain, and from protective to harmful pain are poorly understood. The current understanding of the mechanisms of pathological pain is far from a point where mechanistic therapies can reliably be engineered. However, a few concepts are worth noting. Peripheral and central sensitizations seem to be critical processes of pathological pain. Alterations of the pain pathways lead to hypersensitivity, hyperalgesia (exaggerated pain to painful stimuli), and allodynia (pain response to non-painful stimuli).

Peripheral Sensitization

After a peripheral nerve lesion, aberrant regeneration or change of function may occur (Fig. 4.1). Sensory neurons become abnormally sensitive and develop spontaneous pathological activity, unusual excitability, and augmented sensitivity to chemical, thermal, and mechanical stimuli. The term "peripheral sensitization" is used to describe this phenomenon. It usually involves activation of several types of cells, such as macrophages, mast cells, platelets, endothelial cells, fibroblasts, and other immune cells, in reaction to tissue injury or inflammation. These cells release a milieu of inflammatory factors, which in turn bind to specific receptors of the nerve endings. These factors include cytokines [interleukin-1β (IL-1β), interleukin 6 (IL-6), tumor necrosis factor-α (TNF-α), leukemia-inhibiting factor (LIF)], nerve growth factor (NGF), histamine, bradykinin, prostaglandin E2, ATP, adenosine, and proton. These factors act on specific receptors or channels such as receptor tyrosine kinases (RTK), two-pore potassium (K2P) channels, G protein-coupled receptors (GPCR), transient receptor potential (TRP) channels, acid-sensitive ion channels (ASIC), and purinergic receptors (e.g., P2X) in the sensory nerve endings and lead to increased excitability of the peripheral sensory neurons. In addition, the nerve endings of the nociceptors may release substance P (acting on neurokinin 1 receptor) and calcitonin gene-related peptide (CGRP), both of which have been associated with neurogenic inflammation and possibly peripheral sensitization. Nociceptors are thus often referred to as "bidirectional signaling machine" because they not only release neurotransmitters and neuromodulators at the central ends in the spinal cord but also release active agents from the nerve endings in the periphery.

Central Sensitization

Neuroplasticity also occurs in the central nervous system (Fig. 4.2). The dorsal horn of the spinal cord serves as an interface in pain processing. Increased volley of afferent input from nociceptors can trigger a prolonged but reversible increase in the excitability and synaptic efficacy of neurons in nociceptive pathways. The term "central sensitization" is used to describe this phenomenon. Central sensitization manifests as pain hypersensitivity and may contribute to the pain phenotype in patients with fibromyalgia, osteoarthritis, musculoskeletal disorders with generalized pain hypersensitivity, neuropathic pain, and visceral pain hypersensitivity disorders. At least three interrelated mechanisms have been proposed to explain central sensitization.

1. Glutamate/NMDA receptor-mediated sensitization. Increased nociceptive afferent input leads to a massive release from nociceptor central endings of a variety of neurotransmitters and/or neuromodulators, including glutamate, substance P, CGRP, and ATP, onto output neurons in lamina I of the superficial dorsal horn. Consequently, increased release of glutamate

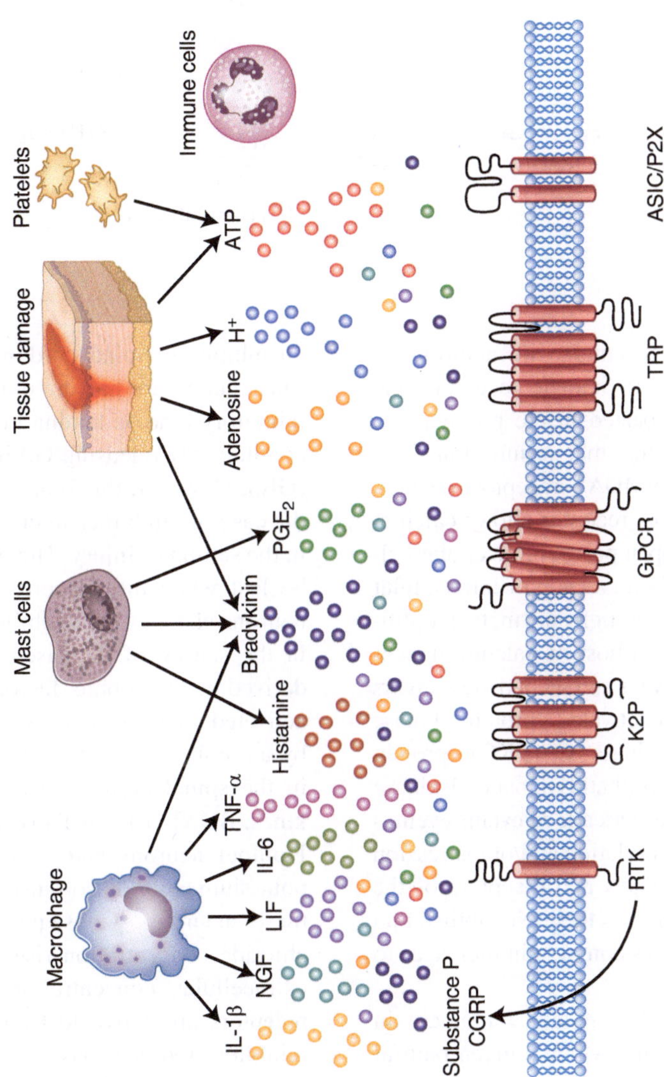

Fig. 4.1 Peripheral sensitization

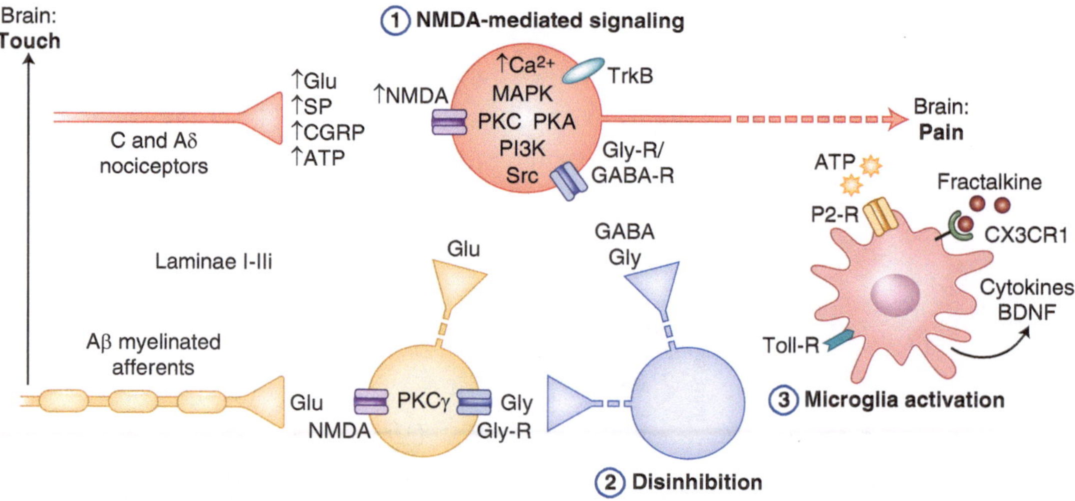

Fig. 4.2 Central sensitization

activates NMDA receptors, in addition to non-NMDA receptors (kainate receptors and AMPA receptors) located in the postsynaptic neuron, by displacing magnesium ions that normally keep NMDA receptors silent. Activation of NMDA receptor allows calcium influx through its open pores. Intracellular calcium in turn triggers a cascade of intracellular signaling processes through enzymatic amplifications that involve a host of calcium-dependent signaling pathways and second messengers including mitogen-activated protein kinase (MAPK), protein kinase C (PKC), protein kinase A (PKA), phosphatidylinositol 3-kinase (PI3K), and Src. This cascade of events eventually leads to phosphorylation and/or expression of relevant ion channels and receptors of the output neurons, increases their excitability, and facilitates the transmission of pain messages to the brain.

Pain windup is the perceived increase in pain intensity over time when a given painful stimulus is delivered repeatedly above a critical rate. It is caused by repeated stimulation of group C peripheral nerve fibers, leading to progressively increasing electrical response in output neurons in lamina I of the superficial dorsal horn. In the spinal cord, windup results in dramatic increase in neuron firing from 1 every 3 s up to 50 per second.

2. Disinhibition. Spinal cord inhibitory interneurons, under normal circumstances, keep an inhibitory tone on lamina I output neurons by continuously releasing GABA and/or glycine (Gly). However, this inhibition can be lost in the case of inhibitory interneuronal cell death in the setting of injury. The inhibition can also be lost when the property of the inhibitory neurons changes from inhibitory to excitatory in the setting of increased release of brain-derived neurotrophic factors (BDNF) from activated microglia (Fig. 4.3). Upon activation by a number of mechanisms, microglial cells in the spinal cord release BDNF and cytokines. BDNF acts on TrkB receptor of lamina I output neurons and leads to inhibition of potassium chloride cotransporter 2 (KCC2) of these neurons. Consequently, intracellular chloride concentration rises and exceeds the extracellular concentration. When GABAa receptors are activated by GABA release of inhibitory interneurons, an outflux of chloride ions occurs, leading to depolarization and excitation of lamina I output neurons.

In addition, disinhibition is believed to contribute to allodynia through activation of the PKCγ-expressing interneurons in inner lamina II. These neurons receive synaptic input from nonnociceptive myelinated Aβ primary afferents and project to excitatory

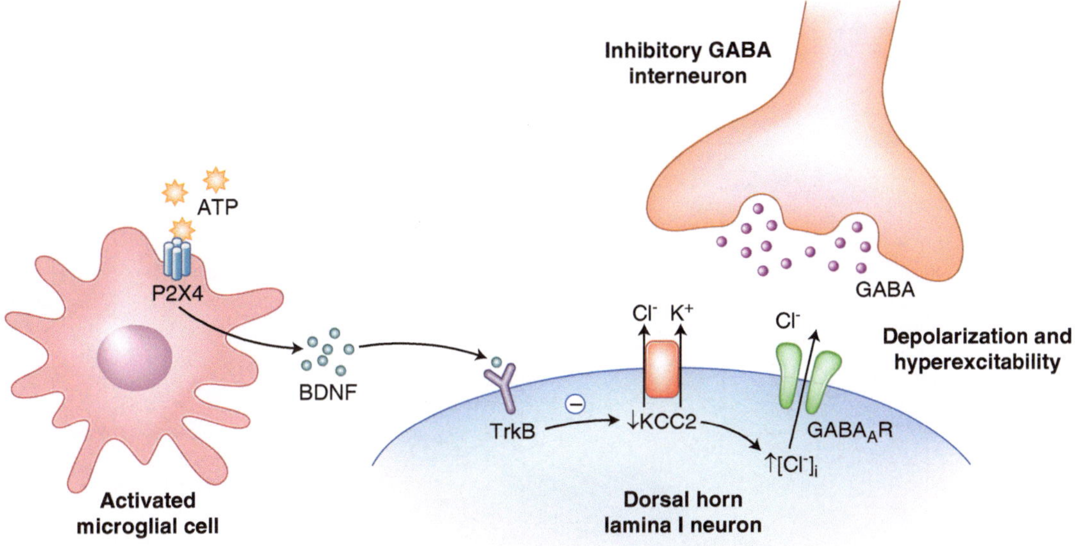

Fig. 4.3 Disinhibition

synaptic output to the lamina I output neurons. However, under normal circumstances, this group of neurons is silent due to strong input from inhibitory interneurons. This pathway can be activated by disinhibition, allowing nonnociceptive myelinated Aβ primary afferents to engage in the pain transmission circuitry. Consequently, normally innocuous stimuli are now perceived as painful (allodynia).

3. Microglial activation and glial-neuron interactions. In addition to glutamate, substance P and CGRP, peripheral nerve injury promotes release of ATP and the chemokine fractalkine that can stimulate microglial cells. Specifically, activation of purinergic P2-R receptors, CX3CR1, and Toll-like receptors on microglia results in the release of BDNF, which through activation of TrkB receptor and inhibition of KCC2, both, expressed by lamina I output neurons, promote increased excitability and enhanced pain in response to both noxious and innocuous stimulation. Activated microglia also release a host of cytokines, such as TNF-α, IL-1β, IL-6, and other factors that contribute to central sensitization, by mechanisms similar to sensitization of the nociceptors.

In addition to peripheral and central sensitization, other factors may contribute to the mechanisms of pathological pain. Such factors include sprouting of afferent fibers in the spinal cord, changes in descending inhibitory and excitatory pathways, and reorganization of the cortical area and their interconnections. These are areas of intense research interest.

Suggested Reading

1. Basbaum AI, Bautista DM, Scherrer G, Julius D. Cellular and molecular mechanisms of pain. Cell. 2009;139(2):267–84.
2. Mifflin KA, Kerr BJ. The transition from acute to chronic pain: understanding how different biological systems interact. Can J Anaesth. 2014 Feb;61(2):112–22.
3. Woolf CJ. Central sensitization: implications for the diagnosis and treatment of pain. Pain. 2011;152(3 Suppl):S2–15.

5 Pain Assessment

Rodrigo Benavides

Key Concepts

- An accurate initial pain assessment is the first step to a successful pain management strategy.
- Given that pain is a subjective experience, there may not be a direct relationship between the amount of physical pathology and the reported pain intensity.
- An effective and trustful patient-physician relationship will facilitate more efficient exchange of information, setting appropriate treatment expectations and a coordinated approach to pain management.
- Elderly patients and patients from different cultural backgrounds may present with barriers to communication, and require the physician to make adjustments in his interaction to meet their specific needs.
- A general physical exam is necessary during the initial pain evaluation, with more detail given to the area where the patient refers his symptoms; the musculoskeletal and neurological systems are usually of particular interest.
- Standardized assessment tools are inexpensive and easy to perform. They can rapidly assess a wide range of behaviors including patient's attitudes, symptoms, coping skills, quality of life, and expectancies. They can also provide guidance if a particular type of intervention may be beneficial and hint to their prognosis.
- The selection of appropriate diagnostic tests will help to accurately confirm the diagnosis and can evaluate the extent of structural pathology associated with the patient's symptoms.

Pain Assessment

Despite the progress in our knowledge of the pathophysiology of pain and the development of potent analgesic and interventional procedures, most patients with chronic pain continue to experience significant impairment in their quality of life, with physical disability and emotional distress. Therefore, the appropriate assessment of a chronic pain patient is essential to determine an accurate diagnosis and the most effective treatment strategies for pain management.

Given the multifactorial nature of chronic pain states, the initial evaluation of these patients requires a comprehensive approach, not only identifying possible organic etiologies but also the emotional and social factors underlying the patients report.

There are a group of variables that the physician should revisit throughout the patient interaction in order to create the optimal parameters for a treatment plan, these include:

R. Benavides, MD (✉)
Alan Edwards Pain Management Unit, McGill Anesthesia Department, McGill University Health Centre, Montreal, QC, Canada
e-mail: rodrigo.benavidescordero@mail.mcgill.ca

J. Cheng, R.W. Rosenquist (eds.), *Fundamentals of Pain Medicine*,
https://doi.org/10.1007/978-3-319-64922-1_5

- The degree of the patient's emotional versus physical illness
- The level of burden that these symptoms have in the patient's life, is there a disproportion?
- The presence of any associated psychological or social factors that could be influencing the patient's degree of suffering or disability

As pain is a subjective experience, there may not be a direct relationship between the amount of physical pathology and the reported pain intensity. For this reason, alongside searching for an objective pathological finding, the physician must also evaluate the patient's mood, expectancies, coping mechanisms, social resources, and interactions with significant others.

To obtain information of relevance in the most efficient way, the assessment of a chronic pain patient will involve:

- Thorough history
- Physical examination
- The use of standardized assessment tools
- Evaluation of diagnostic tests to identify possible structural pathology

Each of these categories will be subsequently analyzed in more detail.

Patient History

The pain history is obtained alongside the patient's general medical history, which must contain the basic components of an H&P, including:

- Past medical and surgical history
- Medications
- Family history
- Social history
- Review of systems

An appropriate pain history will not only help to determine the correct diagnosis but will also prevent the overinterpretation of additional laboratory or diagnostic imaging findings, which should be used for confirmatory purposes, or to guide further aspects of the evaluation. Table 5.1 shows the most relevant information to be obtained from the patient's history.

Throughout the assessment, it is not only essential to obtain the verbal information from a standard pain interview, but also to evaluate the patient's behavior and subjective body language as he delivers his report. It is important to observe the patient's interaction with significant others and their perception of the patient's illness. Also, other maladaptive attitudes may be detected such as disproportionate adherence or avoidance to certain therapeutic choices (medication or interventional), or alternative beliefs about the cause of pain. Identifying these maladaptive thoughts can help avoid hopelessness, frustration, or unwillingness to engage in potentially useful treatment options.

While obtaining the patient's history, there is also opportunity to establish a rapport with the patient and his family. Given that the course of treatment of most chronic pain cases will require frequent follow-ups and reassessment of treatment strategies, an effective and trustful patient-physician relationship will facilitate a more efficient exchange of information. As a consequence, appropriate treatment expectations can be established, and a coordinated multidisciplinary management strategy can be achieved.

Some patients may present with specific situations that could act as barriers for an efficient communication and require the physician to make adjustments in his interaction to meet their specific needs. Table 5.2 shows the most common of these situations and approaches that can improve interacting with these patients.

Physical Examination

The initial physical exam must include the basic aspects of a general exam, in addition to a more detailed evaluation of the specific system related to the patient's symptoms. In combination with the patient's history, an accurate physical examination will help determine the need of fur-

Table 5.1 Relevant information to be obtained from the patient's history

Parameter	Description
Pain characteristics	Onset and duration: Gradual, spontaneous, associated to an injury or any possible triggering event, brief flashes, or rhythmic pulses
	Location and distribution: Localized/radiating, dermatomal patterns, referred pain
	Quality: Sharp, stabbing, burning, tingling, pulsating, aching, dull, cramping, squeezing, stiffness
	Intensity: Increase or decrease over time, fluctuations during the day, higher and lower intensity scores ever achieved
	Associated symptoms: Nausea/vomiting, autonomic symptoms (temperature changes, diaphoresis or skin color changes), trophic changes (skin, hair, nail changes), difficulty with bowel or bladder control, unintentional weight loss, gait difficulty, fevers, chills, or night sweats, arm or leg weakness
	Exacerbating /alleviating factors: Bending forward, sitting, standing, climbing stairs, physical activity, lying down, lifting objects, food intake, sexual intercourse, cold weather, skin contact
Treatment strategies	Past and current medications (OTC, prescription, alternative) and their effectiveness
	Adverse reactions to previous medications (including psychiatric side effects)
	Previous interventional procedures (nerve blocks, epidurals)
	Physical therapy/home exercise (duration, frequency, effectiveness)
	Other alternative therapies such as acupuncture, tai chi, massotherapy
Past medical history	Coexisting acute or chronic illnesses
	Previous surgeries, injuries
	Psychiatric illness
	Alcohol/ tobacco, recreational drugs
	Substance abuse/dependence
	Sleep disturbance
Family history	Family history of chronic pain
	Rheumatologic/autoimmune disease
Social history	Employment, sources of income, disability, current legal process involved (lawsuits, disability claims)
	Marital status
	Social support networks, coping mechanisms, family's perception of the patients' illness, history of domestic violence
	Living situation: Who lives at home?, home assistance resources
	Activities of daily living (ADLs)
	Health insurance issues
Expectations and goals	What are the patients' goals and expectations regarding pain intensity, daily activities, and quality of life?

ther diagnostic testing, evaluate if the existing medical data can explain the patient's symptoms, and evaluate for functional limitations secondary to the patient's current illness.

The following is a list of findings that may be of particular interest in the evaluation of chronic pain by systems:

Vital signs:	Tachycardia, hypertension, fever
General appearance:	Nutritional status, body habitus
	Pain behaviors
	Restlessness, anxiety, somnolence
Generally in the area of pain:	Skin integrity, color
	Skin changes (atrophy, hair/nail growth)
	Temperature changes, edema, diaphoresis
	Allodynia/hyperalgesia/hyperesthesia
	Tenderness, muscle spasms
	Changes in pain intensity with physical factors (motion, heat or cold application, deep breathing, changes in position)
	Evident lesions (rashes, ulcers, open wounds, scars)
	Anatomical deformities (congenital/acquired)
Chest/respiratory:	Labored breathing, pleuritic chest pain
	Costochondral joint tenderness
Abdominal:	Distention, tenderness, muscle spasms, rebound
Peripheral vascular:	Capillary refill, peripheral pulses
	Trophic ischemic changes in lower extremities
	Lymphedema
General musculoskeletal:	Body type, posture, symmetry, spine curvature
	Lower extremity alignment
	Range of motion (spinal/extremities)
	Muscular tone/atrophy
	Muscular trigger points
Neck:	Tenderness over the paraspinal muscles
	Spurling test, axial loading test, Hoffman's sign
	Pain or limitation of neck range of motion (ROM)
Thoracic/lumbar spine:	Tenderness over the paraspinal muscles
	Costovertebral angle tenderness
	Facet loading test, pain or limitation of ROM
	Straight leg raising test
Pelvis (musculoskeletal):	FABER test, thigh thrust, Piriformis test
	PSIS tenderness, ischial tuberosity tenderness
	Pain or limitation of hip ROM
Extremities:	Peripheral joint ROM
	Joint instability/laxity
	Muscular strength
	Peripheral edema
Neurologic:	Mental status changes
	Cranial nerves evaluation
	Sensory abnormalities (paresthesia, allodynia, dysesthesia, hyperpathia)
	Motor deficits (weakness, abnormal reflexes, pathological reflexes)
	Upper and lower extremity coordination
	Gait abnormalities
Psychiatric:	Facial expression, eye contact, cooperative toward exam
	Abnormal mood/affect
	Suicidal ideations

Table 5.2 Common barriers of communication and approaches that can improve interacting with these patients

Patient population	Possible limitations	Recommendations
Elderly patients	Sensory impairments (visual, auditory) Underreporting of pain Cognitive decline, verbal communication impairment	Consider alternative tools such as the faces pain scale Use alternative indicators to measure symptom improvement/deterioration (ADLs) Avoid time pressure
Patients of different cultural backgrounds	Language barriers Cultural differences in pain perception Alternative treatment preferences	Recognize the behavioral responses of pain perception for patients of different cultural backgrounds Provide assessment tools and educational material in the patients native language

Standardized Pain Assessment Tools

The implementation of standardized pain assessment tools has become an invaluable method to asses for possible contributing factors to the patient's illness. Also, they can provide guidance if a particular intervention may be beneficial to the patient. Some of the advantages of the use of these instruments include:

- Inexpensive and easy to administer
- Facilitate obtaining information about behaviors that might be uncomfortable to disclose
- Rapid assessment of a wide range behaviors including patient's attitudes, symptoms, coping skills, quality of life, and expectancies

Rather than replacing the interview, these tools should be used as complement information to help determine if a particular issue should be addressed with greater detail or investigated with different diagnostic measures. Tables 5.3 and 5.4 show the general characteristics of the most commonly used unidimensional and multidimensional pain standardized tools, respectively.

Table 5.3 Common unidimensional pain standardized tools

Standardized tool	Route	Parameter assessed	Comments
Numerical rating scale (NRS)	Verbal or visual	Pain intensity using a numerical scale (0–10, 0–100)	Most commonly used rating scale, simple to explain, less reliable in very young or elderly patients
Visual analogue scale (VAS)	Visual	Pain intensity using a 10 or 100 mm line, anchored with no pain and worst possible pain	Easy to administer, can cause patient confusion if cognitively impairment
Facial pain scale (FPS)	Visual	Pain intensity using a range of facial expressions	Preferred method for pediatric and elder patients, potential for distorted assessment as patients tend to point to the center of the scale
Verbal rating scale (VRS)	Verbal	Pain intensity using verbal descriptors (mild, moderate, severe)	Not recommendable if language barriers exist or cognitively impaired

Table 5.4 Common multidimensional pain standardized tools

Standardized tool	Number of questions	Parameter assessed	Comments
McGill pain questionnaire (MPQ)	20	Pain quality and location	Takes 5–15 min to complete
DN4	4	Neuropathic pain features	Takes less than 5 min to complete
Pain disability index (PDI)	7	Pain disability and interference with family and social life	Useful to evaluate patients with multiple painful conditions
Brief pain inventory (BPI)	32	Pain intensity and interference with functional capacity	Good choice for the follow up of patients with progressive conditions
Beck depression inventory (BDI)	21	Depressive mood	Important adjuvant as pain and depression are often comorbid and potentiate each other
Pain catastrophizing scale (PCS)	13	Catastrophizing related to pain	Can be completed in less than 5 min, requires a sixth-grade reading level
Coping strategies questionnaire (CSQ)	10	Coping strategies for chronic pain	Includes 5 cognitive and 1 behavioral pain coping scale, takes 5 min to complete

Diagnostic Tests in the Assessment of Chronic Pain

The use of diagnostic studies is meant to supplement a comprehensive patient history and physical exam. The selection of an appropriate test will help to accurately confirm a diagnosis and can evaluate the extent of structural pathology associated with the patient's symptoms. A list of the most commonly used diagnostic tests in chronic pain management is shown as follows:

Laboratory test:	CBC, electrolytes, BUN/Cr
	Vitamin D levels, folate, and vitamin B12
	Liver enzymes
	Urinalysis
	Ferritin, Fibrinogen, Haptoglobin, CRP, ESR
	Autoimmune markers (rheumatoid factor, antinuclear antibodies, antiphospholipid antibodies)
Imaging studies:	X-rays
	CT, MRI
	Bone Scans
	Myelography
Electrodiagnostic tests:	Electromyography
	Nerve conduction studies
Diagnostic procedures:	Diagnostic nerve blocks
	Lumbar discography
	Lumbar sympathetic block
	Differential epidural block
	Transversus abdominis plane block

Suggested Reading

1. Colvin LA, Rowbotham D. Postgraduate educational issue managing pain: recent advances and new challenges. Oxford: Oxford University Press; 2013. British Journal of Anesthesiology.
2. Fishman SM, Ballantyne JC, Rathmell JP. Bonica's management of pain. 4th ed. New York: Lippincott Williams & Wilkins; 2010.
3. Flor H, Turk DC. Chronic pain: an integrated biobehavioral approach. Seattle: IASP Press; 2011.
4. Miller A, DiCuccio HK, Davis BA. The 3-minute muscoloskeletal & peripheral nerve exam. 1st ed. New York: Demos Medical Publishing; 2008.
5. Turk DC, Melzack R. Handbook of pain assessment. 3rd ed. New York: Guiford Press; 2011.

Diagnosis of Pain States

6

Jianguo Cheng and Richard W. Rosenquist

Key Concepts

- One of the most important competencies of a pain physician is being able to accurately diagnose pain states. Effective treatments rely on accurate diagnosis.
- Misdiagnosis of pain states is frequently due to clinician's inability to gather adequate clinical information, clinicians' gap of critical knowledge or skill set, or the complexity of a particularly challenging case.
- Localizing the pain and identifying the potential cause of problem are the primary goals of physician-patient interactions for clinical assessment and diagnosis.
- The generator of pain may be any part of the body, and the pain may be localized in a single area, multiple areas, or diffuse areas of the body.
- The causes of pain may be traumatic, ischemic, inflammatory, degenerative, neuropathic, autoimmune, cancer related, genetic, psychogenic, or malingering.
- Differential diagnosis is a key process to minimize misdiagnosis and requires knowledge, skills, and genuine desire to understand the patient's problem.
- It is common to utilize diagnostic tests and diagnostic blocks to help establish or rule out a diagnosis. In many cases, a trial treatment may be necessary to confirm or refute a working diagnosis.

The Significance of Pain State Diagnosis

Accurate and timely diagnosis of pain states is a prerequisite for efficacious and cost-effective management of pain to relieve patients' suffering. Inaccurate diagnosis often leads to treatment failure and patients' dissatisfaction. Delayed diagnosis may cause unnecessary suffering or even make treatment more difficult due to exacerbated peripheral and central sensitizations of pain. Thus physicians' ability to accurately diagnose pain states is a core competency that can't be overemphasized.

Misdiagnosis is not uncommon even in the hands of well-trained and experienced pain physicians. The reasons are multifactorial. Too often, physicians may not spend sufficient time and effort to gather critical information about the

J. Cheng, MD, PhD (✉)
Departments of Pain Management and Neurosciences, Cleveland Clinic Anesthesiology Institute and Lerner Research Institute, Cleveland, OH, USA
e-mail: CHENGJ@ccf.org

R.W. Rosenquist, MD
Department Pain Management, Cleveland Clinic, Cleveland, OH, USA

J. Cheng, R.W. Rosenquist (eds.), *Fundamentals of Pain Medicine*,
https://doi.org/10.1007/978-3-319-64922-1_6

patient and his/her complaints. Remember the answer to the question of what exactly is the patient's diagnosis may be found by closely examining the patient or reviewing the patient's medical, surgical, social, or psychological history. Also common is that the patient may not be able to offer important information for various reasons, such as poor communication skills, cultural predilection, language barriers, educational limitations, or cognitive/mental status changes. A third common cause for misdiagnosis and treatment failure may be due to complexity of the pain condition itself and limitations in our understanding of the underlying causes. Due to the subjective nature of pain, it may be difficult to find objective measures to help localize the pain and determine the underlying causes. With these considerations in mind, it is critical to take a systematic approach to the investigation of the patients' problems and pain states. Localizing the pain and identifying the potential cause of problem are the primary goals of physician-patient interactions for clinical assessment and diagnosis.

Pain Localization Diagnosis

The first step of pain diagnosis is to localize the pain. Since pain has to be generated in a particular structure of the body, it is critically important to localize the pain generator, which may be any part of the body, including the spinal cord and brain (central pain and psychogenic pain). The pain may be localized in a single area, multiple areas, or diffuse areas of the body. Generally speaking, the more areas are involved, the causes are more complex, and the treatments are more challenging.

Single area: The pain is well localized to a specific anatomic location of the body. Examples include specific joint pain, headaches, trigeminal neuralgia, postherpetic neuralgia, well-defined radiculopathy, neuroma, and stump pain.

Two areas: The pain is localized to two areas of the body. Examples include back pain and leg pain, neck pain and headaches, neck pain and arm pain, etc. In such cases, the pain in the two locations may be related or independent. It is important to determine the predominant area of pain in order to set treatment priority. For example, a transforaminal epidural injection may be indicated if a patient presents with predominantly radicular leg pain with a less degree of low back pain. In contrast, a facet joint block may be indicated if the patient presents with axial back pain as the predominant complaint with referred pain to the leg, typically above the knee.

Multiple areas: The pain is localized to more than two areas of the body. Examples include complaint of pain in the feet and hands; pain in the back, neck, and extremities; and pain in the abdomen, pelvis, and head. In such cases, multiple causes of pain are typically present. Treatment usually has to be tailored to the underlying causes that may or may not be interrelated.

Diffuse areas: Diffuse pain means "widespread" and refers to *pain* that is more or less all over or at least in many areas. Examples include fibromyalgia, inflammatory polyarthritis (rheumatoid arthritis, ankylosing spondylitis, psoriatic arthritis), polymyalgia rheumatica, systemic lupus erythematosus, polymyositis/dermatomyositis, generalized osteoarthritis, osteoporosis, cancer-related diffuse bone pain, hypothyroidism, and psychogenic pain [1].

Pain Cause Diagnosis

Once the pain is localized, the underlying cause of pain should be determined. It may be organic, functional, or mixed. It may be nociceptive, neuropathic, or mixed. It may be somatic, visceral, or mixed. For neuropathic pain, it may be peripherally or centrally mediated. Patients' description of the pain and physical findings may provide cues for the cause of the pain. The following are some of the causes that may underlie the patients' pain complaints. These causes may overlap and contribute a specific pain state.

Traumatic injury of organ(s) is the main cause of pain after surgery or trauma. In such cases, determining the extent of injury will help deliver comprehensive and adequate pain treatment in both the acute and possibly chronic phases of traumatic pain. Multimodal analgesia

(MMA) is often preferred as an effort not only to manage the acute pain but also to minimize the likelihood of transitioning to chronic pain state [7].

Ischemic pain is due to imbalance between oxygen supply and demand. It is commonly seen in such tissues as the heart, abdominal visceral organs, or extremities. Identifying such cause of pain often leads to restorative interventions that not only alleviate symptoms but also restore critical functions. In some cases, prolonged ischemia may lead to nerve injury and neuropathic pain. Examples include refractory angina, which encompasses neurological, psychogenic, and mitochondrial dysfunctions that, in addition to tissue ischemia, are responsible for a persistent cardiac pain syndrome. A second example is ischemic demyelinating peripheral neuropathy, which is often associated with *ischemic* vascular disease of the lower extremities [6]. In such neuropathic pain conditions, neuromodulation in the form of spinal cord stimulation may be indicated [3, 5, 8].

Inflammatory causes are responsible for a large number of acute and chronic pain states, including inflammatory polyarthritis (rheumatoid arthritis, ankylosing spondylitis, and psoriatic arthritis), radiculitis, myositis, and complex regional pain syndromes. Anti-inflammatory drugs, including steroids, may be indicated for systemic or targeted delivery to treat such diseases.

Degenerative changes may underlie many chronic pain states, including osteoarthritis, degenerative disc disease, and facet arthropathy. Treatment strategies include behavioral modifications, regenerative therapies, neural ablations, and replacement surgeries.

Lesion or disease of the somatosensory nervous system often leads to neuropathic pain. Examples include trigeminal neuralgia, postherpetic neuralgia, painful diabetic neuropathy, radiculopathy/radiculitis, nerve entrapment and neuromas, and central pain syndromes. There are many causes of neuropathic pain, including infections, nerve injuries, metabolic and endocrine disorders, mechanical compression, chemical irritation, cerebrovascular events, vitamin deficiencies, heavy medal or chemical toxicity, radiation, cancer, and genetic disorders.

Cancers frequently cause pain by direct invasion of tissues, compression of nerves, surgical injury of nerves, chemotherapy neurotoxicity, and radiation-induced neuropathies. Aggressive and effective pain control is one of the primary goals of palliative care in a large number of cases.

Autoimmune disorders may cause neuropathic, musculoskeletal, or visceral pain [4]. Examples include complex regional pain syndrome, multiple sclerosis, Guillain–Barré syndrome, rheumatoid arthritis, polymyalgia rheumatica, dermatomyositis, erythema nodosum, ulcerative colitis, systemic lupus erythematosus, and sarcoidosis. In many of such cases, immune modulatory therapy may prove to be the best strategy. Symptom management is also important to maintain or improve quality of life in such patients.

Genetic variations have been associated with pain disorders [9]. Erythromelalgia and familial migraine with aura are two examples of this category.

Pain Differential Diagnosis

Pain in a particular location may have various causes. It is imperative for clinicians to have an adequate list of differential diagnoses for each pain state and master the skills to differentiate the possible causes for each individual patient. The pain history and characteristics may suggest a particular cause or causes. Physical findings and diagnostic tests, such as imaging, may provide objective support for differential diagnosis under consideration. Diagnostic nerve blocks play a key role in differential diagnosis. In many cases, the validity of a particular diagnosis needs to be tested with a trial treatment because false-positive diagnostic test is not uncommon. Let's use chronic low back pain as an example to demonstrate the complexity of differential diagnosis (Table 6.1).

Chronic low back pain is one of the most common pain states. It is etiology is among the most diverse [2]. Effective treatment relies on accurate

Table 6.1 Differential diagnosis of low back pain

Causes	Examples	Comments on diagnosis/treatment
Myofascial	Muscle strain and sprains	History of injury. Self-limiting in most cases
	Myalgia and myositis	Pain in specific muscle or muscle groups, often with trigger points. TPI, muscle relaxants, and PT may be indicated
	Fibromyalgia	Meet specific diagnostic criteria. Anaerobic excise first-line treatment
Joint	Facetogenic pain	Diagnostic facet medial branch block is confirmatory. RFA of the medial branches often indicated
	Sacroiliac joint pain	Intraarticular injections may be diagnostic and therapeutic. RFA of sacral dorsal branches often indicated
	Hip joint pain	Intraarticular injection may relieve pain for months. RFA of articular branches of the femoral and obturator nerves may produce longer term relief. Joint replacement may be needed
	Spondylolysis (fatigue fracture of the pars interarticularis)	Surgical stabilization of the spine may be indicated
Vertebral disc	Discogenic pain (pain generated within the vertebral disc)	Discography may be needed. Multiple therapies including intradiscal procedures may be attempted
	Disc herniation with radiculopathy/radiculitis (mechanical compression or chemical irritation of the nerve roots)	MRI valuable. Transforaminal epidural injections may provide short-term pain relief and functional improvements. Surgical decompression or endoscopic procedures may be indicated
	Discitis	MRI valuable. Long-term antibiotics are commonly indicated
	Spondylolisthesis (a forward slippage of one vertebra over the one below it)	MRI valuable. Surgery may be indicated in unstable cases
Bone	Osteoporosis	Bone density should be evaluated and treated
	Vertebral compression fracture	MRI valuable to identify acute fracture, which may respond well to vertebroplasty or kyphoplasty
	Osteomyelitis	Antibiotic and surgical treatments are often indicated
	Cancers	CT or MRI may reveal primary or metastatic cancers

(continued)

Table 6.1 (continued)

Causes	Examples	Comments on diagnosis/treatment
Epidural	Epidural adhesion	Epidurography and epidurolysis may be indicated in patients with failed back surgery syndromes
	Epidural abscess	MRI valuable. Spontaneous or secondary to procedures. Surgical drainage and intravenous antibiotics may be indicated
	Epidural hematoma	MRI valuable. May be spontaneous or after procedures. Surgical decompression may be indicated
	Epidural lipomatosis	MRI valuable
Multiple factors	Spinal stenosis	MRI valuable. Epidural injections, minimum invasive lumbar decompression procedure, and surgical decompression are options
	Scoliosis	Often a physical exam finding. May need manipulative or surgical correction. Epidural injections may be indicated when radicular symptoms are present
	Failed back surgery syndrome	Neuromodulation is often a preferred option. Epidural injections or epidurolysis may be efficacious
Back pain referred from the viscera	Abdominal aorta aneurysm	CT valuable. Surgical intervention often indicated
	Kidney, ureter, bladder pain	Urological interventions often indicated. Sympathetic blocks (celiac plexus or splanchnic nerves) may be indicated in refractory cases
	Genital tracts: Prostatitis (male); endometriosis (female)	Urological or gynecological workup and interventions indicated. Superior hypogastric block and/or ganglion impar block may be indicated
	Gastrointestinal tract: Duodenal ulcers, chronic pancreatitis, colonic pain, rectal pain	Gastroenterology evaluation and interventions indicated. Sympathetic nerve blocks and RFA may be indicated (splanchnic nerve/celiac plexus blocks for abdominal pain; superior hypogastric nerve blocks for pelvic pain; ganglion impar blocks for rectal pain and pain in the lower genital and urological tracts)

(continued)

Table 6.1 (continued)

Causes	Examples	Comments on diagnosis/treatment
Uncommon syndromes	Bertolotti's syndrome (lumbosacral transitional vertebra)	Radiography typical sufficient for diagnosis. Treatment may be directed to manage adverse consequences of biomechanical changes (e.g., disc herniation, facet arthropathy) of the transitional vertebra
	Baastrup disease (kissing spine syndrome)	Radiography and MRI valuable. Injections into pseudo bursitis between the adjacent kissing spinal processes or surgical removal may be indicated
	Maigne's syndrome (thoracolumbar junction syndrome)	T12-L2 Lateral branches of dorsal ramus blocks or RFA may be indicated for diagnostic or therapeutic purposes. Cluneal nerve block may be indicated in nerve entrapment cases
	Forestier's disease (diffuse idiopathic skeletal hyperostosis, DISH)	Radiography of the spine is the single most useful imaging modality
	Ankylosing spondylitis	Radiography of the spine is the single most useful imaging modality
Red flags	Infection: Epidural abscess, discitis, and osteomyelitis	MRI critical. Antibiotics and/or surgery
	Cancer: Multiple myeloma, metastatic cancers	Analgesics and/or palliative care
	Cauda equina syndrome	Surgical decompression
Yellow flags	Psychogenic pain (caused, increased, or prolonged by mental, emotional, or behavioral factors)	A form of persistent somatoform pain disorder Psychotherapy, antidepressants, analgesics
	Fictitious disorders	Diagnosis of exclusion and evidence of deceiving
	Malingering for secondary gains (litigation, disability claims)	Inconsistent findings, evidence of intention for secondary gains. Diagnosis of exclusion

CT computed tomography, *MRI* magnetic resonance imaging, *RFA* radiofrequency ablation, *TPI* trigger point injection, *PT* physical therapy

differential diagnosis. Potential causes include discogenic pain, facetogenic pain, sacroiliac joint pain, myofascial pain, compression fracture of the vertebral body, spondylolisthesis, spinal stenosis, lumbar disc herniation with radiculopathy/radiculitis, failed back surgery syndrome, Bertolotti's syndrome (lumbosacral transitional vertebra), Baastrup disease (kissing spine syndrome), Maigne's syndrome (thoracolumbar junction syndrome), Forestier's disease (diffuse idiopathic skeletal hyperostosis, DISH), ankylosing spondylitis, hip arthropathy, fibromyalgia, and referred pain from visceral organs. Additional causes include infection, such as epidural abscess, discitis, and osteomyelitis and cancers, such as multiple myeloma and metastatic cancers. It is also important to keep in mind the possibility of psychogenic pain and malingering for secondary gains (litigation, disability claims). This list of potential causes of low back pain is by no means complete, nor is it intended to be. However, it does make it clear that accurate differential diagnosis holds the key to efficacious and cost-effective treatment of the patient.

It is noteworthy that many of these causes may coexist in a single patient. It is necessary to differentiate these causes by accurately gathering relevant information from patient history, physical findings, imaging and other tests, diagnostic nerve blocks, and even trial treatments. Treatment often has to be individualized because it is often extremely difficult to generalize findings from randomized controlled trials (RCTs), which typically target to study a specific hypothesis in a defined patient population as homogenous as possible, even if evidence from RCTs does exist. Table 6.1 summarizes some of the factors for differential diagnosis of chronic low back pain.

In summary, the formation of a medical diagnosis is imperative to enable a clinician to arrive at a suitable treatment for the pain. Clinicians should be able to first localize the pain and then investigate the causes of the pain. Misdiagnosis is often due to inadequate clinical information, clinician's gap in knowledge and skillset in pain medicine, or the complexity of a particular pain complaint. Differential diagnosis is a key process to minimize misdiagnosis and requires not only knowledge and skills but more importantly a genuine desire to understand the patient's problem. It is common to utilize diagnostic tests and diagnostic blocks to help establish or rule out a diagnosis. In many cases, a trial treatment may be necessary to confirm or refute a working diagnosis.

Suggested Reading

1. Bliddal H, Danneskiold-Samsoe B. Chronic widespread pain in the spectrum of rheumatological diseases. Best Pract Res Clin Rheumatol. 2007;21(3):391–402.
2. Jenkins H. Classification of low back pain. Australasian Chiropr Osteopath J Chiropr Osteopath Coll Australasia. 2002;10(2):91–7.
3. Lapenna E, Rapati D, Cardano P, De Bonis M, Lullo F, Zangrillo A, et al. Spinal cord stimulation for patients with refractory angina and previous coronary surgery. Ann Thorac Surg. 2006;82(5):1704–8.
4. Mifflin KA, Kerr BJ. Pain in autoimmune disorders. J Neurosci Res. 2016;95(6):1282–94.
5. Naoum JJ, Arbid EJ. Spinal cord stimulation for chronic limb ischemia. Methodist Debakey Cardiovasc J. 2013;9(2):99–102.
6. Ugalde V, Rosen BS. Ischemic peripheral neuropathy. Phys Med Rehabil Clin N Am. 2001;12(2):365–80.
7. Vadivelu N, Mitra S, Schermer E, Kodumudi V, Kaye AD, Urman RD. Preventive analgesia for postoperative pain control: a broader concept. Local Reg Anesthesia. 2014;7:17–22.
8. van Kleef M, Staats P, Mekhail N, Huygen F. 24. Chronic refractory angina pectoris. Pain Pract Off J World Inst Pain. 2011;11(5):476–82.
9. Zorina-Lichtenwalter K, Meloto CB, Khoury S, Diatchenko L. Genetic predictors of human chronic pain conditions. Neuroscience. 2016;338:36–62.

Part II

The Management of Pain States

Psychological Management of Pain

7

Sara Davin, Judith Scheman, and Edward Covington

Key Concepts

- Pain is not what occurs at the periphery but what is experienced by the brain. It entails both sensory and emotional processes.
- Cognitive and emotional factors are important modifiers of the pain experience: Hopelessness, helplessness, anger, fear, and other distressing emotions increase both acute and chronic pain.
- Chronic non-cancer pain carries staggering individual and societal costs. Pain persists for the majority, despite the availability of advanced procedures, surgeries, and new pharmacological treatments. It often remains unchanged despite the expenditure of vast amounts of healthcare resources.
- *Chronic pain syndrome* is a term that refers to severe persistent pain, accompanied by significant functional impairment/disability, behavioral changes, and psychological comorbidity.
- Substantiated non-pharmacological treatments include education, exercise/physical therapy, cognitive behavioral therapy, mindfulness-/acceptance-based therapies, and biofeedback therapy/relaxation training. These are often used in combination.
- Interdisciplinary pain rehabilitation programs (IPRPs) are a cost-effective treatment of persistent, disabling pain. Such programs integrate physical reconditioning, education, medication management, and psychological interventions.

Significance

Most of those who experience painful illnesses or trauma (including surgery) are able to obtain satisfactory analgesia during the acute and convalescent stages with pharmacological or other interventions. However, for many, these approaches are either ineffective or insufficient when used in isolation, so that they must be supplemented or even replaced with alternative strategies to optimize patient comfort and function. Many of the most effective approaches are psychological in nature. This is even truer in the case of chronic non-cancer pain (CNCP), which is rarely fully responsive to pharmacotherapy.

Psychosocial variables have been repeatedly demonstrated to predict pain-related outcomes in situations as diverse as joint replacement surgery, back strain, and arthritis [1–3]. Investigations of pain-relieving procedures such as lumbar discectomy and spinal cord stimulation have

S. Davin, PsyD, MPH (✉) • E. Covington, MD
Center for Neurological Restoration, Cleveland Clinic, Cleveland, OH, USA
e-mail: davins@ccf.org

J. Scheman, PhD
Digestive Disease and Surgery Institute, Cleveland Clinic, Cleveland, OH, USA

J. Cheng, R.W. Rosenquist (eds.), *Fundamentals of Pain Medicine*,
https://doi.org/10.1007/978-3-319-64922-1_7

demonstrated that psychological variables are major predictors of their effectiveness. Additionally, psychosocial variables have often been found to predict pain-related disability better than physical pathology in those with persistent pain [4]. Since not all patients achieve acceptable relief from medical or surgical interventions, it is essential that healthcare providers identify those in need of more comprehensive treatment and direct them to providers who can deliver it. Fortunately, psychological therapies tend to be economical when compared with other treatments and may therefore become increasingly important.

Psychosocial Modulation of Pain

Negative emotions and thoughts about pain have a direct effect on its perception, and failure to address them can impede relief. The fact that pain is both an emotional and sensory experience, rather than a simple perception, suggests the need for a multidimensional approach. Pain is a complex phenomenon that is modified by neurobiology, psychology, environment, and prior experiences. These components must be considered to fully understand and mitigate difficult cases of pain and dysfunction [5, 6].

Pain is dramatically altered by such internal factors as fears, beliefs/cognitions and mood, and by external factors, including stressors and incentives/disincentives for health versus sick-role behavior. Attention and distraction demonstrably amplify and attenuate pain, respectively. Numerous investigations have showed reduced brain activity in areas related to pain perception, such as the somatosensory cortex and dorsal horn (DH), with distraction [7–9]. Similarly responding to chronic pain with social isolation and disengagement from occupational and recreational activities lessens the opportunity for competing outside stimulation. Anticipating pain and guarding against it activate cells in the rostroventral medulla that amplify incoming pain signals at the level of the DH. Animal models suggest that the simple facts of anticipating a pain and expecting it to be important are sufficient to trigger these "on cells," in essence activating the "amplifiers" before the pain stimulus has begun [10].

Emotions contribute substantially to the pain experience, as is demonstrated by compelling evidence of their precipitating, moderating, and perpetuating influences on pain [11]. Negative emotional states such as depression, fear/anxiety, and anger amplify pain, hinder coping, and lessen overall treatment response in both acute and chronic pain [12–15]. Furthermore, emotional states may maintain many problematic behaviors, such as regression and overreliance upon medications that perpetuate a disabled lifestyle.

Anger is associated with exacerbation of both acute and chronic pain. A number of authors have found associations between anger regulation, both expression and suppression, and severity of chronic pain [16–18]. Burns et al. found that patients with chronic low-back pain who were told to suppress their anger toward a study confederate exhibited more pain behaviors and reported more pain than those who did not suppress their anger [19].

Pain catastrophizing is a term used to denote a negative cognitive–affective response to anticipated or actual pain [20]. It has been shown to markedly amplify pain. It is common in chronic pain patients and is associated with poorer outcome, heightened pain sensitivity, and impaired functioning [21]. It is therefore imperative that the healthcare provider not promote catastrophizing by using dramatic descriptions of pathology, such as, "you have the spine of a 90 year-old," or "your nerves are being crushed." This is even more true in light of the poor correlation between imaging findings and patient's pain and associated disability. Beliefs that pain must seriously impact one's life are associated with higher levels of pain, suffering, and disability [22].

The Role of Past and Current Stressors

Prior emotional trauma has long been associated with somatization and chronic pain in later life. Factors such as early childhood neglect, abandonment, abuse, or loss are more common in individuals with fibromyalgia or somatoform pain disorders [23]. Additionally, there is evidence that individuals with histories of childhood abuse may have more pain [24]. Other childhood traumas, such as loss, are associated with poorer outcome in terms of pain and social adjustment [25]. These studies are further supported by recent animal models demonstrating that rats exposed to stress as pups demonstrate lowered pain thresholds [26].

Psychological Management of Pain

Interventions for chronic non-cancer pain (CNCP) largely follow from the psychosocial factors that exacerbate or mitigate pain and functional impairment. They include education, cognitive behavioral therapy, relaxation/meditation training techniques, behavior modification, and treating concurrent psychological symptoms such as anxiety and depression [27].

Education

Catastrophizing can be mitigated by reassuring information. For example, a statement such as, "Your spine shows some degenerative changes, but then everyone's spine shows some changes after age 40 or so, and people with far worse imaging are often still able to bike, ski, garden, and otherwise enjoy life while feeling useful," can both validate the patient's pain complaints and invalidate their catastrophic beliefs and expectations of debility. Other pain-related beliefs, such as "avoiding activity helps prevent further harm and pain," promote deconditioning and a cycle of "fear avoidance," typified by progressively lessened participation in rewarding experiences and subsequent loneliness, depression, and fear. This "chronic pain cycle" is obviously not resolved by medical interventions.

Misunderstanding the causes and expected course of pain significantly affects the pain experience. Uncertainty, fear, helplessness, and hopelessness often derive from inaccurate beliefs about the meaning of pain. Almost three decades of literature support the usefulness of education in chronic disease management. Interventions that maximize self-efficacy and challenge faulty pain-related beliefs have demonstrable impacts on pain and disability. Some of the earliest and strongest evidence for this was demonstrated with arthritis patients, who showed improvements in perceived control of disease/illness, depression, health-promoting behaviors (relaxation, exercise), and lessened healthcare utilization after participating in a group-based educational program [28].

Family Education

Since chronic pain does not exist in isolation, education of the family system is crucial. It affects relationships in pronounced and often harmful ways. Misconceptions and faulty beliefs promote helplessness and confusion. Family members often assume a care-giving role, inadvertently promoting debility. *Hostile dependency* (a phenomenon in which the person experiences considerable anger toward those who are providing care) can significantly impair communication and intimacy. Family education can not only help maintain the emotional support that is essential but can also guide them in strategies likely to promote improved function and quality of life instead of debility.

Families are typically torn about how to respond to their loved ones. They've found that pampering was nonproductive, ignoring seemed callous and nonproductive, and criticism was toxic. They don't know how to react. Fortunately, there is now sufficient data to inform their behavior [29–31].

1. Support, validation, and positive regard are essential.
2. Rewarding "pain behavior" promotes its increase; thus, positive statements and attention should be contingent on healthy behaviors rather than "sick-role" behaviors; e.g., comments about emotions or current life events should receive more response than comments about pain, medications, and treatments.

3. Overprotection promotes invalidism. Attempts at normal behavior should elicit encouragement, not cautions. Suggestions for rest and inactivity are toxic.
4. Criticizing "pain behavior" is likely to make it worse and promotes depression.
5. It may be helpful for those who have become caretakers to think in terms of replacing this role with that of companion, friend, lover, or playmate.

Important Educational Points for the Patient and Family

- Chronic pain, unlike acute pain, is usually more a reflection of neurological sensitization than of tissue pathology or fragility.
- Hurt does not imply harm.
- In the long term, exercise helps pain and mood (even in small quantities).
- Pacing activities and working to quota (not tolerance) is an important part of managing pain.
- Emotions and beliefs about pain are an integral part of the pain experience.
- Attempts to protect the person with pain often reinforce dependency, disability, and negative emotions such as anger and resentment.

In order for families to accept and act on this advice, they must first understand that these responses are both safe and compassionate, which require understanding the medical basis for the patient's pain.

Cognitive Behavioral Therapy (CBT)

CBT for pain (CBT-P) is predicated on the influence of maladaptive cognitions and emotional states on pain. Thoughts, beliefs, and interpretations about oneself, others, and the world directly impact emotional state and behaviors. In CBT-P the goal is to modify maladaptive thoughts or beliefs related to pain and one's ability to cope with it. Alternative cognitions, along with adaptive behavioral and emotional responses, are trained with a resultant decrease in pain and disability. Systematic reviews and meta-analyses over 15 years demonstrate substantial improvements in pain, mood, and function across a variety of pain conditions, and these improvements persist up to 5 years following treatment [7]. In cases of degenerative disc disease and so-called "failed back syndrome," CBT-P was shown to be as effective as lumbar fusion in two randomized controlled trials [32].

The techniques utilized in cognitive behavioral therapy vary widely but generally involve teaching individuals to identify and monitor unhelpful patterns of thinking that contribute to poor coping and disability. For example, a patient might be asked to challenge the belief, "I will suffer for the rest of my life because of my pain," and to develop healthy coping statements such as, "My pain does not control me." Such education may mitigate such beliefs as "I will never recover normal function without surgery." This type of reframing can empower patients to take control of their lives and reduce feelings of helplessness, hopelessness, and dread of the future.

A consistent finding across systematic reviews of psychological approaches for chronic pain is that the effectiveness of CBT is best demonstrated for pain-related mood and function, with somewhat less of an effect on pain severity [33].

Mindfulness Meditation and Acceptance-Based Therapies

Mindfulness- and acceptance-based therapies generally emphasize adaptation and lessened resistance to the pain experience. Mindfulness, a construct rooted in Buddhist philosophy, teaches individuals to adapt a nonjudgmental and curious awareness toward one's thoughts, feelings, and body. The ironic processes model posits that intentional attempts to suppress unwanted thoughts may paradoxically increase them and amplify the corresponding emotional reaction

[34]. Furthermore, suppression of negative emotions increases self-reported pain and pain behaviors [35]. Following from this line of thinking, mindfulness- and acceptance-based therapies teach that efforts to control or avoid unwanted experiences may actually increase suffering. To this degree, mindfulness-/acceptance-based therapies for pain teach individuals to "befriend" their bodies, thoughts, and emotional reactions.

Over the past decade, various adaptations of mindfulness- and acceptance-based therapies have evolved, including mindfulness-based stress reduction (MBSR), mindfulness-based cognitive therapy (MBCT), and acceptance and commitment therapy (ACT). They have been adapted to a variety of somatic and stress-related conditions. These therapies emphasize formal and informal meditation practice, psychological "flexibility," and also incorporate some of the central tenants of CBT.

Evidence for the efficacy of mindfulness-based treatments is still preliminary, due to small to modest treatment effects, methodological limitations of studies (no control group, lack of control for non-specific effects). One recent systematic review and meta-analysis of meditation programs that included only randomized controlled trials and accounted for placebo effect found moderate evidence for its effects on mood and pain but no evidence that such benefits exceed those obtained from other psychological and medical treatments [36]. A review of mindfulness-based therapies specifically for chronic pain reported small non-specific improvements in pain and depression, across ten studies reviewed; however, significant and sustained improvements were demonstrated in pain acceptance, quality of life, and stress [37].

In a meta-analysis of 22 acceptance-based studies, including mindfulness and ACT, significant improvements were found for pain, depression, anxiety, physical well-being, and quality of life [38]. Thus, these relatively new therapeutic approaches appear to be a viable option that offers patients an alternative way to conceptualize, understand, and cope with their pain experience, with comparable benefits to other treatment approaches. Such therapies have the potential to help patients let go of expectations for a pain-free or stress-free life and to understand that pain and periods of emotional distress are components of the human experience, which do not necessarily dictate a life of suffering.

Healing Old Wounds

Psychodynamic psychotherapy is one psychological approach that may be useful to help individuals who have history of extensive childhood trauma heal emotionally. In general psychodynamic therapy emphasizes relationships and attachment patterns, with a focus on early childhood experiences. There is evidence that psychodynamic approaches produce improvements in psychiatric and somatic symptoms, as well as reduce healthcare utilization among patients with a variety of somatic medical conditions [39]. However, there is limited empirical support of its efficacy in chronic pain [40].

Relaxation/Biofeedback Training

Chronic uncontrolled stress amplifies pain and associated emotional distress. Relaxation with or without the assistance of biofeedback training aim to modify the stress response and the associated physiological indicators. The benefits of relaxation training are well established. A recent study showed reductions in cortisol, ACTH, and norepinephrine and perceived psychophysiological distress in a group of participants after listening to a CD designed to elicit the relaxation response [41].

Relaxation techniques vary in nature but include deep breathing, progressive muscle relaxation, guided imagery, and visualization. Relaxation techniques can have a direct effect on tense muscles and heightened arousal that is accompanied by the stress of pain, as well as decrease any limbic augmentation that may be contributing to the pain experience. Relaxation training offers a quick, simple, and drug-free method for slowing the cascade of stress hormones that often accompanies chronic pain.

Biofeedback training uses electronic feedback to demonstrate changes in various physiological indices of stress (muscle tension, palmer sweat response, heart rate, hand temperature), in conjunction with the use of relaxation techniques facilitate self-regulation of the stress response [42].

Biofeedback training has been studied in a variety of pain conditions with variable evidence of efficacy. However it is an intervention that continues to be utilized, perhaps due to its unique ability to objectify the stress response in a fairly simple, noninvasive manner. This may be particularly useful with those patients who are skeptical about the connection between the mind and body.

Clinically, many of the techniques discussed here are combined, e.g., it would be common to combine biofeedback training with progressive muscular relaxation and guided imagery and to utilize cognitive approaches at the same time. In such use, it is likely that the combination of therapies, modified according to the patient's apparent needs, is more effective than any individual component.

Fitness

This chapter on the psychological management of pain addresses the issue of fitness for several reasons. Psychological issues impact functional abilities, and fitness impacts psychological status. Many patients with chronic pain develop a fear of movement, so-called kinesophobia. Having become deconditioned due to rest following the onset of their pain, they hurt more whenever they attempt activities, leading to the false belief that activity is hazardous and should be avoided. This leads to more inactivity. Breaking this cycle is critical for rehabilitation to take place. A number of studies have addressed kinesophobia [43–45]. Patients who have this trait report more pain and disability and engage in more self-protective behaviors [46]. A graded exercise program gradually reduces this fear and promotes increased function and a reduction in the self-perception of fragility [47]. Exercise is an important component of psychological treatment of pain. It is a powerful antidote to "learned helplessness" and directly reduces such symptoms as anxiety and depression [48–50].

Key Points

- Deconditioning promotes self-perceptions of helplessness and physical fragility. Reconditioning reverses both.
- Aerobic exercises reduce anxiety, depression, and pain (even in brief duration) [1].
- Reconditioning restores access to life activities that provide joy and increases self-esteem.
- As people learn that exercise is safe, vigilance to symptoms decreases, which decreases pain.

Behavior Modification/Operant Conditioning

"Behavior rewarded is behavior repeated." This common saying has great significance in the management of chronic pain, where overt and covert reinforcements for "illness behavior" commonly exist, often along with aversive consequences of "wellness behavior," e.g., a person seen mowing the lawn risks loss of disability income [51]. Maladaptive pain behaviors generally include excessive dependence upon others, disability, and other behaviors typifying the "sick role." Operant conditioning aims to maximize reinforcements for healthy/non-pain behavior and minimize reinforcement for such "pain behaviors" as excessive somatic conversation, reclining, isolation, etc. Behavior modification can occur in a variety of contexts, including physical therapy, family therapy, group psychotherapy, patient–provider interactions, and IPRPs. Numerous studies confirm that operant conditioning is an important agent of change, with benefits demonstrated in function/activity, pain intensity, and analgesic use [52].

Treatment of Comorbid Psychiatric Illness

Comorbid psychiatric disorders are very common in those with chronic pain and may either precede the pain or arise as a response to it. Rates of depression among individuals with chronic pain range from 30 to 60%, and more than one-third meet criteria for an anxiety disorder [53].

Major depression can present with pain, in which case treatment of the mood disorder often provides relief. More commonly, however, depression appears as a direct or indirect consequence of pain. Rudy et al. showed that the link between pain and depression could be mediated by perceived life interference (loss of gratifying activities) and loss of self-control [54]. Moreover, Strigo et al., in a study of the association of major depressive disorder and experimental pain, observed that anticipation of pain was associated with increased activity in the amygdala, anterior insula, and anterior cingulate cortex in patients with major depressive disorder when compared with normals [55]. This suggests that depressed patients experienced an affective response even before they experienced the painful stimulus. This reaction was also associated with greater perceived helplessness. They posit that patients with major depressive disorder have an altered functional response within specific neural networks during the anticipation of pain that may lead to an impaired ability to modulate the painful experience as well as their emotional response to the pain.

Post-traumatic stress disorder (PTSD) is highly comorbid in chronic pain, with up to 66% of a sample of veterans with PTSD also suffering from chronic pain [56]. Importantly, anxiety and depressive disorders predict outcome in chronic pain [57]. Psychiatric disorders limit the successful treatment of pain, and pain reciprocally impedes the treatment of psychiatric disturbance [58, 59].

The pronounced interaction between psychiatric illness and chronic pain and disability requires that these conditions be treated concurrently for optimum benefit. The fact that many of the psychiatric symptoms result from such factors as learned fear and helplessness, loss of life activities that provide joy and a sense of self-esteem, and such other losses as social, financial, and sexual, probably explains the observation that pharmacological treatment is usually insufficient to resolve them and that psychotherapeutic interventions are essential.

Substance use disorders, involving drugs initially used recreationally, as well as those used medically, are highly prevalent among those with chronic pain and must be appropriately treated in conjunction with other pain-related treatments. A separate chapter in this volume is dedicated to this issue.

Interdisciplinary Chronic Pain Rehabilitation Programs

When chronic non-cancer pain (CNCP) is refractory to traditional treatments and is associated with significant functional impairment or psychological distress, IPRPs provide an option with well-demonstrated and durable outcomes [60]. Due to the nature of the treatment, controlled studies are limited [61]. ICPRPs focus on functional restoration and improved quality of life and typically combine physical reconditioning, psychological rehabilitation, and pharmacotherapy. They encourage patients to accept and manage their pain in a way that maximizes their ability to enjoy life and contribute to it, despite having a distressing symptom that cannot fully be eliminated. They attempt to minimize sick-role behavior and nonproductive healthcare utilization. These programs vary in intensity from several hours of care and several days a week for several weeks all the way to inpatient care. Day care or so-called partial hospitalization programs are common. IPRPs are supported by compelling research demonstrating sustainable improvements in pain, mood, and function that lasts up to 10 years [62].

Summary

The Psychological Management of Pain Includes

- Challenging faulty beliefs related to pain and forming new expectations
- Reengaging in life's activities, including socialization, fun, and work and understanding that this process helps control pain
- The abandonment of passive dependency on others
- Learning the difference between hurt and harm
- Believing in and experiencing the benefits of exercise in terms of pain and mood
- Learning to relax so as to stop the exacerbation of pain by stressors, including pain itself
- Learning that emotions have a direct effect on pain
- Being able to attenuate central amplification of pain through techniques such as those utilized in cognitive behavioral therapy (CBT)
- Healing from past traumas and learning how to get physical and emotional needs met in a healthy manner
- Gaining a sense of mastery and control in the management of chronic pain

References

1. Celestin J, Edwards RR, Jamison RN. Pretreatment psychosocial variables as predictors of outcomes following lumbar surgery and spinal cord stimulation: a systematic review and literature synthesis. Pain Med. 2009;10(4):639–53.
2. Katz J, Seltzer Z. Transition from acute to chronic postsurgical pain: risk factors and protective factors. Expert Rev Neurother. 2009;9:723–44.
3. Masselin-Dubois A, Attal N, Fletcher D, Jayr C, Albi A, Fermanian J, Bouhassira D, Baudic S. Are psychological predictors of chronic postsurgical pain dependent on the surgical model? A comparison of total knee arthroplasty and breast surgery for cancer. J Pain. 2013;14(8):854–64.
4. Carragee EJ, Alamin TF, Miller JL, Carragee JM. Discographic, MRI and psychosocial determinants of low back pain disability and remission: a prospective study in subjects with benign persistent back pain. Spine J. 2005;5(1):24–35.
5. Seebach CL, Kirkhart M, Lating JM, Wegener ST, Song Y, Riley LH 3rd, Archer KR. Examining the role of positive and negative affect in recovery from spine surgery. Pain. 2012;153(3):518–25.
6. Campbell P, Bishop A, Dunn KM, Main CJ, Thomas E, Foster NE. Conceptual overlap of psychological constructs in low back pain. Pain. 2013;154(9):1783–91.
7. Bushnell MC, Duncan GH, Hofbauer RK, Ha B, Chen JI, Carrier B. Pain perception: is there a role for primary somatosensory cortex? Proc Natl Acad Sci U S A. 1999;96(14):7705–9.
8. Sprenger C, Eippert F, Finsterbusch J, Bingel U, Rose M, Büchel C. Attention modulates spinal cord responses to pain. Curr Biol. 2012;22(11):1019–22.
9. Petrovic P, Petersson KM, Ghatan PH, et al. Pain-related cerebral activation is altered by a distracting cognitive task. Pain. 2000;85:19–30.
10. Duncan GH, Bushnell MC, Bates R, Dubner R. Task-related responses of monkey medullary dorsal horn neurons. J Neurophysiol. 1987;57(1):289–310.
11. Gatchel RJ, Peng YB, Peters ML, Fuchs PN, Turk DC. The biopsychosocial approach to chronic pain: scientific advances and future directions. Psychol Bull. 2007;133(4):581–624.
12. Fernandez E, Turk DC. The scope and significance of anger in the experience of chronic pain. Pain. 1995;61(2):165–75.
13. Berna C, Leknes S, Holmes EA, Edwards RR, Goodwin GM, Tracey I. Induction of depressed mood disrupts emotion regulation neurocircuitry and enhances pain unpleasantness. Biol Psychiatry. 2010;67(11):1083–90.
14. Stewart SH, Asmundson GJ. Anxiety sensitivity and its impact on pain experiences and conditions: a state of the art. Cogn Behav Ther. 2006;35(4):185–8.
15. Thompson T, Keogh E, French CC, Davis R. Anxiety sensitivity and pain: generalisability across noxious stimuli. Pain. 2008;134(1–2):187–96.
16. Kerns RD, Rosenberg R, Jacob MC. Anger expression and chronic pain. J Behav Med. 1994;17:57–67.
17. Burns JW, Johnson BJ, Mahoney N, Devine J, Pawl R. Anger management style, hostility and spouse responses: gender differences in predictors of adjustment among chronic pain patients. Pain. 1996;64:445–53.
18. Bruehl S, Burns JW, Chung OY, Ward B, Johnson B. Anger and pain severity in chronic low back pain patients and pain free controls: the role of endogenous opioid blockade. Pain. 2002;99:923–33.
19. Burns JW, Quartana P, Gilliam W, Lofland K, Gray E, Matsuura J, Nappi C, Wolf B. Effects of anger suppression on pain severity and pain behaviors among

chronic pain patients: evaluation of and ironic process model. Health Psychol. 2008;27(5):645–52.
20. Quartana PJ, Campbell CM, Edwards RR. Pain catastrophizing: a critical review. Expert Rev Neurother. 2009;9(5):745–58.
21. Weissman-Fogel I, Sprecher E, Pud D. Effects of catastrophizing on pain perception and pain modulation. Exp Brain Res. 2008;186(1):79–85.
22. Roth RS, Punch MR, Bachman JE. Patient beliefs about pain diagnosis in chronic pelvic pain: relation to pain experience, mood and disability. J Reprod Med. 2011;56(3–4):123–9.
23. Imbierowicz K, Egle UT. Childhood adversities in patients with fibromyalgia and somatoform pain disorder. Eur J Pain. 2003;7(2):113–9.
24. Sachs-Ericsson N, Kendall-Tackett K, Hernandez A. Childhood abuse, chronic pain, and depression in the National Comorbidity Survey. Child Abuse Negl. 2007;31(5):531–47.
25. Mallouh SK, Abbey SE, Dillies LA. The role of loss in treatment outcomes of persistent somatization. Gen Hosp Psychiatry. 1995;17:187–91.
26. Coutinho SV, Plotsky PM, Sablad M, Miller JC, Zhou H, Bayati AI, McRoberts JA, Mayer EA. Neonatal maternal separation alters stress-induced responses to viscerosomatic nociceptive stimuli in rats. Am J Physiol Gastrointest Liver Physiol. 2002;282(2):G307–16.
27. Kerns RD, Sellinger J, Goodin BR. Psychological treatment of chronic pain. Annu Rev Clin Psychol. 2011;7:411–34.
28. Marks R, Allegrante JP, Lorig K. A review and synthesis of research evidence for self-efficacy-enhancing interventions for reducing chronic disability: implications for health education practice (part I). Health Promot Pract. 2005;6:148–56.
29. LM MC. Social context and acceptance of chronic pain: the role of solicitous and punishing responses. Pain. 2005;113:155–9.
30. Raichle KA, Romano JM, Jensen MP. Partner responses to patient pain and well behaviors and their relationship to patient pain behavior, functioning, and depression. Pain. 2011;152(1):82–8.
31. Alschuler KN, Hoodin F, Murphy SL, Rice J, Geisser ME. Factors contributing to physical activity in a chronic low back pain clinical sample: a comprehensive analysis using continuous ambulatory monitoring. Pain. 2011;152(11):2521–7.
32. Brox JI, Reikerås O, Nygaard Ø, Sørensen R, Indahl A, Holm I, Keller A, Ingebrigtsen T, Grundnes O, Lange JE, Friis A. Lumbar instrumented fusion compared with cognitive intervention and exercises in patients with chronic back pain after previous surgery for disc herniation: a prospective randomized controlled study. Pain. 2006;122(1–2):145–55.
33. Eccleston C, Morley SJ, Williams AC. Psychological approaches to chronic pain management: evidence and challenges. Br J Anaesth. 2013;111(1):59–63.
34. Wegner DM. Ironic processes of mental control. Psychol Rev. 1994;101(1):34–52.
35. Burns JW, Quartana P, Gilliam W, Gray E, Matsuura J, Nappi C, Wolfe B, Lofland K. Effects of anger suppression on pain severity and pain behaviors among chronic pain patients: evaluation of an ironic process model. Health Psychol. 2008;27(5):645–52.
36. Goyal M, Singh S, Sibinga EM, Gould NF, Rowland-Seymour A, Sharma R, Berger Z, Sleicher D, Maron DD, Shihab HM, Ranasinghe PD, Linn S, Saha S, Bass EB, Haythornthwaite JA. Meditation programs for psychological stress and well-being: a systematic review and meta-analysis. JAMA Intern Med. 2014; 174(3):357–68.
37. Chiesa A, Serretti A. Mindfulness-based interventions for chronic pain: a systematic review of the evidence. J Altern Complement Med. 2011;17(1):83–93.
38. Veehof MM, Oskam MJ, Schreurs KM, Bohlmeijer ET. Acceptance-based interventions for the treatment of chronic pain: a systematic review and meta-analysis. Pain. 2011;152:533–42.
39. Shedler J. The efficacy of psychodynamic psychotherapy. Am Psychol. 2010;65(2):98–109.
40. Turk DC, Swanson KS, Tunks ER. Psychological approaches in the treatment of chronic pain patients--when pills, scalpels, and needles are not enough. Can J Psychiatr. 2008;53(4):213–23.
41. Chang BH, Dusek JA, Benson H. Psychobiological changes from relaxation response elicitation: long-term practitioners vs. novices. Psychosomatics. 2011;52(6):550–9.
42. Glick RM, Greco CM. Biofeedback and primary care. Prim Care. 2010;37(1):91–103.
43. Vlaeyen JWS, Linton SJ. Fear avoidance and its consequences in treatment for chronic musculoskeletal pain: a state of the art. Pain. 2000;85:317–32.
44. Wertli MM, Rasmussen-Barr E, Weiser S, Bachmann LM, Brunner F. The role of fear avoidance beliefs as a prognostic factor for outcome in patients with nonspecific low back pain: a systematic review. Spine J. 2013;pii:S1529-9430(13)01576-3.
45. Sullivan MJL, Thorn B, Haythornwaite JA, Keefe F, Martin M, Bradlet LA, Lefebvre JC. Theoretical perspectives in the relationship between catastrophizing and pain. Clin J Pain. 2001;17:52–64.
46. Trost Z, France CR, Thomas JS. Exposure to movement in chronic pain: evidence of successful generalization across a reaching task. Pain. 2008;317:26–33.
47. De Jong JR, JWS V, Onghena P, et al. Fear of movement/(re)injury in chronic low back pain education or exposure in vivo as mediator to fear reduction? Clin J Pain. 2005;21:9–17.
48. Dimeo F, Bauer M, Varahram I, et al. Benefits from aerobic exercise in patients with major depression: a pilot study. Br J Sports Med. 2001;35(2):114–7.
49. Herring MP, Puetz TW, O'Connor PJ, Dishman RK. Effect of exercise training on depressive symptoms among patients with a chronic illness: a systematic

review and meta-analysis of randomized controlled trials. Arch Intern Med. 2012;172(2):101–11.
50. Herring MP, Jacob ML, Suveg C, Dishman RK, O'Connor PJ. Feasibility of exercise training for the short-term treatment of generalized anxiety disorder: a randomized controlled trial. Psychother Psychosom. 2012;81(1):21–8.
51. Gatzounis R, Schrooten MG, Crombez G, Vlaeyen JW. Operant learning theory in pain and chronic pain rehabilitation. Curr Pain Headache Rep. 2012;16(2):117–26.
52. Sanders SH. Operant therapy with pain patients: evidence for its effectiveness. In: Lebovits AH, editor. Seminars in pain medicine, vol. 1. Philadelphia: W.B. Saunders; 2003. p. 90–8.
53. Bair MJ, Wu J, Damush TM, Sutherland JM, Kroenke K. Association of depression and anxiety alone and in combination with chronic musculoskeletal pain in primary care patients. Psychosom Med. 2008;70(8):890–7.
54. Rudy TE, Kerns RD, Turk DC. Chronic pain and depression: toward a cognitive-behavioral mediation model. Pain. 1988;35(2):129–40.
55. Strigo IA, Simmons AN, Matthews SC, Craig AD, Paulus MP. Association of major depressive disorder with altered functional brain response during anticipation and processing of heat pain. Arch Gen Psychiatry. 2008;65(11):1275–84.
56. Shipherd JC, Keyes M, Jovanovic T, Ready DJ, Baltzell D, Worley V, Gordon-Brown V, Hayslett C, Duncan E. Veterans seeking treatment for posttraumatic stress disorder: what about comorbid chronic pain? J Rehabil Res Dev. 2007;44(2):153–66.
57. Edwards RR, Klick B, Buenaver L, et al. Symptoms of distress as prospective predictors of pain-related sciatica treatment outcomes. Pain. 2007;130(1–2):47–55.
58. Williams LS, Jones WJ, Shen J, Robinson RL, Kroenke K. Outcomes of newly referred neurology outpatients with depression and pain. Neurology. 2004;63(4):674–7.
59. Kroenke K, Shen J, Oxman TE, et al. Impact of pain on the outcomes of depression treatment: results from the RESPECT trial. Pain. 2008;134(1–2):209–15.
60. Schatman ME. Interdisciplinary chronic pain management: international perspectives. Pain Clinical Updates. 2012;20(7):1–5. Accessed 2/1/14 at http://www.iasp-pain.org/AM/AMTemplate.cfm?Section=Pain_Clinical_Updates1&CONTENTID=16590&SECTION=Pain_Clinical_Updates1&TEMPLATE=/CM/ContentDisplay.cfm.
61. Gatchel RJ, McGeary DD, Peterson A, Moore M, LeRoy K, Isler WC, Hryshko-Mullen AS, Edell T. Preliminary findings of a randomized controlled trial of an interdisciplinary military pain program. Mil Med. 2009;174(3):270–7.
62. Patrick LE, Altamaier EM, Found EM. Long-term outcomes in multidisciplinary treatment of chronic low back pain: results of a 13-year follow-up. Spine. 2004;8:850–5.

The Management of Pain States: Pharmacologic Treatment

8

Robert Bolash

Abbreviations

CNS	Central nervous system
COX	Cyclooxygenase
EKG	Electrocardiogram
GABA	Gamma-aminobutyric acid
NMDA	N-methyl-D-aspartate
NSAID	Nonsteroidal anti-inflammatory drug
SIADH	Syndrome of inappropriate antidiuretic hormone
SNRI	Serotonin-norepinephrine reuptake inhibitor
TCA	Tricyclic antidepressant
WBC	White blood cell

Key Concepts

- Nonsteroidal anti-inflammatory drugs (NSAIDs) are first-line agents for the treatment for nociceptive pain. They exert their action by inhibiting cyclooxygenase and blocking the production of inflammatory mediators. Common adverse effects of NSAIDs include gastrointestinal irritation, impaired coagulation, and renal insufficiency.
- Anticonvulsants can be employed in the treatment of neuropathic pain conditions and act to decrease pathological nerve firing. Gabapentin and pregabalin block calcium channels, while carbamazepine and lidocaine block sodium channels that transmit painful impulses to the brain. Sedation is the most common side effect of anticonvulsant use.
- Select antidepressants provide pain relief even in the absence of a coexisting mood disorder. Tricyclic antidepressants and serotonin-norepinephrine reuptake inhibitors are used for a variety of neuropathic and chronic musculoskeletal conditions. Anticholinergic and antihistaminergic side effects seen with tricyclic agents are largely avoided with newer serotonin-norepinephrine reuptake inhibitors.
- Advanced pharmacotherapy administered intravenously such as ketamine, as well as agents delivered intrathecally, such as ziconotide, are available for refractory chronic pain conditions.
- Topical agents such as capsaicin and local anesthetics work at the site of application. Systemic side effects are largely avoided through the use of topiceuticals. This is in contrast to a transdermal agent such as the fentanyl patch which is absorbed at the site of

R. Bolash, MD (✉)
Department of Pain Management, Cleveland Clinic, 9500 Euclid Ave / C25, Cleveland, OH 44195, USA
e-mail: robert@bolash.org

J. Cheng, R.W. Rosenquist (eds.), *Fundamentals of Pain Medicine*,
https://doi.org/10.1007/978-3-319-64922-1_8

application but travels through the bloodstream and acts systemically.
- Opioids are useful for the treatment of acute pain and represent a therapeutic option for cancer, nociceptive, and neuropathic pain complaints. Opioids primarily work as agonists of the mu opioid receptor in the brain and spinal cord. Adverse effects include constipation, sedation, and respiratory depression.

Introduction

Selecting medications to address pain states requires an appreciation of the nature of the patient's complaint, as well as an understanding of the pharmacology and limitations of the prescribed medications. While the pain assessment remains subjective, the clinician must glean some understanding of the pathology from the history, physical examination and advanced diagnostic tests before designing a treatment plan. In fact, making the correct diagnosis is more important than selecting therapies, since an inappropriately selected medication is unlikely to result in therapeutic benefit, irrespective of a comprehensive knowledge of the pharmaceutical. For this reason, it will be useful to refer back to this chapter as you navigate through the disease-specific chapters later in this book.

This chapter is designed to expose the reader to the diversity of agents available and provide a view of the indications, contraindications, and adverse effects for clinical practice. Each agent's mechanism of action, adverse effects, drug-drug interactions, and patient-specific considerations are presented in brief.

Perhaps the easiest way to appreciate the diversity of pharmacological agents used in the treatment of chronic pain is to consider each drug by its mechanism of action. Agents such as NSAIDs and opioids are often supplemented with adjunctive agents both in the acute and chronic settings and form the basis for a multimodal pain treatment regimen. The discussion of opioids is intentionally placed at the end of this chapter to trigger the reader to consider alternative agents first. Whereas opioids were once considered the "gold standard" for treating pain, an increasing body of evidence has failed to demonstrate functional improvement with chronic opioid therapy and has prompted the use of a more diverse group of agents in the treatment of chronic pain conditions.

Nonsteroidal Anti-inflammatory Drugs

Nonsteroidal anti-inflammatory drugs (NSAIDs) including diclofenac, naproxen, ketorolac, and meloxicam represent a first-line therapeutic option for nociceptive pain caused by conditions such as arthritis, gout, bone metastasis, or acute tissue injury. NSAIDs exert their actions peripherally, inhibiting the cyclooxygenase (COX) enzymes. COX is responsible for the conversion of arachidonic acid to thromboxane and prostaglandins, mediators of the inflammation. NSAIDs also work to prevent hyperalgesia centrally by inhibiting prostaglandins and preventing the production of inflammatory mediators in response to tissue injury. NSAIDs are highly protein bound and eliminated by hepatic oxidation, and therefore caution should be exercised in the presence of hypoalbuminemia or hepatic dysfunction.

COX variants have been the subject of recent investigation with the advent of agents specific to the COX-2 variant (Table 8.1). COX-2 is predominantly induced with inflammatory states, whereas COX-1 is constitutively active. In addition to the action of COX in generating inflammatory mediators, COX-1 also plays a role in platelet aggregation, renal autoregulation, and maintaining the gastric mucosa. With the

Table 8.1 Cyclooxygenase variants

	Role	Inhibitors
COX-1	Gastric protection Platelet aggregation Renal autoregulation	Nonselective NSAIDs
COX-2	Induced with inflammatory states	Nonselective NSAIDs Celecoxib
COX-3	CNS prostaglandin synthesis	Acetaminophen

exception of celecoxib, many commercially available NSAIDs indiscriminately inhibit COX variants. Initially, COX-2-specific agents such as celecoxib were hypothesized to target inflammatory pain without the platelet, renal, and gastric effects of COX-1. This excitement diminished when post-marketing studies revealed an increasing number of adverse cardiac events in patients taking the COX-2-specific agents. Celecoxib's predecessor rofecoxib was removed from the market due to an increased incidence of myocardial infarction.

NSAIDS act within hours of administration and are generally administered orally, though formulations of ketorolac and ibuprofen are available for intravenous use. Topical NSAIDs such as diclofenac in the form of a gel or spray are efficacious for acute musculoskeletal pain and chronic pain conditions such as knee osteoarthritis. Since systemic absorption is minimal, many of the adverse effects are diminished with topical NSAID preparations. Given the need to apply topical diclofenac gel four times a day to achieve efficacy, a continuous release transdermal patch formulation of diclofenac is available to facilitate administration.

Side effects of NSAIDs include gastrointestinal irritation, impaired platelet aggregation, and a potential to compromise glomerular filtration in those with renal insufficiency. NSAID gastropathy can be mitigated by coadministration of a proton pump inhibitor or by selecting a COX-2-specific agent. NSAID-related impairment in renal function is limited to patients dependent upon preglomerular prostaglandin-mediated vasodilation to maintain perfusion as is seen in prerenal azotemia or congestive heart failure. Because NSAIDs inhibit the production of COX, prostaglandin-dependent glomerular vasodilation is similarly blunted, and thereby blood flow to the nephron can be compromised.

Acetaminophen deserves special consideration since it lacks the peripheral anti-inflammatory effects seen with NSAIDs and acts centrally to produce analgesia. Despite its widespread use, the mechanism of pain relief is not entirely understood but is likely attributable to inhibition of COX-3 in the brain. With COX-3 inhibited, prostaglandin synthesis is similarly blocked resulting in centrally mediated analgesia. Oral, rectal, and intravenous forms of acetaminophen are available, and the time between acetaminophen administration and therapeutic effect is brief.

The antipyretic effects of acetaminophen are attributable to the drug's action on the hypothalamus where it facilitates peripheral vasodilation. Heat is subsequently lost through increased sweating. While acetaminophen lacks the adverse effects on the gastric mucosa and platelets seen with nonspecific NSAIDs, hepatotoxicity is the most noteworthy side effect. Acetaminophen toxicity is implicated as the number one cause of acute liver failure in the United States. Acetaminophen undergoes hepatic metabolism generating toxic by-products that are inactivated by glutathione. If glutathione stores are depleted, these by-products accumulate and can cause hepatic injury.

Anticonvulsants

Anticonvulsants can be employed as first-line agents for neuropathic pain conditions such as diabetic peripheral neuropathy, multiple sclerosis, and spinal cord injury. Anticonvulsants are also useful for the treatment of fibromyalgia, as well as the prevention of headache disorders.

Gabapentin and pregabalin act on the alpha-2-delta subunit of voltage-gated calcium channels to prevent aberrant neurotransmitter discharge and increase the threshold for depolarization. Achieving therapeutic efficacy with anticonvulsants requires a gradual dose titration that limits the usefulness of these agents in the treatment of acute pain. Even with pregabalin, a lipophilic formulation that passes more rapidly into the CNS, patients often require at least 1 week of therapy before realizing a reduction in pain. Both gabapentin and pregabalin are excreted in the urine and require dose adjustments in the presence of compromised renal function. Common adverse effects include dizziness and sedation that can be mitigated by slowly increasing the dose.

Carbamazepine is an anticonvulsant indicated for the treatment of trigeminal neuralgia and acts to prevent the rapid opening of voltage-gated sodium channels. It is administered orally and undergoes hepatic metabolism where it induces cytochrome P450. Induction of cytochrome P450 can result in drug-drug interactions including increased clearance of warfarin, phenytoin, and oral contraceptives. Adverse effects include bone marrow suppression which can range from mild decreases in WBC count to complete bone marrow suppression. Syndrome of inappropriate antidiuretic hormone (SIADH), Stevens-Johnson syndrome, and congenital anomalies are seen in those treated with carbamazepine. Oxcarbazepine shares the same mechanism of action as carbamazepine but avoids the potential adverse effect of bone marrow suppression. Adverse effects of oxcarbazepine include the potential for development of hyponatremia, teratogenicity, and the craving of salty foods.

Topiramate is an anticonvulsant often used for the prevention of migraine and cluster headaches. It acts to block voltage-gated sodium channels but also acts to enhance GABA and antagonize the NMDA receptor. Topiramate blocks carbonic anhydrase and has been associated with the development of metabolic acidosis, kidney stones, and glaucoma. Loss of appetite is commonly observed and can be utilized as a favorable side effect in overweight patients.

Lidocaine has been used both topically and parenterally for the treatment of chronic pain conditions including neuropathic pain due to peripheral neuropathy and postherpetic neuralgia. Lidocaine blocks voltage-gated sodium channels creating a local area of anesthesia when used topically with limited systemic absorption. Intravenous lidocaine is thought to blunt spontaneous neural firing seen in neuropathic pain conditions at concentrations lower than those that would affect cardiac conduction. Somnolence, seizure, and cardiovascular collapse occur sequentially with the development of lidocaine toxicity. Topical lidocaine patches are generally well tolerated, though efficacy can be variable.

Antidepressants

While concurrent depressive disorders can exist in patients suffering from chronic pain, tricyclic antidepressants and serotonin-norepinephrine reuptake inhibitors possess analgesic properties separate from their antidepressant effects. Because of this, these agents can be useful even in the absence of a coexisting mood disorder.

Tricyclic antidepressants including amitriptyline, nortriptyline, and desipramine are effective adjuncts in the treatment of neuropathic pain when used at doses lower than those required to treat depression. The primary mechanism of action of the tricyclic antidepressants is via inhibition of the reuptake of both serotonin and norepinephrine. These agents may also act as NMDA receptor antagonists and can potentiate the effects of endogenous opiates.

The effective analgesic dose for tricyclic antidepressant agents varies among patients, and pain relief only occurs after reaching an effective dose. One strategy is to begin 10 mg of amitriptyline or nortriptyline at night and titrate the dose upward every week until pain relief is achieved. Tricyclic antidepressants can produce undesirable adverse effects that can limit their usefulness. Anticholinergic effects are most commonly seen with amitriptyline, while desipramine has the least anticholinergic effects. Doxepin has the most antihistaminergic effects. The numerous adverse effects seen with the use of tricyclic antidepressants including orthostatic hypotension, cardiac conduction abnormalities, gastrointestinal, and sedating effects have fueled the increased use of serotonin-norepinephrine reuptake inhibitors for chronic pain (Table 8.2).

Serotonin-norepinephrine reuptake inhibitors (SNRI) possess the same favorable treatment effects as tricyclic antidepressants but lack many of the anticholinergic and antihistaminergic adverse effects of their predecessors. Venlafaxine, duloxetine, and milnacipran act at the level of the synapse to inhibit the reuptake of both serotonin and norepinephrine into the synaptic cleft, potentiating neurotransmitter availability at the nerve terminal. Venlafaxine and duloxetine are more selective reuptake inhibitors of serotonin, while

Table 8.2 Adverse effects of antidepressants used for chronic pain

	Anticholinergic	Neurologic	Cardiovascular	Gastrointestinal
Tricyclic antidepressants (TCA)	Dry mouth Urinary retention Blurry vision	Sedation Dizziness Restlessness Confusion	QT prolongation Orthostatic hypotension Conduction abnormalities	Nausea Vomiting Constipation
Serotonin-norepinephrine reuptake inhibitors (SNRI)		Insomnia Headache	Hypertension Conduction abnormalities	Nausea Dry mouth Constipation

milnacipran is more selective for norepinephrine. Duloxetine has indications for both peripheral neuropathy and chronic musculoskeletal pain, while milnacipran is useful for fibromyalgia

Ketamine

Ketamine is a synthetic agent used in refractory chronic pain conditions including complex regional pain syndrome. By acting on the N-methyl-D-aspartate (NMDA) receptor, low doses of ketamine can be used to provide analgesia, while high doses can be used for the induction and maintenance of general anesthesia. Intraoperative ketamine may decrease postoperative opioid consumption in select populations.

Ketamine can be administered intravenously, intramuscularly, orally, or topically and lacks the respiratory depressant effects seen with opioids. Conversely ketamine acts on the respiratory system as both a bronchodilator and respiratory stimulant. Ketamine is a sympathomimetic and may cause tachycardia and hypertension by blocking the reuptake of norepinephrine, necessitating caution in patients with cardiovascular disease.

Outpatient administration of ketamine for chronic pain conditions remains controversial, and variable evidence for its use in refractory pain conditions, as well as for the treatment of addiction and depression, is emerging. Nonmedical use as a recreational psychotropic agent has led to increased oversight by both US and international regulatory bodies.

Ziconotide

Ziconotide is a peptide derived from the cone snail and is used for the treatment of chronic refractory pain conditions. Ziconotide is administered directly into the cerebrospinal fluid and blocks N-type voltage-gated calcium channels thereby preventing the transmission of painful signals. Because of the requirement for continuous intrathecal delivery, it is typically reserved for those patients who have failed a multitude of other treatment modalities. Creatine kinase increases are seen in some patients treated with ziconotide. Because of a narrow therapeutic window and the potential for severe adverse CNS effects including psychosis, hallucinations, and delirium, careful patient selection is required. Despite the challenges, patients treated with ziconotide do not develop tolerance to the drug, and ziconotide does not cause respiratory depression.

Botulinum Toxin

The use of botulinum toxin in the treatment of chronic pain conditions is growing. Onabotulinumtoxin A is approved for chronic migraine prophylaxis, and efficacy has been demonstrated in neuropathic pain conditions such as postherpetic neuralgia and diabetic peripheral neuropathy, as well as chronic pelvic pain conditions. Botulinum toxin is administered intramuscularly or subcutaneously and acts at the neuromuscular junction to prevent the presynaptic release of acetylcholine. Mild adverse effects include headache and a flu-like syndrome, while severe adverse effects are typically attributable to the sequelae of botulinum toxin's spread to distant muscle groups.

Topical Agents

In addition to topiceutical formulations of ketamine, local anesthetics, and NSAIDs mentioned previously, capsaicin is a compound with an exclusively topical route of delivery. Topical agents must be applied directly to the painful area, and systemic absorption is minimized when compared to other routes of delivery. Because blood levels of these agents are low, many side effects of systemic administration can be avoided.

Capsaicin is available as a cream, lotion, or patch and is used in the treatment of musculoskeletal and neuropathic pain conditions including postherpetic neuralgia. It is extracted from chili peppers and binds to the TRPV1 receptors, which are found on thermal sensing peripheral nerves. The binding of capsaicin to TRPV1 results in depletion of presynaptic substance P, a chemical important to the transmission of painful signals from the peripheral to central nervous system. The most noteworthy adverse effects of capsaicin are the development of a local area of erythema upon application and a transient increase in pain, while substance P is depleted.

A topical agent must be differentiated from a transdermal medication, the latter of which requires achieving a therapeutic bloodstream level before providing analgesia. Transdermal agents are carried from their site of application, into the bloodstream, and throughout the body resulting in systemic effects similar to those seen with oral or intravenous formulations. The fentanyl patch is one example of a transdermal preparation of the synthetic opiate that is used for the treatment of chronic pain.

Opioids

Opioids are a class of agents that share a common mechanism of action as agonists at mu receptors located within the brain and spinal cord. Both short-acting and sustained release formulations are available. Opioids can be administered via oral, subcutaneous, intravenous, transdermal, rectal, sublingual, buccal, intranasal, intrathecal, and epidural routes.

Short-acting opioids are often combined with other analgesics such as acetaminophen or an NSAID and provide pain relief at a dose lower than that which can be achieved with the opioid alone. When considering the use of these combination agents, prescribers should be cautious about the potential to reach toxic doses of all components of a combination tablet. The use of combination agents becomes particularly concerning with more frequent daily use. Hepatic injury can develop with high doses of acetaminophen, and adverse gastric and renal effects can be seen with high doses of NSAIDs.

Morphine is often considered the prototypical opioid with which all others are compared. When administered orally, morphine has a gradual onset and a sustained duration of action lasting approximately 4 h. With intravenous administration, onset occurs more rapidly, and bioavailability is increased. The primary action of morphine is via direct action on the mu opioid receptors located in the CNS. Agonism of the mu receptors results in analgesia, sedation, and respiratory depression. Morphine is metabolized in the kidney before undergoing renal excretion. One notable metabolite of morphine is morphine 3-glucoronide which is responsible for the adverse effects on CNS excitability including seizure and myoclonus. The antitussive and analgesic medication codeine undergoes hepatic conversion to morphine, and similar caution should be exercised in patients when administering codeine to patients with renal insufficiency.

Because the adverse effects of sedation, nausea, and vomiting occur less often, hydromorphone is becoming increasingly utilized in place of morphine. Gastrointestinal side effects occur less frequently with hydromorphone, while its onset is more rapid after oral administration. Hydromorphone is more lipid soluble than morphine, and bioavailability is increased necessitating smaller milligram-per-milligram dosing. Hydromorphone undergoes metabolism via hepatic glucoronidation to form the metabolite hydromorphone 3-glucoronide, though in much lower quantities than its morphine 3-glucoronide counterpart. Levels of hydromorphone 3-glucoronide remain clinically insignificant making hydromorphone a reasonable choice for patients with acute or chronic kidney disease. The widely used short-acting oral agent, hydrocodone, is metabolized to hydromorphone to exert its analgesic effects.

Oxycodone is a synthetic oral opioid with a more favorable side effect profile. Sedation and pruritus are minimized when compared to morphine. Oxycodone is available in both short-acting and sustained release formulations, as well as preparations combined with acetaminophen and aspirin. Oxycodone undergoes hepatic metabolism via the cytochrome P450 system to form oxymorphone, a mu opioid agonist. Synthetic oxymorphone is also available in oral and intravenous forms and bypasses cytochrome P450 which may be useful in those patients whose cytochrome P450 enzymes are genetically or pharmacologically inhibited.

Fentanyl is a lipophilic opioid with widespread use for operative analgesia but important uses in pain management as well. Notably the transdermal, buccal, and transmucosal forms do not require the presence of an intact digestive tract and can be used in patients with dysphagia or advanced gastrointestinal pathologies. Transdermal fentanyl is formulated as a patch which is applied to the skin, and the analgesic is continuously released for 72 h. Though it avoids the alimentary canal, transdermal fentanyl is metabolized by the cytochrome P450 system in the liver. Perspiration and fluctuations in skin temperature can result in variability in the rate of transdermal fentanyl absorption, and heat-based therapies should not be applied in close proximity to the patch. Dosing transdermal fentanyl requires some patience when commencing or adjusting therapy since it takes 3 days to attain steady state. In contrast, the oral transmucosal and buccal formulations act rapidly, but have a short duration, and are useful for the treatment of acute or breakthrough pain.

Tramadol is somewhat unique among the opioids since it acts as both as a mu opiate receptor agonist and a serotonin and norepinephrine reuptake inhibitor. Because of its mixed action, it has been used for the treatment of neuropathic pain and fibromyalgia, conditions that are typically considered poorly responsive to pure mu opioid agonists. Tramadol is metabolized in the liver and has been associated with the risk of seizure activity and serotonin syndrome, especially with the concurrent use of antidepressants.

Though much stigmatized for its association with heroin detoxification programs, methadone is prescribed for chronic pain conditions due to its low cost and rapid onset after oral administration. Methadone acts as an opioid receptor agonist and a serotonin and norepinephrine reuptake inhibitor but exhibits variable bioavailability and a long half-life which makes achieving a steady-state difficult. Additionally, methadone can prolong the QTc interval resulting in *torsade de pointes*, and a baseline EKG should be obtained prior to administration. These complexities, combined with the disproportionate incidence of overdose-related deaths associated with methadone, often result in avoidance of the agent by inexperienced prescribers.

Several adverse effects are shared by all opioids. Gastrointestinal side effects including nausea and vomiting are caused by opioid activation of medullary chemoreceptors, and constipating effects are due to an increase in vagal output. These side effects can either be mitigated with opioid rotation or treated with an antiemetic, stool softener, or prokinetic agent. Sedation or delirium is often treated by reducing the dose of an opioid or by rotating to an alternative opioid or non-opioid analgesic. Respiratory depression remains a rare but potentially catastrophic side effect of opioid use. Many cases of respiratory depression are associated with the concomitant use of opioids and benzodiazepines. Naloxone antagonizes the effects of opioids and is a valuable rescue medication to treat opioid-induced respiratory depression.

Conclusion

Selecting pharmacotherapy for the treatment of both acute and chronic pain requires an understanding of not only the analgesic agents but also the nature of the patient's pain complaint and comorbidities. It requires diligence on the part of the physician to differentiate the nature of the patient's pain and prescribe an agent tailored to their pathology. If an agent selected for nociceptive pain such as an NSAID is administered for neuropathic pain, the patient will ultimately fail pharmacotherapy, regardless of the agent, route, or dose. This again underscores the importance of understanding the pathophysiology before delving into pharmacotherapy.

Despite the progress in developing new techniques and interventions discussed later in this book, pharmacotherapy remains a therapeutic option that is widely acceptable to patients and often represents their first entry into a pain treatment algorithm. Though pharmacotherapy is no longer viewed as a panacea, it retains an important adjunctive role when designing a multimodal treatment plan.

Suggested Reading

1. Dworkin RH, O'Connor AB, Backonja M, Farrar JT, Finnerup NB, Jensen TS, Kalso EA, Loeser JD, Miaskowski C, Nurmikko TJ, Portenoy RK, Rice AS, Stacey BR, Treede RD, Turk DC, Wallace MS. Pharmacologic management of neuropathic pain: evidence-based recommendations. Pain. 2007;132(3):237–51.
2. Finnerup NB, Sindrup SH, Jensen TS. The evidence for pharmacological treatment of neuropathic pain. Pain. 2010;150(3):573–81.
3. McNicol ED, Midbari A, Eisenberg E. Opioids for neuropathic pain. Cochrane Database Syst Rev. 2013;29:8.
4. Roelofs PD, Deyo RA, Koes BW, Scholten RJ, van Tulder MW. Non-steroidal anti-inflammatory drugs for low back pain. Spine (Phila Pa 1976). 2008;33(16):1766-74.
5. Saarto T, Wiffen PJ. Antidepressants for neuropathic pain: a Cochrane review. J Neurol Neurosurg Psychiatry. 2010;81(12):1372–3.
6. Silberstein SD, Lipton RB, Dodick DW, Freitag FG, Ramadan N, Mathew N, Brandes JL, Bigal M, Saper J, Ascher S, Jordan DM, Greenberg SJ, Hulihan J. Topiramate chronic migraine study group. Efficacy and safety of topiramate for the treatment of chronic migraine: a randomized, double-blind, placebo-controlled trial. Headache. 2007;47(2):170–80.
7. Staats PS, Yearwood T, Charapata SG, Presley RW, Wallace MS, Byas-Smith M, Fisher R, Bryce DA, Mangieri EA, Luther RR, Mayo M, McGuire D, Ellis D. Intrathecal ziconotide in the treatment of refractory pain in patients with cancer or AIDS: a randomized controlled trial. JAMA. 2004;291(1):63–70.

Interventional Approaches

9

Jianguo Cheng

Key Concepts

- Interventional pain medicine uses minimally invasive techniques to block, ablate, or modulate pain pathways for diagnostic and therapeutic purposes.
- Proper patient selection based on accurate diagnosis and benefit/risk analysis is critically important to ensure safety, efficacy, and cost-effectiveness. It is imperative for pain physicians to understand the relevant anatomy, pharmacology, and toxicity of local anesthetic and other agents, as well as the essential equipment used in the procedures.
- Proper use of sedation, adequate monitoring, efficient imaging guidance, and proficient technical skills are required to safely perform interventional procedures. Pain physicians must be cognizant of potential complications and be able to recognize and manage various complications associated with each specific procedure.
- Blocking specific cranial nerves and their branches, spinal nerves and their branches, or visceral nerves with a local anesthetic with or without steroid is an important and commonly accepted technique in pain medicine. Extended pain relief may also be achieved by radiofrequency ablation, cryoneurolysis, or chemical neurolysis of specific peripheral nerves.
- Intramuscular injections may be used to treat myofascial pain, usually in combination with physical therapy, transcutaneous electrical stimulation, and massage and relaxation therapy.
- Joint and/or bursa injections are used to treat joint pain due to arthritis, bursitis, and tendonitis with variable levels of evidence supporting the therapeutic efficacy.
- A number of intradiscal procedures have been designed to manage discogenic pain or radicular pain due to disc herniation with variable levels of evidence. The long-term outcomes of these procedures remain to be determined by rigorously designed clinical studies.
- Vertebroplasty and kyphoplasty are procedures used to percutaneously inject bone cement into the vertebral body to treat compression fractures due to osteoporosis or metastatic cancer, usually in the acute phase after a trial of conservative treatment has failed.

Definition of Interventional Pain Management

Interventional pain management or interventional pain medicine refers to the use of invasive techniques to block, destruct, or modulate pain

J. Cheng, MD, PhD (✉)
Departments of Pain Management and Neurosciences, Cleveland Clinic Anesthesiology Institute and Lerner Research Institute, Cleveland, OH, USA
e-mail: CHENGJ@ccf.org

J. Cheng, R.W. Rosenquist (eds.), *Fundamentals of Pain Medicine*,
https://doi.org/10.1007/978-3-319-64922-1_9

pathways and pain perception for diagnostic and therapeutic purposes. Originated from regional anesthesia and neural blockade, interventional pain medicine has evolved into a distinct subspecialty that has received a specific specialty designation by the US National Uniform Billing Committee to allow its practitioners to bill Federal healthcare programs such as Medicare and Medicaid. Interventional pain management is an integral and significant component in the continuum of pain management. Here, we will focus on the common interventional procedures that are utilized to manage a wide range and variety of pain conditions. These procedures include nerve blocks, nerve ablation, intramuscular injections, intra-articular injections, intradiscal interventions, and vertebroplasty and kyphoplasty. It is important to recognize the significance of understanding the principles and techniques of image guidance by ultrasound, fluoroscopy, or computed tomography, as well as patient sedation, monitoring, and safety during and after these minimally invasive interventional procedures, even though these are beyond the focus of this chapter. Surgical interventions, such as spinal cord stimulation, peripheral nerve stimulation, brain stimulation, and intrathecal drug delivery techniques, will be discussed in the following chapter.

Nerve Blocks

Blocking nerves with local anesthetics with or without steroid is a technique widely used for diagnostic and therapeutic purposes in pain management. Cranial nerves and their branches, spinal nerves and their branches, and sympathetic nerves can be blocked. For example, trigeminal nerve (or ganglion) block is used for refractory trigeminal neuralgia, postherpetic neuralgia, and other facial pain conditions. Branches of the trigeminal nerve can also be blocked to relieve pain localized in specific area of its innervation. For instance, the supraorbital nerve can be blocked to relieve pain in the frontal area due to entrapment of this nerve at or around the exit site of the supraorbital foramen. Blocking the sphenopalatine ganglion is effective in reducing the frequency and intensity of cluster headaches.

The spinal nerves are blocked through many procedures in many pain conditions. Epidural blocks through interlaminar, transforaminal, or caudal approaches may be used to block multiple nerve roots and ganglia to provide diagnostic and/or therapeutic pain relief from acute, subacute, and chronic pain conditions. These blocks are used predominately to manage surgical and traumatic pain in acute setting. For chronic pain, these blocks are most commonly performed for radicular pain in the upper and lower extremities or the trunk due to herniated disc, spinal stenosis, and other conditions. Selective nerve root blocks are used to block one or two nerve roots for diagnostic and therapeutic purposes. It may be used to determine the specific spinal nerve involved in the pain condition and help locate the pathology such as a pain generating intervertebral disc. When one of the spinal nerve roots is irritated, patients may experience pain, numbness, tingling, and sometimes weakness down an arm or a leg. A diagnostic selective block can be used to indicate that a pinched nerve is the problem. Nerve blocks may be done more distally, such as paravertebral block, intercostal nerve block, and transverse abdominis plane (TAP) block. Blocks are also performed for specific nerves such as the lateral femoral cutaneous nerve, genitofemoral nerve, pudendal nerve, and coccygeal nerve. Terminal nerves innervating the joints may be blocked for diagnostic and therapeutic purpose, such as the medial branches of the dorsal rami innervating the facet joints, the lateral branches of the sacral dorsal rami innervating the sacroiliac joints, and genicular nerves innervating the knee joints.

The sympathetic nerves may be blocked for diagnostic and therapeutic purposes. For instance, the stellate ganglion or the lumbar sympathetic chain may be blocked in the setting of complex regional pain syndrome; the celiac plexus or splanchnic nerves are blocked to reduce visceral abdominal pain, the hypogastric nerve plexus for pelvic visceral pain, and the ganglion impar to manage sympathetically mediated rectal pain or coccydynia. Blocking the afferent sensory, as well as the efferent, fibers may contribute to pain relief in these conditions.

Mechanisms of Nerve Block

The duration of pain relief varies from hours, days, and weeks to months after each block. The mechanisms of these effects are poorly understood. Local anesthetics typically provided blockade of sodium channels of nerve cells for durations ranging from minutes to hours. Adding corticosteroids may prolong the sensory and motor blockade by hours. Apparently, none of these effects could explain the relief of pain for days, weeks, and months. Other mechanisms must be in play. One potential mechanism may be related to the anti-inflammatory effects of corticosteroids as well as local anesthetics. The anti-inflammatory effects of local anesthetics have been recognized and demonstrated in many studies. The potential long-term effects of local anesthetics on the excitability of neurons in the peripheral and central nervous systems also remain to be investigated.

Indications

Nerve blocks find extensive diagnostic and therapeutic applications. It is an essential skillset for pain specialists and anesthesiologists. The essence of these applications is that pain signals have to be conducted, transmitted, and modulated in the peripheral and central nervous systems. Blocking these processes in the peripheral or central nervous system would lead to pain relief or prevent pain signals from reaching the cortical level. For diagnostic purpose, specific nerves can be blocked to test if pain is generated from a particular anatomical structure/region such as the facet joints or sacroiliac joints. For therapeutic purpose, nerve blocks are often used to manage acute pain from medical procedures, surgeries, and trauma. In subacute and chronic pain settings, nerve blocks are performed to provide pain relief for days, weeks, or months. Nerve blocks are often used to relieve pain conditions that can be somatic or visceral, nociceptive or neuropathic, and acute or chronic. Therapeutic blocks usually involve more medications and larger volumes.

Contraindications

There is a set of contraindications that are common to all nerve blocks, such as:

- Local and systemic infection
- Coagulopathy and anticoagulation therapy
- Hemodynamic instability
- Lack of patient consent

There are contraindications that are specific to particular nerve blocks. For example, elective nerve block for chronic pain should not be performed in pregnant women; generally speaking, stellate ganglion block should not be performed in patients with glaucoma, pneumothorax, or severe COPD. Some of these conditions may be considered as relative contraindications. Decisions are usually made for each individual case after careful evaluation of the potential benefit, risks, and alternative approaches. Sound clinical judgment is required of the practitioners.

Complications

Most of the nerve block procedures carry intrinsic risks of complications. The most common is pain at the procedural site, which is usually transient and self-limited. Other complications include infection, bleeding, nerve injury, paralysis, blindness, or even death. Interventional pain physicians must possess the essential skills of cardiopulmonary resuscitation and advanced cardiovascular life support and be able to recognize and manage life-threatening complications. This set of skills include airway management, sedation/analgesia, fluoroscopic imaging and radiation safety, pharmacology of local anesthetics and treatment of its systemic toxicity, and safety of other injectable medications including radiographic contrast agents and corticosteroid preparations.

In summary, nerve blocks play an indispensable role in pain management. Selecting the appropriate procedure for the proper patient is critically important for successful block and desired outcomes. Most nerve blocks require the interventionist to have adequate knowledge of the anatomy and the ability to read and interpret medical images before and during the procedure. Successful blocks demand the practitioner to have experiences and skills to effectively and safely use the needles, injectates, and other relevant equipment. Above all, the practitioner should know by heart the indications, contraindications, and potential complications of each procedure he/she performs and be prepared for managing complications should they occur.

Nerve Ablation (Neurolysis)

Nerve blocks typically provide pain relief for limited duration. When a longer term of pain relief is desired, nerve ablation may be performed to provide pain relief for an extended period of time. It is usually employed when more conservative modalities of treatment have failed to effectively manage severe and debilitating pain conditions. Clinically, it is achieved by chemical neurolysis, radiofrequency ablation, or cryoneurolysis. These interventions cause degeneration of the nerve fibers and interference with the transmission of pain signals. In these procedures, the basal lamina (a thin protective layer around the nerve fiber) is preserved so that, as a damaged fiber regrows, it travels within its basal lamina tube and connects with the correct target of innervation, and function may be restored. In contrast to neuroablation, surgical cutting of a nerve (neurectomy) severs these basal lamina tubes. Without intact basal lamina to channel the regenerating fibers, a painful neuroma or deafferentation pain may develop over time. Another disadvantage of neurectomy is that surgical lesion usually requires an incision and is much traumatic to tissues surrounding the target nerve. This is why the neurolytic approach is usually preferred over surgical intervention.

Chemical Neurolysis

Application of chemicals (such as alcohol, phenol, or glycerol) to a nerve, a plexus of nerves, or a nerve ganglion can cause degeneration of the nerve fibers. Neurolysis of the sympathetic nerve with alcohol or phenol is a useful tool in managing cancer pain. Sympathetic nerves may regenerate over a course of 3–5 months or longer. Repeat injections may be necessary. Glycerol is primarily used to treat medically refractory trigeminal neuralgia.

Alcohol, at a concentration of 50–100%, produces destruction of nerve fibers by extracting neural cholesterol, phospholipids, and cerebrosides and by precipitating lipoproteins and neuropeptides. Injection into a peripheral nerve results in Wallerian degeneration, with damage to the nerve cell and the Schwann cells. Alcohol injection may produce severe pain. Thus, it is recommended to first inject a local anesthetic (5–10 ml of 0.25% bupivacaine) 5 min prior to alcohol injection or to dilute 100% alcohol by 50% with local anesthetic (0.25% bupivacaine). In contrast, injection of phenol in a 10% final concentration is painless. Both agents seem to have the same efficacy.

Phenol (carbolic acid) is a potent proteolytic agent. Concentrations of phenol of 5–10% are proteolytic and dissolve tissues on contact. When injected immediately adjacent to a nerve, phenol produces a chemical neurolysis. The effects are nonselective across nerve fiber size and are most prominent on the nerve's outer aspect. Local anesthetic effects are observed within 5–10 min following an injection of a neurolytic dose of phenol. The long-term effects of neurolysis typically occur after 24 h. The duration of analgesia is typically several months and may be related to the length of the denervated nerve.

Clinical application of chemical neurolysis is primarily limited to cancer pain management because it is generally not recommended for the treatment of noncancer pain. It may be advantageous to use chemical neurolysis to denature nerve plexuses that are diffuse and difficult to target with radiofrequency ablation needles or cryoneurolysis probes. Targets for chemical neurolysis include the following structures, with respective applications:

- Celiac plexus, most commonly for cancer of the gastrointestinal tract up to the transverse colon and cancer of the pancreas, stomach, gall bladder, and common bile duct; also used for chronic pancreatitis, active intermittent porphyria, and adrenal mass
- Splanchnic nerve, for retroperitoneal pain and similar conditions to those addressed by the celiac plexus block but, because of its higher rate of complications, used only if the celiac plexus block is not producing adequate relief
- Hypogastric plexus, for cancer affecting the descending colon, sigmoid colon, and rectum, as well as cancers of the bladder, prostatic urethra, prostate, seminal vesicles, testicles, uterus, ovary, and vaginal fundus
- Ganglion impar, for cancer affecting the perineum, anus and distal rectum, vulva and distal third of the vagina, and distal urethra
- Stellate ganglion, usually for head and neck cancer or sympathetically mediated arm and hand pain (rarely)

Glycerol, a trihydric alcohol that absorbs water from the atmosphere, is a mild neurolytic agent. It has been applied percutaneously to the retrogasserian rootlets to alleviate trigeminal neuralgia, often with preservation of facial sensation. The exact mechanism of action remains unknown. Its surfactant property may alter the axon cell membrane, inhibiting propagation of action potentials without necessarily destroying the nerve fibers. Alternatively, it may produce focal demyelination, axonal swelling, and neuronal loss as shown in an experimental model. Gasserian ganglion block is performed using 100% glycerol.

Other applications include cervical paravertebral sympathetic neurolysis, intercostal and thoracic paravertebral sympathetic neurolysis, lumbar paravertebral sympathetic neurolysis, and peripheral nerve neurolysis of the cranial and spinal nerves.

Complications

Chemical neurolysis can potentially be associated with a number of complications:

- Injection into epidural, subdural, and subarachnoid spaces or spinal cord, causing spinal cord injury, paralysis, or death
- Intravascular injection causing high spinal block (radicular artery), convulsions (vertebral artery), or death
- Hypotension and cardiac arrest
- Retroperitoneal hematoma/aortic wall dissection due to neurolytic solution diffusion
- Renal trauma/puncture of ureter/hematuria
- Neuralgia/anesthesia of lumbar plexus and genitofemoral nerves, due to diffusion of neurolytic solution
- Hematoma
- Pneumothorax
- Exacerbated pain
- Sexual impairment (bilateral block of hypogastric plexus)

Radiofrequency Ablation (RFA)

Tissues of the heart, tumor, or nerve can be ablated using the heat generated from high-frequency alternating current (in the range of 350–500 kHz). Compared to chemical neurolysis, an important advantage of RFA is that it can be very specific for treating the desired tissue in a controlled manner without significant collateral damage. Consequently, it is widely used in many medical specialties during the last 15 years. In pain management, RFA procedures are typically performed under image guidance (such as X-ray screening, CT scan, or ultrasound) with mild sedation at an outpatient setting. Clinical applications are extensive and expanding. Various modalities of RF treatment have been used.

The traditional thermal RFA is achieved by a voltage gradient generated between the active electrode and a disperse ground plate, placed at a body part distant to the active electrode. The lesion is created around the active electrode. The size of the lesion depends on the temperature generated at the tip of the probe, the size of the electrode, and the rate of heat "washout" by conductive hear loss and blood circulation. This modality of RFA is widely used to manage pain generated from the facet joints and the sacroiliac joint. It is also used to treat visceral abdominal pain (splanchnic nerve RFA), trigeminal neuralgia (trigeminal nerve RFA), and other neuropathic conditions.

Bipolar RFA is accomplished by placing two active electrodes adjacent to each other without using a disperse ground plate. The circuitry is completed between the two active electrodes, and a lesion is created between and around the two electrodes. This approach is used to create a larger lesion that is determined by the size of the electrodes, the distance between the electrodes, the temperature of the tip, and the duration of the ablation. These parameters can be optimized to create a desirable and controlled lesion in shape and size. Bipolar RFA is more energy efficient and cost-effective. It also minimizes the risk of interference with other implanted devices such as pacemakers and defibrillators. Bipolar RFA is most commonly used in the management of sacroiliac joint pain.

Cooled RFA is similar to traditional thermal RFA with the exception that a special cooling apparatus is used to prevent overheating and charring of the tissues surrounding the active electrode. This mechanism employs circulation of cooling water during RF delivery and allows increased power delivery to create larger lesions that are sometimes required to cover specific target tissues. It is particularly suitable for nerves with large anatomical variations. However, the larger lesions are achieved at the cost of longer procedure time and higher costs for equipment and disposables. Comparative advantage of this approach remains to be demonstrated in pain management. Cooled RFA has been used in the management of pain generated from the sacroiliac joint (sacral lateral branches), the thoracic facet joint (medial branches), the knee joint (genicular nerves), and the intervertebral disc (biacuplasty).

Pulsed Radiofrequency (PRF) In contrast to continuous radiofrequency, PRF delivers bursts of electrical pulses (500 kHz), with burst duration of 20 ms. The tip of the electrode is controlled at 42 °C. Two mechanisms have been considered to explain the PRF effects observed clinically. One concerns the possibility that a mild ablative effect of PRF may lead to lesions of the thin nerve fibers related to pain sensation. A second explanation is that PRF may activate afferent neurons, cause a transsynaptic effect on the dorsal horn neurons, and lead to induction of gene expression of these neurons in both the short and long term. These changes may modulate the conduction and transmission of pain signals in the central nervous system. Clinical applications include cervical radicular pain (dorsal root ganglion PRF), shoulder pain (suprascapular nerve PRF), occipital neuralgia (greater occipital nerve PRF), and facial pain and cluster headaches (sphenopalatine PRF).

Cryoneurolysis

Cryoneurolysis, also referred to as *cryoanalgesia* or *cryoneuroablation*, uses cold to cause controlled nerve destruction. It is performed by inserting a small probe to locate and freeze the nerve. The minimally invasive procedure allows for regeneration of the damaged nerve, as well as function of the nerve. It could significantly reduce pain in patients with many different conditions.

Principles of Cryoneurolysis

Cold temperature (−70 °C) at the tip of a cryoprobe is produced by rapid expansion of a gas (N_20 or CO_2) through a micropore outlet or by phase changes of liquid nitrogen. Application of the cold cryoprobe to the nerve disrupts nerve function and leads degeneration of the axons and myelin sheaths. However, the basal lamina, as well as the epineurium and perineurium, is maintained intact, thus leaving a "tube" which may serve as tracks to guide nerve regeneration and allowing for a precise return of preexisting structure. Theories as to how cryoneurolysis works include ischemic necrosis, physical destruction through large ice crystals, damage to proteins, alterations in cell volume, production of autoimmune antibodies, and membrane disruption caused by rapid water loss. As there is minimal inflammatory reactions, regeneration of axons is unlikely to form neuromas. Since the rate of axonal regeneration is essentially constant, between 1 and 3 mm per day, the return of baseline sensorimotor function is dependent on the distance between the cryolesion and the end organ. In addition to the degree of low temperature, successful analgesia is also affected by the duration of application of the cryoprobe, the rate at which the tissue thaws, and the size attained by the cryoprobe. Thus, cryoneurolysis is best utilized in conditions in which the nerve is small and well localized.

Indications

Various conditions with persistent, intractable pain can be managed with cryoneurolysis. A working diagnosis of the painful condition should be established prior to the cryoneurolysis. A diagnostic block of the target nerve with local anesthetics should produce at least 50% pain reduction. Equivocal results should be challenged with a repeat block.

Common Targets of Cryoneurolysis

- Intercostal nerves for pain of the chest wall and abdominal wall
- Iliohypogastric nerves and the ilioinguinal nerves for pain in the inguinal area
- Genitofemoral nerves for pain in scrotum and inner thigh
- Lateral femoral cutaneous nerves for lateral thigh pain (meralgia paresthetica)
- Pudendal nerves for vaginal, penoscrotal, perianal, and rectal pain
- Sacral nerve roots (S4 and S5) for perineal pain and coccydynia

The efficacy of cryoneurolysis has been supported by multiple clinical studies in a period of over several decades even though randomized controlled trials are scarce for practical reasons. The safety is acceptable when caution is exercised to avoid complications such as pneumothorax, bleeding, infection, unintended nerve injury, and damage to adjacent structures. When utilized appropriately with careful case selection, neurolysis appears to be a cost-effective treatment.

Techniques of Cryoneurolysis

The cryosystem consists of a cryoprobe (as described above), a cryoneurolysis machine with a built-in stimulator, and gas cylinders. Liquid nitrogen is most commonly used to cool the probe to −70 °C. The cryoneurolysis machine has indicators for "freeze" and "defrost," a flowmeter to monitor and control high-pressure gas flow, and a pressure gauge to monitor cylinder content.

Patients are positioned to facilitate localization of the target nerve. Minimal or no sedation is recommended so that the patient is able to respond to nerve stimulation and provide reliable feedback. Ultrasound guidance (or fluoroscopy guidance where applicable) is often useful to accurately identify the nerve and placing the probe. The operating site is prepared with sterile technique. A local anesthetic is used to numb the skin overlying the target nerve. A small incision (~5 mm) is made to facilitate insertion of the probe, and then a 10 gauge, 3 in. angiocatheter (3.4 × 76 mm) is inserted and directed at the target nerve. The stylet is removed and replaced by a cryoprobe, which is further advanced slowly and carefully with intermittent test stimulation. Electrical stimulation at low intensities (0.1–0.4 V) helps confirm precise placement of the probe in proximity to the target nerve. Ultrasound guidance can be valuable in this process. Two freeze-thaw cycles are usually carried out to increase the destructive effects.

Side Effects and Complications

As with all invasive procedures, side effects and complications such as post-procedural pain, bleeding, infection, and damage to adjacent structures can occur. Pneumothorax or hemothorax is of particular concern with procedures around the pleural space. Other complications include frostbite or skin lesion due to the probe being too close to the skin surface, nerve damage by introducer cannula or by removing the probe before the ice ball at the tip of the probe thaws, neuritis or persistent dysesthesia, and undesirable numbness in the scalp (occipital nerve), nipples (third and fourth intercostal nerve), and clitoris (pudendal nerve).

In summary, cryoanalgesia is an effective technique that can be considered in various intractable pain conditions, especially with nerves which are relatively small and superficial. Cryoanalgesia appears to be a relatively inexpensive technique to provide intermediate-term pain relief without long-term histological nerve damage. Solid anatomy knowledge and adequate training of procedural skills are required to safely and effectively perform the procedure.

Intramuscular Injections

Myofascial pain syndrome is often associated with a hypersensitive palpable nodule, called a myofascial trigger point. It is a hyperirritable point in skeletal muscle in patients with chronic disorders of the musculoskeletal system. A trigger point is usually within a taut band of skeletal muscle or in the muscle fascia. Compression of trigger point can reliably give rise to characteristic referred pain, which follows a consistent and reproducible pattern but not necessarily in dermatomal distributions. In addition to pain and hypersensitivity, myofascial pain syndrome may also be associated with motor and autonomic symptoms such as changes in skin temperature, sweating, piloerection, and erythema. The mechanisms of trigger point formation are poorly understood. Traumatic events or repetitive microtrauma to the muscles may lead to chronic stress, tension, and fatigue of the muscles, resulting in hypersensitivity to compression (the injury pool theory). A diagnosis of myofascial pain is often based on the pain history, consistent physical examination, and careful exclusion of other types of musculoskeletal diseases.

Intramuscular (trigger point) injection is one of the several treatment modalities for myofascial pain, such as physical therapy, transcutaneous electrical stimulation, ultrasound, massage, and ischemic compression therapy. Trigger point injection remains the treatment with the most scientific evidence support. Various injected substances and techniques have been investigated, including local anesthetics, corticosteroids, botulinum toxin, sterile water, sterile saline, and dry needling. The duration of pain relief after the procedure typically outlasts the duration of action of the injected medication for reasons that are poorly understood.

Techniques for Trigger Point Injection

The patient is often situated in a recumbent position to prevent syncope, assist in patient relaxation, and decrease muscle tension. The trigger point is identified by the palpable band. Then, the skin is prepared in a sterile fashion. A 25 gauge needle with length appropriate for the depth of the muscle is recommended. After the trigger point is entered, the needle should be aspirated to avoid intravascular injection. A small volume should be injected if the physician chooses to inject an agent. The needle may be withdrawn to the subcutaneous level and redirected to the trigger point, repeating the process and attempting to contact as many sensitive loci as possible. The patient is encouraged to stretch the muscle group that was injected as an integral part of trigger point therapy.

Local anesthetics are commonly used and have been shown to improve measures on a pain scale, range of motion, and algometry pressure thresholds. Small volumes are considered the most effective. Typically less than 1 ml of local agent, such as 1% lidocaine, is injected. *Local steroid injections* offer the potential advantage of reducing a local inflammatory response. However, a trigger point is typically non-inflammatory, and the use of steroid may be associated with local myotoxicity, subcutaneous tissue damage, and skin discoloration. *Local injection of botulinum toxin A* relaxes an overactive muscle by blocking the release of acetylcholine at the neuromuscular junction. However, the high cost of the agent limits its use. The physician should be careful to localize the trigger point since the toxin does not discriminate between trigger points and normal motor end plates. *Dry needling* involves multiple advances of a needle into the trigger point, similar to acupuncture. Its use in myofascial pain syndrome in the lower back appears to be a useful addition to standard therapies.

Complications of Trigger Point Injections

Infection is uncommon when sterile techniques are properly observed. Injection over an area of infected skin is contraindicated. Care should be taken to avoid pneumothorax when the injection is close to the lungs. Hematoma formation can be minimized with proper injection technique and holding pressure over site after withdrawal of the needle. Syncope or vasovagal response may happen in some individuals and require attention, monitoring, and proper responses from the practitioner.

Joint and Bursa Injections

Joint diseases affect an estimated 46 million (22%) of adults in the United States. For example, radiographic evidence of knee osteoarthritis (OA) increases with age, from 27% in subjects younger than age 70 to 44% in subjects age 80 or older. Nearly half of all adults will develop symptomatic knee OA by the age of 85. Rheumatoid arthritis (RA) and juvenile rheumatoid arthritis (JRA, also called juvenile idiopathic arthritis (JIR), juvenile chronic polyarthritis, and Still's disease) are also common and affect millions of children and adults in the United States. In addition, traumatic joint disease from sports and other injuries further adds to this large population of patients. Almost all joints of the body can be affected.

Intra-articular or periarticular injections of local anesthetics, corticosteroids, viscosupplements (hyaluronate), or other agents (such as botulinum toxin type A and tropisetron) are an integral part in the continuum of care from physical therapy and pharmacotherapy to joint replacement. These injections are commonly performed by physicians of various specialties in the management of patients with pain in their joints caused by arthritis, bursitis, or tendonitis.

Techniques for Joint Injections

Intra-articular injection is a common practice for noninfectious arthritis, such as rheumatoid arthritis and osteoarthritis affecting the hip, knee, shoulder, facet, and sacroiliac joints. High levels of evidence support for knee injection have been systematically reviewed. The findings may be applicable to other major joints such as the hip and shoulder even though the same rigorous review has yet to be performed for these joints. It is a common observation that intra-articular injections provide significant pain relief, improved functionality, and reduced medication requirement for durations ranging from weeks and months to a year after each injection. The injection techniques are relatively straightforward. Ultrasound or fluoroscopy guidance facilitates and helps confirm needle placement in the hip, shoulder, and other joints. Sterile technique is critical to minimize the risk of infection. Patient positioning is usually joint specific. Sedation is rarely needed.

Bursa injection can be performed for noninfectious bursitis. Bursitis is inflammation of one or more bursae that are small sacs lined with a synovial membrane that secretes a lubricating synovial fluid. The bursae rest at the points where the muscles and tendons slide across the bone. Healthy bursae create a smooth gliding surface and allow for normal movement frictionless and painless. However, the joint becomes painful at rest or during movement when bursitis occurs. Movement of tendons and muscles over the inflamed bursa further aggravates its inflammation, perpetuating the problem. Localized warmth, erythema, joint pain, and muscle stiffness are common. Pressure over the bursa by palpation often reproduces focal tenderness.

Common locations of bursitis include the subacromial, olecranon, greater trochanteric, ischial, iliopsoas, prepatellar, infrapatellar, pes anserinus, Achilles, and retrocalcaneal bursae. Bursitis is most commonly caused by repetitive movement and excessive pressure, among other etiologies such as trauma, autoimmune disorders, and infection. The injection techniques are similar to intra-articular injection even though the target is the inflamed bursa. A local anesthetic and corticosteroid combination is most commonly used. Ultrasound or fluoroscopy guidance may be required for some procedures. In addition to injections, bursitis may also be treated with rest, ice, elevation, physical therapy, anti-inflammatory drugs and other pain medications, and surgeries such as bursectomy and aspiration.

Injections for tendinitis and tendinosis. Tendinitis is inflammation of a tendon that follows larger-scale acute injuries. It is common in the upper and lower extremities, including tendinitis in the rotator cuff attachments, Achilles tendinitis, and patellar tendinitis (jumper's knee). Tendinosis (chronic tendinitis) occurs as the acute phase of healing has ended (6–8 weeks) but has left the area insufficiently healed. Tendinosis is caused by microtears in the connective tissue in and around the tendon. This may lead to reduced tensile strength, thus increasing the chance of tendon rupture. Treatment of tendinitis helps reduce some of the risks of developing tendinosis. Steroid injections to the close proximity of the injured tendon have been shown to be more effective than NSAIDs in the short term, but the long-term benefits have not been demonstrated. Steroid injection for tendinosis is generally not recommended because of concerns of risks of tendon rupture. Both platelet-rich plasma (PRP) injections and prolotherapy (injection of non-pharmacological and non-active irritant solution into the region of tendons or ligaments) are being used frequently for the purpose of strengthening weakened connective tissue and alleviating musculoskeletal pain with good clinical short- and long-term outcomes in tendinosis. However, more rigorously designed outcomes research is needed to establish evidence-based practice.

Complications of Joint Injections

The most common complication associated with joint injections is infection that includes spondylodiscitis, septic arthritis, epidural abscess, necrotizing fasciitis, osteomyelitis, gas gangrene, and albicans arthritis. Other complications include spinal cord injury and peripheral nerve injuries, pneumothorax, air embolism, pain or swelling at the site of injection, skeletal muscle toxicity, and tendon and fascial ruptures. Many of the infectious complications may be preventable by strict adherence to aseptic techniques. Some other complications may be minimized by refining the procedural techniques with a clear understanding of the relevant anatomies.

Intradiscal Interventions

A number of intradiscal interventions have been developed to treat discogenic pain or radiculopathy/radiculitis due to intervertebral disc herniation. However, the efficacy, safety, and cost-effectiveness of these procedures remain to be established by well-designed outcomes research. Some of the procedures, such as intradiscal electrothermal annuloplasty (IDET), have already been out of favor due to inadequate or inconsistent outcomes research support. Here we describe briefly some of the options for diagnosing and treating discogenic pain and/or disc herniation-related radiculitis.

Discography

Discography is also referred to as discogram. It is used for evaluation of intervertebral disc pathology. It can be considered for patients with persistent, severe low back pain or neck pain who have abnormal disc morphology on magnetic resonance imaging (MRI). It is usually reserved for situations where a disc (or discs) is suspected as the source of pain, other diagnostic tests have failed to confirm, and surgical intervention is being considered.

Under strict sterile condition, needles are inserted through the back into the center of the disc near the suspect area, guided by fluoroscope imaging. A contrast is then injected to pressurize the disc and to show the diffusion pattern of the contrast under fluoroscopy. The pain responses are recorded. Injection-induced pain that is similar or identical to the patient's usual painful symptoms in location and nature is considered concordant pain. Otherwise, it is considered discordant pain.

The interpretation of the test is based on the level of pressure, above the open pressure within the disc, at which concordant pain is reported by the patient.

- Concordant pain reported at <15 psi above open pressure is regarded as positive response and interpreted as chemically induced discogenic pain.
- Concordant pain reported at 15–50 psi above open pressure is regarded as positive response and interpreted as mechanically induced discogenic pain.
- Concordant pain reported at 51–90 psi is considered indecisive response.
- Pain reported at >90 psi above open pressure is considered as negative response.

These interpretations can only be regarded in relative terms. The specificity and sensitivity of discography based on these criteria is still open to debates. It is also important to include at least one control disc (normal disc) adjacent to the symptomatic disc, in which pressure of >90 psi above open pressure yields negative response or discordant pain. The provocative test is repeated in random order for the various discs, without the patient knowing which disc is pressurized so as to maximize objectivity.

The morphology of the disc and the contrast diffusion pattern is also valuable. Under fluoroscopy, a normal disc maintains normal height on both anteroposterior and lateral views. Injected contrast fills the nucleus pulposus, showing either unilobular or bilobular shape. A degenerated disc may show a reduced disc height and complex or multiple irregular fissures in the annulus fibrosis with, or without, contrast leakage through annular tears into the epidural space (fistula). CT images obtained following discography can further provide much details of the contrast spread in the nucleus pulposus and annular fibrosis. Based on the patterns of contrast spread, the degree of disruption of the annular fibrosis ranging from mild fissure to full-thickness fistula can be determined.

More recently, analgesic discography has been tested. In lieu of, or in addition to, provocative discography, a local anesthetic is injected to test the pain relief. It is an additional way of assessing discogenic pain. However, the specificity and sensitivity of discography remains to be determined. Possible complications of discography include nerve damage and discitis. Sterile techniques and pre-procedure use of antibiotics are necessary.

Intradiscal Injections

Intradiscal injections of a number of agents have been tested. These agents include methylene blue or jellified alcohol to denature nociceptors within the disc, chymopapain or ozone to break proteoglycan (the major matrix of the nucleus pulposus) (chemonucleolysis) and reduce the volume of nucleus pulposus, and steroids to reduce inflammatory mediators released from the disc. The clinical outcomes have been reported in forms of case series, prospective cohort studies, or randomized clinical trials. The efficacy, safety, and cost-effectiveness of these injections remain to be determined. The evidence supporting these practices in the United States is still limited even though some of the procedures, such as ozone intradiscal injection, have been widely used in many countries in Europe and Asia. The techniques and precautions are similar to what has been described for discography.

Biacuplasty

Biacuplasty is a new technique that applies radiofrequency energy to heat and decompress the posterior portion of the annulus fibrosus through two probes placed about 1.5 cm apart in the posterior part of the annulus fibrosus. It is intended to ablate the nociceptors invading the annulus fibrosus and coagulate fissures of the annulus. It is achieved by cooled radiofrequency electrodes which may regulate the temperature of the probes through an embedded cooling system and increase the size of the lesion. It may be used for patients with chronic discogenic pain, originating from annular fissures or contained disc herniation as suggested by a positive discography with concordant pain. The use of this technique is supported by a randomized controlled trial with intermediate-term pain relief. Clearly, more outcome research is needed before this procedure can be considered standard of care.

Percutaneous Disc Decompression

Percutaneous disc decompression is a technique to physically remove some of the disc content and reduce the volume of the nucleus pulposus and pressure on the affected nerves. A probe (titanium auger) is introduced through a cannula and is connected to a disposable rotational motor, which mechanically aspirates nucleus pulposus toward a proximal chamber. A herniated disc is decompressed for about 3 min and 0.75–2 ml disc material is removed. The probe is then removed along with the cannula.

The evidence supporting application of this technique is limited to a number of case series. It may be considered for patients with radicular pain that failed to respond to conservative therapy for >6 months, with MRI-documented contained disc herniation ≤6 mm, with positive discogram and concordant axial and/or leg pain, and with a confirmatory selective spinal nerve root block that achieves >80% relief of radicular pain.

Nucleoplasty

Nucleoplasty is also known as percutaneous discectomy. It is another procedure used to treat patients with back and leg pain caused by a herniated disc. Under fluoroscopy guidance, a coblation technology is used to remove nucleus pulposus tissue from the center of the disc to relieve pressure on the affected nerves. A PERC-D wand is introduced into the disc, and radiofrequency energy is delivered to generate a focused plasma field and break down pulposus tissue to smaller molecules and gases that escape from the introducer. In coblation mode, a series of six channels are created, removing about 1 ml of pulposus tissue. In coagulation mode, the channels are sealed. It may reduce pain and restore mobility. A recent systematic review concluded that "Nucleoplasty significantly reduces pain in patients with symptomatic contained disc herniation and also increases their functional capacity. According to currently available data from RCTs, it can be confirmed that nucleoplasty is an effective, safe, and minimally invasive treatment option in cervical, thoracic, and lumbar contained disc herniations."

Percutaneous Transforaminal Endoscopic Discectomy

Percutaneous transforaminal endoscopic discectomy is a technique that utilizes a rod endoscopy to visualize the herniated disc and assist the removal of the herniated nucleus pulposus and/or annulus fibrosus, decompress affected nerves, and relieve radicular or discogenic pain. It employs a combination of methods to directly visualize the disc, epidural space, and the neural structures in the foreman, remove the pathological tissues and decompress the affected nerves using a rongeur, seal or ablate the defected part of the annulus using bipolar radiofrequency probes, and irrigate the surgical field and washout the debris using an irrigation port. All of these operations are achieved under real-time visualization through a cannula that contains channels specific for these functions.

Briefly, under fluoroscopy guidance, the target disc is approached through the foreman from a posterolateral angle with a needle that is inserted without causing leg pain. A guide wire is inserted through the needle into the disc. The needle is replaced by a dilating tube to facilitate insertion of the cannula, which has a beveled edge to allow expanded visualization of the surgical field. A cavity is created in the disc to allow visualization and removal of the pathological tissue. Staining of the degenerated disc fragments with indigo carmine dye further facilitates differentiation of degenerative tissue from normal tissue. The instruments are removed when the procedure is completed. An important advantage of the endoscopic approach is that the instrument can also be directly placed in the epidural space, outside of the disc, to remove an extruded fragment of a disc that is completely isolated from or barely connected with the disc through a narrow neck. A holmium YAG laser can be used through the cannula to divide thick collagenous tissue and ablate cortical bone, allowing better instrument access to the disc and/or the epidural space.

This endoscopic approach also allows for the visualization of foraminal and intradiscal pathology that is not appreciated by the traditional approach and may help reduce surgical morbidity to the dorsal muscle column. Because of the minimal damage to bone and muscle tissue, patient undergoing this procedure typically experience less surgical trauma than those with more extensive procedures, allowing reduced recovery times and a quicker return to normal activities. Lumbar endoscopic discectomy may also result in a lower rate of serious complications during or after surgery. However, these potential benefits remain to be demonstrated by rigorously designed, comparative outcomes research. Evidence-based practice of this procedure remains to be established on the safety, efficacy, and cost-effectiveness.

Vertebroplasty/Kyphoplasty

Vertebroplasty and *kyphoplasty* are similar procedures to treat compression fracture of the spinal vertebral body by percutaneously injecting bone cement to relieve back pain and improve mobility. These are minimally invasive procedures for compression fracture that is frequently caused by osteoporosis or metastatic cancer. When performed in the acute phase of vertebral compression fracture (in the first 6 weeks of fracture with MRI evidence of edema), vertebroplasty or kyphoplasty is typically effective in reducing back pain and improving mobility. However, when patients with subacute or chronic vertebral fractures were included in placebo-controlled and randomized clinical trials, vertebroplasty was not more effective than placebo control. Therefore, appropriate patient selection is extremely important. These procedures may be considered for patients who have failed to improve after a trial of conservative treatment, which is effective in two-thirds of the cases.

Vertebroplasty is typically performed by a spine surgeon, interventional radiologist, or pain specialist. With fluoroscopy guidance, a bone access needle is placed into the fractured vertebra typically through a transpedicular approach, either unilaterally or bilaterally. Bone cement (2–6 ml) is injected through a coaxial cement cannula into the vertebra under continuous fluoroscopy monitoring. The cement quickly hardens and forms a support structure within the vertebra that provides stabilization and strength. The bone needle is removed without leaving any cement in the needle track outside of the vertebral bone. It makes a small puncture through the skin that is easily covered with a small bandage after the procedure. Before discharge, the patient should be evaluated for potential complications, particularly those associated with leakage of bone cement to outside of the vertebral body such as pulmonary embolism and spinal cord injury.

Kyphoplasty is a variation of a vertebroplasty. It includes the use of a small balloon that is inflated in the vertebral body to create a void within the cancellous bone prior to cement injection. It may partially restore the height and angle of kyphosis of a fractured vertebra. Once the void is created, bone cement is delivered directly into the newly created void in a similar manner as a vertebroplasty. The outcomes of vertebroplasty and kyphoplasty are still open to debates. In one study, both vertebroplasty and kyphoplasty are effective at improving pain, functional disability, and quality of life. However, kyphoplasty provides better results, which are maintained over long-term follow-up. Also, kyphoplasty is believed to be advantageous over vertebroplasty in restoring lost vertebral height and in safety issues like cement extravasation. But, kyphoplasty is performed at significantly higher cost.

Suggested Reading

1. Atallah JN. Management of cancer pain. In: Vadivelu N, Urman RD, Hines RL, editors. Essentials of pain management. New York: Springer; 2011.
2. Caracas HC, Maciel JV, Martins PM, de Souza MM, Maia LC. The use of lidocaine as an anti-inflammatory substance: a systematic review. J Dent. 2009;37(2):93–7.
3. Cassuto J, Sinclair R, Bonderovic M. Anti-inflammatory properties of local anesthetics and their present and potential clinical implications. Acta Anaesthesiol Scand. 2006;50:265–82.
4. Cheng J, Abdi S. Complications of joint, tendon and muscle injections (invited review). Tech Reg Anesth Pain Manag. 2007;11:141–7.
5. Cheng OT, Souzdalnitski D, Vrooman B, Cheng J. Evidence based knee injections for the management of arthritis. Pain Med. 2012;13:740–53.
6. Chua NH, Vissers KC, Sluijter ME. Pulsed radiofrequency treatment in interventional pain management: mechanisms and potential indications-a review. Acta Neurochir. 2011;153:763–71.
7. de Leon-Casasola OA. Critical evaluation of chemical neurolysis of the sympathetic axis for cancer pain. Cancer Control. 2000;7:142–8.
8. Gleich GJ. Treatment of asthma with nebulized lidocaine: a randomized, placebo-controlled study. J Allergy Clin Immunol. 2004;113:853–9.
9. Hollmann MW, Durieux ME. Local anesthetics and the inflammatory response: a new therapeutic indication? Anesthesiology. 2000;93(3):858–75.
10. Hunt LW, Frigas E, Butterfield JH, Kita H, Blomgren J, Dunnette SL, Offord KP, Movafegh A, Razazian M, Hajimaohamadi F, Meysamie A. Dexamethasone added to lidocaine prolongs axillary brachial plexus blockade. Anesth Analg. 2006;102:263–7.
11. Manchikanti L, Glaser SE, Wolfer L, Derby R, Cohen SP. Systematic review of lumbar discography as a diagnostic test for chronic low back pain. Pain Physician. 2009;12(3):541–59.
12. Trescot AM. Cryoanalgesia in interventional pain management. Pain Physician. 2003;6:345–60.
13. Yeung AT, Yeung CA. Minimally invasive techniques for the management of lumbar disc herniation. Orthop Clin North Am. 2007;38(3):363–72.

Surgical Approaches to Chronic Pain

10

Sean J. Nagel, Bryan S. Lee,
and Andre G. Machado

Key Concepts

- The surgical treatments for refractory chronic pain are underutilized despite a growing body of literature favoring their use for long-term pain control.
- The continuous infusion of intrathecal opioid medication through a programmable pump is a mainstay in controlling malignant and nonmalignant pain in patients with expected survival greater than 1 year who are on high-dose opioid medication.
- Patients with malignant pain and a short life expectancy who are not responding to narcotic medication should be evaluated for an ablative cranial or spinal procedure.
- Spinal cord stimulation is a safe, reversible, and cost-effective way to significantly reduce pain related to failed back surgery syndrome, complex regional pain syndrome, and other painful neuropathic conditions.
- Neuromodulation, including deep brain stimulation, motor cortex stimulation, and peripheral nerve stimulation, has been shown to control pain in some studies and should be considered when other surgical therapies are not indicated or have failed.
- Trigeminal neuralgia is a unique pain syndrome that can be effectively treated with microvascular decompression as well as neuroablative procedures including balloon compression, glycerol rhizolysis, radiofrequency thermocoagulation, and stereotactic radiosurgery.

Neuroablative Procedures of the Brain and Spinal Cord

Prior to the widespread marketing and distribution of commercial neurostimulation devices and opioid medications, patients with refractory chronic pain were often treated with irreversible, destructive brain and spinal cord procedures. Although these operations were initially intended to treat both malignant and nonmalignant pain, they remain an effective option in a subset of patients with malignant pain and expected short

S.J. Nagel, MD (✉)
Department of Neurological Surgery, Center for Neurological Restoration, Cleveland Clinic, Cleveland, OH, USA
e-mail: nagels@ccf.org

B.S. Lee, MD
Department of Neurological Surgery, Cleveland Clinic, Cleveland, OH, USA

A.G. Machado, MD, PhD
Department of Neurological Surgery, Center for Neurological Restoration, Cleveland Clinic, Cleveland, OH, USA

Department of Neurosciences, Lerner Research Institute, Cleveland Clinic, Cleveland, OH, USA

J. Cheng, R.W. Rosenquist (eds.), *Fundamentals of Pain Medicine*,
https://doi.org/10.1007/978-3-319-64922-1_10

survival. Delayed complications and loss of efficacy may occur, but patients with terminal diseases may not live long enough to see these adverse effects.

Percutaneous Cordotomy/Spinothalamic Tractotomy/Anterolateral Cordotomy

Background

Since Spiller first described cordotomy in 1912, over 3600 treated patients have been reported in the literature. The anterolateral spinal cord is composed of fibers that carry nociceptive signals, temperature feedback, and nondiscriminative touch from the contralateral side of the body to thalamic nuclei including the ventroposterolateral nucleus, ventroposteromedial nucleus, and intralaminar nuclei of the thalamus. Lesioning of this spinothalamic tract in the spinal cord disrupts pain processing before it is integrated in the brain.

Indications

Patients with nociceptive cancer pain localized to one half of the body below the C5 dermatome may benefit from cordotomy especially those with unilateral chest wall pain, pulmonary malignancy, compression of the plexus, or malignancy of an extremity. Patients with survival less than 3 months, poor pulmonary function, and pure neuropathic pain are in general not candidates for cordotomy.

Technique

The procedure is completed with patient awake so that they are able to provide feedback. A needle is directed under CT guidance following intrathecal contrast administration into the C1-C2 interspace *contralateral* to the side of the pain. Following the flow of cerebrospinal fluid, a stimulating electrode is then advanced into the lateral spinothalamic tract. After electrophysiologic verification, 2–3 lesions are made until the patient reports diminished sensation in the area of pain.

Outcomes

Although no controlled studies are available, initial pain relief is greater than 90% with recent estimates that approximately 80% of patients report a satisfactory reduction in pain at 6 months. In patients with bilateral pain, cordotomy should be staged to minimize the risk of Ondine's curse if done at all. Other complications include Horner's syndrome, transient or permanent ipsilateral weakness (with injury of the corticospinal tracts), and urinary retention.

Commissural Myelotomy

Background

Commissural myelotomy was first proposed by Greenfield in 1926 as a method to abolish midline visceral pain and first performed 1 year later by Armour [1]. By transecting the ascending visceral pain fibers and spinothalamic tract fibers that cross midline from the dorsal horn to the contralateral spinothalamic pathway, painful bilateral signals from the viscera are interrupted.

Indications

Patients with midline or bilateral abdominal or pelvic pain from cervical, pancreatic, or gastric cancers as well as sacral or bilateral leg pain are potential candidates for commissural myelotomy.

Technique

Both CT-guided percutaneous and open myelotomy techniques are described. In the open operation, a midline incision is made and a laminectomy performed usually from T10 to L1. The thecal sac is opened, the midline septum is exposed, and a radiofrequency or mechanical lesion is made through the dorsal median sulcus.

Outcomes

A 60–70% success rate is reported but recurrence of pain is common. Dysesthesias, bowel and bladder dysfunction, and reduced proprioception are described complications.

Dorsal Root Entry Zone Lesioning

Background

Sindou, in 1974, first described lesioning in the dorsal root entry zone. This was subsequently revised by Nashold in 1976 [3]. DREZ lesioning interrupts pain signals as they enter the posterolateral spinal cord at the lateral portion of dorsal roots and at the excitatory region of Lissauer's tract.

Indications

Because the DREZ procedure is capable of controlling topographically limited pain, especially neuropathic pain, it is still used to control nonmalignant deafferentation pain from brachial plexus injuries and avulsion in addition to its use in brachial plexus malignancy, radiation plexopathy, and Pancoast tumors.

Technique

A laminectomy or hemilaminectomy at the site of the pain is performed initially. The dura is opened in the midline, and an electrode is inserted at the DREZ. Multiple lesions 1–2 mm apart are made targeting dorsal rootlets, substantia gelatinosa, and Lissauer's tract.

Outcomes

Nearly 66% of patients reported good to excellent relief of pain with follow-up of more than 1 year after DREZotomy for brachial plexus avulsion. Ipsilateral lower limb weakness and sensory changes as well as bladder incontinence have been reported complications (Fig. 10.1).

Cingulotomy

Background

The anterior cingulate gyrus is a limbic structure located superior to the corpus callosum. It is part of the circuit of Papez and participates in the processing of behavior and emotion, including the affective sphere of chronic pain. It was first reported by Foltz and White [2].

Indications

Cingulotomy is usually reserved for patients with metastatic cancer and medically refractory pain at multiple sites who are not candidates for other surgical interventions.

Technique

The anterior cingulate is stereotactically targeted with MRI guidance and lesioned bilaterally with

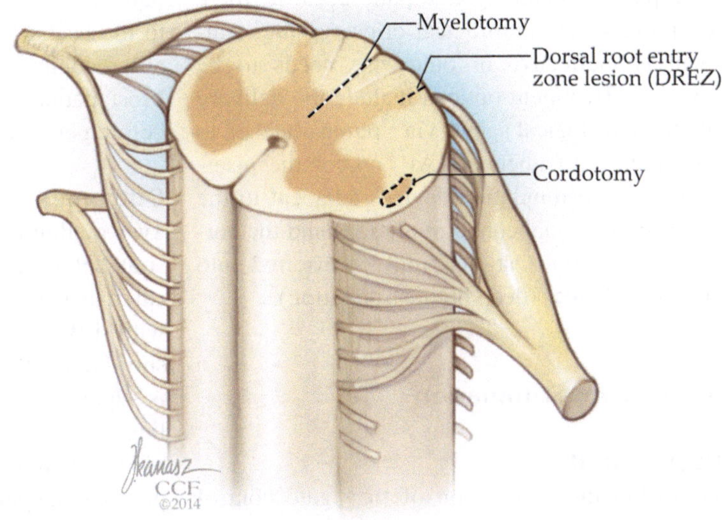

Fig. 10.1 Illustration showing the approximate location of lesions in the spinal cord for treatment of intractable cancer pain (Reprinted with permission, Cleveland Clinic Center for Medical Art & Photography © 2014. All Rights Reserved)

a radiofrequency thermocoagulation electrode passed through paramedian burr holes.

Outcome

Approximately 50% of patients will experience pain relief at 6 months. Complications include seizures and behavioral changes characterized by cognitive decline and behavioral changes. Cingulotomy is used infrequently to control pain.

Other Ablative Lesions

Patients with cranial facial cancer pain are especially challenging. However, lesioning of the ipsilateral spinal trigeminal tract and nucleus caudalis has been reported to control pain in 80% of patients at 6 months. Unfortunately only limited data is available to support its use. Similarly, lesioning the spinothalamic tract as it ascends into the brain at the thalamus (thalamotomy) and in the mesencephalon or pons (mesencephalotomy/pontine tractotomy) may also reduce pain but is rarely attempted any longer.

Neuromodulation Procedures of the Brain and Spinal Cord

Neuromodulation has replaced neuroablation as the preferred treatment of medically refractory neuropathic, nonmalignant pain because there are no residual neurological effects if the treatment is ineffective or otherwise needs to be reversed. Treatment options include the delivery of pharmacological agents via a pump attached to an intrathecal catheter (ITAP) and/or the insertion of neurostimulation devices adjacent to the spinal cord (spinal cord stimulation) and the cortex (motor cortex stimulation) or inserted into subcortical areas (deep brain stimulation).

Spinal Cord Stimulation

Background

Following the publication of the "gate control theory" of pain in 1965 by Melzack and Wall, Shealy described electrical stimulation of the dorsal columns of the spinal cord to attenuate chest pain from a bronchiogenic carcinoma in 1967. It is hypothesized that electrical stimulation of the dorsal columns depolarizes large A-β fibers that activate inhibitory interneurons and "close the gate" to prevent the transmission of pain-inducing nociceptive signals from A-delta and C-fibers which are afferent fibers.

Indications

Continuous SCS reduces chronic neuropathic pain as well as ischemic pain. Persistent pain after spine surgery or failed back surgery syndrome (FBSS) is the most common indication for SCS in the United States. Complex regional pain syndrome (CRPS) has also been shown to improve in a single randomized controlled trial. Other causes of peripheral neuropathy have been shown to respond to SCS but are less well studied. Refractory angina pectoris and, to a lesser extent, ischemic pain arise from peripheral vascular disease and have also been effectively treated with SCS. Additional trials are ongoing.

Technique

Stimulation electrodes are implanted into the thoracic epidural space by a percutaneous approach (cylindrical lead) or open surgical approach via laminotomy (paddle lead). A patient-controlled implanted pulse generator (IPG) inserted into the buttocks or abdominal region is then connected to the leads. Neuropsychological testing is usually recommended before implantation approval. Most patients are trialed first with stimulation before permanent implantation.

Outcomes

Two randomized controlled trials have demonstrated that SCS is superior to conventional medical management alone or reoperation for patients with FBSS. One randomized controlled trial showed that SCS combined with physical therapy is superior to physical therapy alone in controlling pain in patients with CRPS. Complications of SCS include pain induced in the region of SCS placement, spinal cord or peripheral nerve injury, hardware failure, migration, and infection. A

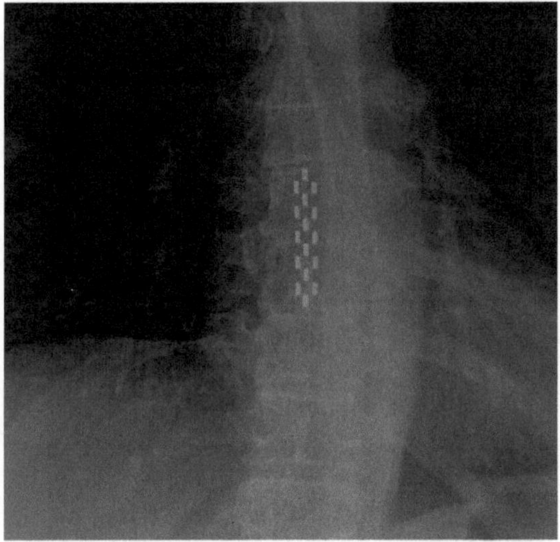

Fig. 10.2 Thoracic radiograph demonstrating a multi-contact paddle electrode overlying the mid-thoracic spinal cord. Wires can be seen coursing caudally

meta-analysis of 18 studies reported an average complication of 34% (Fig. 10.2).

Intrathecal Analgesic Pumps (ITAP)

Background

ITAP delivers analgesics such as morphine into the cerebrospinal fluid (CSF). By directly infusing the medication into CSF, the dose is significantly reduced as many of the side effects are from systemic exposure. The pump stores the analgesic medication which is then refilled percutaneously. The pump controls the rate at which analgesic is delivered. The only FDA-approved medications for intrathecal administration through a pump are morphine, baclofen, and ziconotide. There is a high initial cost of the implant that is recovered when the device is used in the long term.

Indications

Patients with both malignant and nonmalignant pain may respond favorably to intrathecal therapy. ITAP is an option for patients who do not achieve adequate pain relief or those who cannot tolerate the side effects of systemic pharmacotherapy.

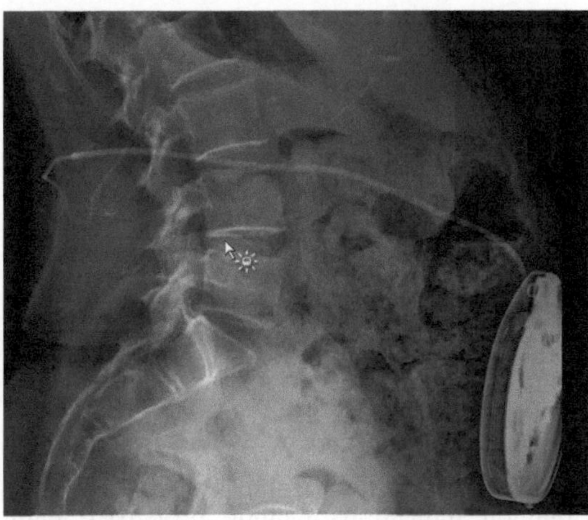

Fig. 10.3 Lateral lumbar radiograph demonstrating a programmable pump with a tunneled intrathecal catheter. The tip of the catheter is in the low thoracic spine

Technique

ITAP is delivered into the intrathecal space via a tunneled catheter that is connected to a programmable pump inserted in the abdomen.

Outcomes

A randomized control study involving 202 patients with cancer pain reported that ITAP together with comprehensive pain management improved pain control compared to comprehensive pain management alone. In addition, patients with ITAP had a decrease in the risk of drug toxicities and depressed levels of consciousness. Hardware-related complications including catheter breakage or blockage are common but easily repaired. Other risks of surgery include CSF fistula, pseudomeningocele, infection and pocket seromas, hematomas, and neurological deficits. Patients are instructed on signs of toxicity and withdrawal. Patients with a history of poor compliance with medical care may not be good candidates as the frequent follow-up visits for refills and drug titration may be onerous (Fig. 10.3).

Deep Brain Stimulation

Background

Although DBS has been validated as an effective treatment for movement disorders, its use in the treatment of chronic pain began prior to this landmark discovery. The earliest reports that describe using electrical stimulation for pain modulation were in 1954 (Heath) and 1956 (Pool) although the targeting was not refined until the 1970s. Two inconclusive multicenter studies in the 1990s tempered enthusiasm for this treatment and its use began to decline.

Indications

DBS is considered an investigational *off*-label surgical option for patients with refractory pain to both pharmacologic and surgical therapies. Common indications include poststroke pain, phantom limb pain/stump pain, and history of spinal injury or brachial plexus injury.

Technique

A stimulating electrode is implanted through a burr hole using stereotactic navigation. The most commonly targeted regions currently are the periventricular gray/periaqueductal gray and the ventral posterior lateral and medial thalamus. Once the electrode is in place, it is secured and connected to an implantable pulse generator that delivers electrical impulses to the brain at a set frequency, pulse width, and intensity.

Outcomes

The response of patients with refractory pain following DBS has been variable. In the largest recent prospective study, 66% of patients improved following DBS. Potential complications of DBS include stroke, intracranial hemorrhage, neurologic deficits, hardware failure/infection, lead dislocation/fracture, and unintentional motor or sensory disturbances.

Motor Cortex Stimulation

Background

Following his observations that deafferentation of the spinothalamic tract in cats led to thalamic hyperactivity that could be abolished by stimulation of the motor cortex, Tsubokawa postulated that chronic motor cortex stimulation might suppress central pain signals in patients. The first study of MCS was published in 1991 by Tsubokawa.

Indications

Patients with trigeminal neuropathy, poststroke pain syndromes (lateral medullary and thalamic infarction), anesthesia dolorosa, spinal cord injury, and peripheral nerve injuries, such as limb stump pain and postherpetic neuralgia, may respond to MCS.

Technique

A minimal access craniotomy is planned over the motor cortex contralateral to the side of pain using neuronavigation. A plate electrode is inserted into the epidural space overlying the region of the motor cortex that corresponds to the location of neuropathic pain and can usually be identified preoperatively with functional MRI. Motor-evoked responses can be used intraoperatively to confirm the location. The electrode is generally tested externally for several days before returning to the operating room for internalization and connection to an implantable pulse generator.

Outcomes

Although MCS has been studied in the treatment of both central and peripheral pain syndromes, inconsistent results have limited its adoption as a salvage procedure for most cases of refractory pain. The results are at least somewhat related to the highly variable patient selection in these studies and small sample size. The one bright spot are those patients with neuropathic face pain who seem to respond better perhaps related to the proportionally large motor representation of the face in the convexity. Hardware-related complications, stroke, abscess, seizures, and intracranial bleeding have all been reported following MCS.

Trigeminal Neuralgia

Background

Patients with trigeminal neuralgia complain of unilateral, paroxysmal, stabbing face pain that will typically follow one or more of the sensory dermatomes of the trigeminal nerve (see Chap. 27 for details). In its classical or typical manifestation, the triggered pain is interrupted by pain-

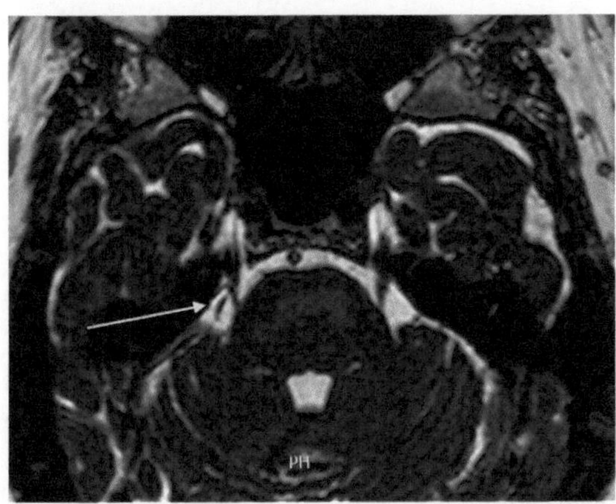

Fig. 10.4 MRI constructive interference in steady-state sequence (CISS) illustrating neurovascular compression of the trigeminal nerve just distal to the root entry zone

free intervals. The pain is most commonly associated with vascular compression at the root entry zone by the superior cerebellar artery and less commonly the anterior inferior cerebellar artery or the superior petrosal vein.

Indications

Failure of or intolerance to medication therapy in patients with TN will usually prompt referral for surgery. Younger patients with MRI evidence of vascular compression with few or no medical comorbidities are often offered MVD. However, posterior fossa exploration for possible MVD can also be considered in patients with no MRI-visible neurovascular conflicts. Likewise, patients who prefer to avoid more invasive procedures can opt for other surgical interventions for TN (Fig. 10.4).

Microvascular Decompression

Technique

Microvascular decompression is the most invasive treatment option for patients with TN, but it has also been shown to provide long-lasting relief. It is generally considered the preferred option in those younger patients with few comorbidities and evidence of neurovascular compression. Patients are operated on under general anesthesia. A retrosigmoid craniectomy is used to gain entry into the posterior fossa. After opening the dura, the offending vessel is dissected off the trigeminal nerve, and a piece of Telfa or other nonabsorbent material is put in its place. Patients often report significant improvement of their pain shortly after surgery, but more delayed improvements may also be seen. Repeat MVD surgery is less likely to be effective and has increased risk of facial weakness.

Outcomes

MVD is associated with long-term pain relief and a low rate of pain recurrence compared to other modalities along with a relatively low risk of complications. In studies with follow-up of up to 10 years, 65–70% is still pain-free. Sensory loss is reported to be 5–10%, and cerebrospinal fluid leak occurs in 7% of patients. Hearing loss and facial weakness may be seen. The mortality rate has been reported to be 0.37%.

Ablative Surgical Options for Trigeminal Neuralgia

Unlike MVD, which has nondestructive goals, the goal of trigeminal rhizotomy is to selectively damage the pain fibers of the nerve to induce partial sensory loss. The procedures discussed below, balloon compression (BC), glycerol rhizotomy (GR), and radiofrequency (RF) rhizotomy, have procedure-specific advantages and disadvantages that should be considered for each patient. Often, however, it is surgeon experience that guides the ultimate decision.

Balloon Compression

Technique

Balloon compression is usually performed under general anesthesia. Using fluoroscopic guidance, a needle is advanced starting 2.5 cm lateral to the ipsilateral corner of the mouth until the foramen ovale is cannulated. The stylet is withdrawn and replaced with a balloon embolectomy catheter. The balloon is inflated until it shows a characteristic pear shape and left up for 60–90 s. BC may elicit transient hypotension and bradycardia that requires a period of transcutaneous pacing in some.

Outcomes

Approximately 90% of patients report pain relief at 6 months. This percentage of patients falls to approximately 70% at 3 years with a recurrence rate generally in the 25% range. Masseter weakness is common (up to 66%) but may be subclinical. Numbness is seen in 2%. BC selectively injures medium and large myelinated pain fibers and thus may spare corneal reflex.

Glycerol Rhizotomy

Technique

The landmarks and entry point for glycerol rhizotomy are the same as for BC. The foramen ovale is cannulated under fluoroscopic guidance. Once the foramen is entered, the patient is moved to a sitting position and contrast is administered followed by the glycerol. The patient is kept upright for 2 h to prevent drainage of glycerol into the posterior fossa.

Outcomes

Most studies report that the pain relief following glycerol injection is less durable than that for the other procedures with estimates approaching 90% at 6 months to above 50% at 3 years. However, sensory loss may be less common than for the other procedures. Dysesthesias and corneal numbness are seen in fewer than 9%, and the incidence of masseter weakness is around 3%.

Radiofrequency Thermocoagulation

Technique

Under monitored anesthesia care, a stimulating electrode is introduced through a needle placed in the foramen ovale with the aid of fluoroscopy. The patient is awoken from anesthesia for mapping of the sensory and motor responses. A thermocouple lead is used to lesion the nerve. The advantage of dermatomal mapping in RF is that it is more selective than BC.

Outcomes

Pain relief following RF approaches 90% with nearly 60% of patients still pain-free at 60 months. The estimated recurrence rate of 25% is likely lower than for glycerol rhizotomy. There is a high incidence of complications with RF, especially masticatory weakness, dysesthesia, and corneal numbness. The increased risk of corneal numbness may be due to injury of the small, unmyelinated pain fibers. The risk of vascular injury is also increased. RF is a good option in a patient unable to undergo general anesthesia or for selective root destruction.

Stereotactic Radiosurgery

Technique

Stereotactic radiosurgery using a Gamma Knife, LINAC, or CyberKnife system is a noninvasive technique used to control refractory TN. The trigeminal nerve is lesioned at the root entry zone using focused radiation with doses between 70 and 90 Gy.

Outcomes

Pain relief is delayed several weeks unlike the other procedures that may acutely relieve the pain. Most studies report that 50–75% of patients achieve good pain control at long-term follow-up with recurrence rates in the range of 5–42%. Increased radiation doses are associated with an increase in paresthesias or dysesthesias. Repeat treatment with GK is an option for recurrent or refractory cases. Overall, the low complication rate coupled with the short recovery makes this an excellent option for higher-risk surgical patients or for those who prefer to avoid more invasive surgical options.

Glossopharyngeal Neuralgia

Glossopharyngeal neuralgia is a rare craniofacial pain syndrome sometimes confused with TN characterized by excruciating pain in the throat and ear. Neurovascular compression is sometimes seen and the pain is typically relieved with MVD of CN IX. In refractory cases, sectioning of the nerve and several of the rootlets of the vagus nerve (X) may abolish the pain.

References

1. Armour D. Surgery of the spinal cord and its membranes. Lancet. 1927;1:691–7.
2. Foltz EL, White LE Jr. Pain "relief " by frontal cingulumotomy. J Neurosurg. 1962;19(2):89–100.
3. Thomas DGT, Kitchen ND. Longterm followup of dorsal root entry zone lesions in brachial plexus avulsion. J Neurol Neurosurg Psychiatry. 1994;57:737–8.

Suggested Reading

1. Boccard SGJ, Pereira EAC, Aziz TZ, Green AL. Long-term outcomes of deep brain stimulation for neuropathic pain. Neurosurgery. 2013;72:221–31.
2. Broggi G, Broggi M, Ferroli P, Frnazini A. Surgical technique for trigeminal microvascular decompression. Acta Neurochir. 2012;154:1089–95.
3. Cheng JS, Lim DA, Chang EF, Barbaro NM. A review of percutaneous treatments for trigeminal neuralgia. Oper Neurosurg. 2013;10(1):25–33.
4. Kanapolat Y, Ugur HC, Ayten M, Elhan AH. Computed tomography-guided percutaneous cordotomy for intractable pain in malignancy. Neurosurgery. 2009;64(3):187–94.
5. Kemler MA, Barendse GAM, van Kleef M, de Vet HCW, Rijks CPM, Furnée CA, van den Wildenberg FAJM. Spinal cord stimulation in patients with chronic reflex sympathetic dystrophy. N Engl J Med. 2000;343(9):618–24.
6. Kumar K, Hunter G, Demeria DD. Treatment of chronic pain by using intrathecal drug therapy compared with conventional pain therapies: a cost-effectiveness analysis. J Neurosurg. 2002;97(4):803–10.
7. Kumar K, Taylor RS, Jacques L, et al. Spinal cord stimulation versus conventional medical management for neuropathic pain: a multicentre randomized controlled trial in patients with failed back surgery syndrome. Pain. 2007;132(1–2):179–88.
8. North RB, Kidd DH, Farrokhi F, Piantadosi SA. Spinal cord stimulation versus repeated lumbosacral spine surgery for chronic pain: a randomized, controlled trial. Neurosurgery. 2005;56(1):98–1067.
9. Raslan AM, Cetas JS, McCartney S, Burchiel KJ. Destructive procedures for control of cancer pain: the case for cordotomy. J Neurosurg. 2011;114:155–70.
10. Sindou MP, Blondet E, Emery E, Mertens P. Microsurgical lesioning in the dorsal root entry zone for pain due to brachial plexus avulsions: a prospective series in 55 patients. J Neurosurg. 2005;112(6):1018–28.
11. Smith TJ, Staats PS, Deer T, Stearns LJ, Rauck RL, Boortz-Marx RL, Buchser E, Català E, Bryce DA, Coyne PJ, Pool GE. Implantable drug delivery systems study group randomized clinical trial of an implantable drug delivery system compared with comprehensive medical management for refractory cancer pain: impact on pain, drug-related toxicity, and survival. J Clin Oncol. 2002;20(19):4040–9.
12. Tsubokawa T, Katayama Y, Yamamoto T, Hirayama T, Koyama S. Chronic motor cortex stimulation for the treatment of central pain. Adv Stereotact Funct Neurosurg. 1991;52:137–9.
13. Viswanathan A, Burton AW, Rekito A, McCutcheon IE. Commisural myelotomy in the treatment of intractable visceral pain. Stereotact Funct Neurosurg. 2010;88:374–82.
14. Yen C, Shlesinger D, Sheehan JP. Gamma knife radiosurgery for trigeminal neuralgia. Expert Rev Med Devices. 2011;8(6):709–21.
15. Yen CP, Kung SS, Su YF, Lin WC, Howng SL. Stereotactic bilateral anterior cingulotomy for intractable pain. J Clin Neurosci. 2005;12(8):886–90.

11 Acupunture and Complementary Integrative Approaches in Pain Management

Lucy Chen

Key Concepts

- *Complementary medicine* refers to unconventional healthcare practice or products that are used in combination with conventional medicine, while *alternative medicine* refers to unconventional healthcare practice or products that are used as an independent treatment modality to replace conventional medicine. *Integrative medicine* is used to describe a discipline that combines conventional therapies with complementary therapies.
- Approximately 38% of adults and 12% of children in the United States used CAM. In 2007, 3.2 million visits were for acupuncture treatment. The other most commonly used CAM therapies include natural products, deep breathing, meditation, chiropractic or osteopathic practice, and massage. Low back pain is among the most common medical conditions treated by CAM. With increasing demand for CAM therapies, the majority of medical schools in the United States have added coursework on integrative medicine.
- Acupuncture is perhaps the most studied both preclinically and clinically and is one of the most commonly practiced among the five major categories of CAM: whole medical systems, mind-body medicine, biologically based practices, manipulative and body-based practices, and energy therapies.
- The safety, efficacy, and cost-effectiveness of acupuncture are gaining support, and the neurohumoral mechanisms are beginning to be understood.
- With the aging population and ever-growing healthcare cost in the United States, more emphasis is being placed on preventive and alternative measures. Many CAM therapies may add value as primary treatments or as useful adjuncts to conventional treatment to allow us to reach the goal of maintaining health, reducing costs, and improving patient satisfaction.

L. Chen, MD (✉)
Associate Professor, Harvard Medical School, MGH Center for Translational Pain Research, MGH Center for Pain Medicine, Department of Anesthesia, Critical Care and Pain Medicine, Massachusetts General Hospital, Harvard Medical School, Boston, MA 02114, USA
e-mail: llchen@mgh.harvard.edu

Introduction

In contrast to conventional medicine, complementary and alternative medicine (CAM) is a group of healthcare practices and products that are not a part of western medicine. Although complementary and alternative medicine has been practiced since ancient times, it did not

J. Cheng, R.W. Rosenquist (eds.), *Fundamentals of Pain Medicine*,
https://doi.org/10.1007/978-3-319-64922-1_11

grow at a remarkable pace in western countries until the 1970s. Over the last several decades, the advancement of both basic science and clinical research in this field has substantially increased the awareness of CAM modalities in western countries.

Complementary medicine refers to unconventional healthcare practice or products that are used in combination with conventional medicine.

Alternative medicine refers to unconventional healthcare practice or products that are used as an independent treatment modality to replace conventional medicine.

Integrative medicine is a term used to describe a discipline that combines conventional therapies with complementary therapies. Integrative medicine has become part of medical practice, which also has been taught in many medical schools. Integrative medicine may have a unique role in clinical pain management because of the multidimensional nature of pain experiences that often require multimodality approaches for successful management.

Current Use of CAM

Over the last few decades, office visits for alternative therapies were two times as many as the visits to primary care physicians as reported in a nationwide survey conducted in 1998; in 2007, approximately 38% of US adults and 12% of children used CAM therapies [1]. Among those visits, 3.2 million visits were for acupuncture treatment alone (2007 NCCAM). The total out-of-pocket expenditures relating to alternative therapies were estimated at $27 billion in 1997, and this figure was comparable to that for all US physician services and has further increased to $33.9 billion in the next 10 years. Third-party reimbursements for alternative therapies have also increased at the patients' request. The most commonly used CAM therapies include natural products, deep breathing, meditation, chiropractic or osteopathic practice, and massage. Low back pain is the most common medical condition for which CAM is frequently used. Due to a significant increase in the demand for CAM therapies, the majority of medical schools in the United States have added coursework on integrative medicine.

Major Categories of CAM

A variety of practices are included in CAM, which can be divided into five major categories based on the information provided by the National Center of Complementary and Alternative Medicine.

- *Whole medical systems*: homeopathy, naturopathy, traditional Chinese medicine, and ayurveda.
- *Mind-body medicine*: meditation, relaxation technique, prayer, mental healing, yoga, Pilates, tai chi, art therapy, music therapy, and dance therapy.
- *Biologically based practices*: dietary supplements, herbal supplements, and scientifically unproven therapies such as shark cartilage.
- *Manipulative and body-based practices*: spinal manipulation (both chiropractic and osteopathic) and massage.
- *Energy therapies*: qigong, reiki, therapeutic touch, and electromagnetic therapy.

Acupuncture is perhaps the most studied both preclinically and clinically and is one of the most commonly practiced among many different modalities of CAM. With the ever-growing demand for acupuncture, FDA classified acupuncture needles as medical equipment subject to the same strict standards for medical needles, syringes, and surgical scalpels in 1996. At a Consensus Development Conference on Acupuncture in 1997 organized by the National Institutes of Health, acupuncture was recognized an extensively practiced modality by medical physicians, dentists, non-MD acupuncturists, and other practitioners. A major reason for patients to seek acupuncture treatment is a remarkably low incidence of adverse effects compared to that of many drugs and commonly accepted medical procedures. Due to a broad range of CAM contents, it will not be possible to cover every modality in this chapter.

Instead, the focus will be placed on acupuncture to illustrate how to integrate this modality into clinical practice of pain management based on up-to-date information in this field.

Acupuncture Theory

Acupuncture is a form of traditional Chinese medicine and has been used in China for more than 3000 years. In the ancient theory of Chinese medicine, human health is maintained through a delicate balance of two opposing but inseparable elements: *yin* and *yang*. Accordingly, human internal "organs" are also divided into the *yin and yang* organs. Yin symbolizes "cold, slow, and passive elements," whereas yang symbolizes "hot, exciting, and active elements." This theory believes that *qi* (pronounced as "chee") is the life force or vital energy. Qi is thought to flow through specific pathways, the so-called *meridians*, in a human body to influence health. Human body consists of 12 main meridians and 8 secondary meridians. Since the balance of the opposing forces of yin and yang is considered to be the basis for the healthy flow of *qi*, any imbalance in this system would disrupt or block the flow of *qi* leading to a state of disease or pain. Technically, acupuncture involves the insertion of fine sterilized needles through specific skin points (so-called acupoints) that are mostly located along the meridians. Acupuncture treats a state of disease or pain through strengthening the weakened q*i*, releasing excessive *qi*, and/or removing the blockage from the flow of *qi* in order to restore the normal balance of the yin and yang system.

Mechanisms of Acupuncture

Although the mechanisms of acupuncture remain unclear, a number of studies have revealed different biological effects on the peripheral or central nervous system. Neurohumoral factors, neurotransmitters, and other chemical mediators have been indicated in acupuncture's therapeutic effects.

Peripheral and Central Nervous System

Studies have shown that the analgesic effect of acupuncture relies on an intact peripheral nervous system because if the acupuncture site is affected by postherpetic neuralgia or local anesthetics, the analgesic effect of acupuncture can be abolished. Earlier studies also showed that electrical acupuncture (EA) at different frequencies could have different effects on the synthesis and release of neuropeptides, particularly the synthesis of several opioid peptides in the central nervous system. In addition, cholecystokinin-like immune reactivity was increased within the medial thalamic area after EA, and EA also enhanced or restored the activity of natural killer cells.

Studies by using functional magnetic resonance imaging (fMRI) and positron emission topographic (PET) scan have made it possible to further understand the effects of acupuncture on neuronal activities of the brain. It has been revealed that acupuncture attenuated neuronal activity activated by nociceptive input in the periaqueductal gray (PAG), thalamus, hypothalamus, somatosensory cortex, and prefrontal cortex regions in humans. Stimulation at different acupuncture points evoked changes in neuroimaging signals (increase or decrease) in specific areas within the central nervous system, and each meridian is connected to a representative area in the cerebral cortex. EA, particularly at a low frequency, produced more widespread fMRI signal changes in the anterior insula area (signal increase) as well as in the limbic and para-limbic structures (signal increase) than manual acupuncture. The data suggest a possible correlation between the effects of acupuncture and neuronal changes in the brain. Also the meridian system defined in the theories of Chinese medicine may be connected to distinct supraspinal regions. These findings may help understand the neural mechanisms of acupuncture treatment and meridian phenomena.

Humoral Factors and Neurotransmitters

Humoral factors may mediate acupuncture analgesia through acupuncture-induced release of substances into the cerebrospinal fluid, a notion supported by a cross-perfusion experiment. It has been shown that acupuncture significantly increased the endorphin production and anandamide (an endogenous cannabinoid) level. These effects can be blocked by the opioid receptor antagonist naloxone or by a specific cannabinoid (CB2) receptor antagonist. EA also decreased the release of gamma-aminobutyric acid (GABA, an inhibitory neurotransmitter), upregulated nitric oxide, and modulated the production and release of neurotransmitters such as epinephrine, norepinephrine, dopamine, and 5-hydroxytryptamine (5-HT). Of interest, selective activation of supraspinal structures and resultant neurotransmitter release may be linked to a particular frequency of EA. For instance, the analgesic effect from EA at 4 Hz was mediated through endogenous opioids, while the analgesic effect from EA at 2 Hz may involve substance P as its mediator.

Clinical Data

Although acupuncture has become popular among patients and medical professionals, controversy remains over its application and overall efficacy. The challenges in acupuncture studies are related to several unique issues such as placebo control, crossover design, and individualization. Nonetheless, it is encouraging to see that an increasing number of controlled, randomized clinical studies of acupuncture have replaced anecdotal case reports regarding the role of acupuncture in clinical pain management.

Low Back Pain

Chronic low back pain is one of the most common health problems associated with high medical expenses and disability. Of more than $90 billion annual healthcare expenses, approximately $26 billion may be directly attributable to the treatment of back pain. Although there are many medical or interventional treatment options, few have a long-term therapeutic effect without side effects. Thus, CAM becomes an option for many patients who suffer from low back pain. In 1993, a national survey revealed that low back pain (36%) is on the top of a list of medical conditions requiring CAM therapy. Recently, acupuncture has become one of the most frequently used CAM therapies for the treatment of low back pain. In a large study involving 1162 patients with chronic low back pain, acupuncture therapy was shown to improve low back pain for at least 6 months. The effectiveness of acupuncture, either real (47.6%) or sham (44.2%) needle, was almost twice than that of conventional therapy (27.4%) [41]. In another large-scale clinical trial, 3093 patients with chronic low back pain were randomly assigned into two groups: acupuncture and conventional medical care. Back function (Hannover Functional Ability Questionnaire), pain, and quality of life were assessed at the baseline, 3 and 6 months. In addition, the cost-effectiveness was also analyzed. The results showed that acupuncture plus routine care was associated with a marked clinical improvement as compared to conventional medical care in these patients and was relatively cost-effective.

The clinical practice guideline from the American College of Physicians and the American Pain Society recommends physicians to consider acupuncture as an addition to non-pharmacologic therapy for low back pain management. In addition, the duration of acupuncture in a single session appeared to be an independent parameter to the treatment outcome. For example, a 30-min acupuncture session was more effective than a 15-min session although a 45-min session did not further improve the outcome [38]. Similar finding was also found in electrical acupuncture stimulation. A 30- or 45-min treatment duration results in similar improvements in the visual analog pain scale, physical activity, quality of sleep scores, and a reduction in the oral analgesic requirements, which is better than 0 (no treatment) or 15-min duration. Of interest to note is that both acupuncture and transcutaneous electrical stimulation (TENS) showed significant effects on pain reduction, although acupuncture appeared to be more effective than TENS in the improvement of lumbar spine range of motion. Acupuncture not only improved back pain intensity but also showed superior effects than conventional medication and physical therapy regarding pain-related disability, quality of sleep, returning to work, and reduced use of analgesics. When compared with sham acupuncture, acupuncture was also superior in the reduction of psychological stress.

Chronic Neck and Shoulder Pain

There are promising results on the treatment of chronic neck and shoulder pain using acupuncture. For neck pain from cervical spondylosis, one study enrolled 106 subjects and randomly divided these subjects into real acupuncture group and control sham acupuncture group. The effective rate was 75.5% in the acupuncture group and 52.8% in the control group ($P < 0.05$). Several other clinical trials of acupuncture on chronic neck pain with sample sizes from 115 to 177 patients also have positive results. These studies demonstrated that acupuncture was superior to controls in reducing neck pain and improving the overall range of motion. In one study, the acupuncture treatment reduced chronic pain in neck and shoulders for at least 3 years with a concomitant improvement in depression, anxiety, sleep quality, pain-related activity impairment, and quality of life. Moreover, in patients with balance disorders caused by cervical torsion after whiplash injuries, acupuncture was effective in reducing their symptoms. If combined with physical therapy, the combination therapy was superior to acupuncture or physical therapy alone in pain reduction and functionality. Beside physical therapy, chronic myofascial neck pain has been frequently treated with trigger point injection either with local anesthetics or using dry needling technique. One prospective, randomized, double-blind, sham-controlled crossover study compared acupuncture, sham acupuncture, and dry needling of local myofascial trigger points in patients with chronic neck pain and limited cervical spine function. Acupuncture showed better results in reducing motion-related pain and improving range of motion. To investigate the effectiveness of acupuncture in addition to routine care as compared to routine care alone in patients with chronic neck pain, a randomized controlled multicenter trial with a total of 14,161 patients with chronic neck pain (duration >6 months) was randomized to an acupuncture group (1880 subjects, 15 acupuncture sessions over 3 months) or a control group receiving no acupuncture (1886 subjects). The results showed a significant improvement in neck pain and disability in the acupuncture group ($P < 0.001$). This large-scale clinic trial demonstrates that integrating acupuncture with routine medical care in patients with chronic neck pain may result in both pain improvement and a reduction of disability.

The cost-effectiveness of acupuncture in treatment of neck pain was analyzed in two meta-analysis studies with 10–14 clinical trials included. There was moderate evidence that acupuncture was more effective for pain relief than sham controls. Overall, the short-term effectiveness and efficacy of acupuncture in the treatment of neck pain appear to be present. However, the cost-effectiveness of additional acupuncture treatment in patients with chronic neck pain as compared to patients receiving routine care alone remains to be determined. More interestingly, in another study with a total of 3451 patients (1753 acupuncture group, 1698 control group), acupuncture treatment was associated with higher costs over the first 3-month duration as compared to routine care. Beyond the 3-month study duration, acupuncture might be associated with further health economic effects. According to international cost-effectiveness threshold values, this study concludes that acupuncture is a cost-effective treatment strategy in patients with chronic neck pain.

Headache

Although new medications, such as selective serotonin receptor agonist sumatriptan, have reduced migraine symptoms in many patients, there are patients who are refractory to such treatment. Alternatively, acupuncture has become a new modality of treatment for those patients with tension headache, migraine, or other types of headaches. In a randomized multicenter study with 302 patients suffering from migraine headache, acupuncture has shown significant therapeutic effects. As a prophylactic measure of migraine without aura, acupuncture treatment for 2–4 months can significantly reduce the number of migraine attacks compared to oral therapy with flunarizine. For many patients, acupuncture not only has a similar, if not better, efficacy as compared with sumatriptan in preventing full migraine attack; acupuncture has unique benefits over sumatriptan-related medications because of its negligible side effects. In a systematic review of 22 trials of 4419 participants, there is consistent evidence that acupuncture provides additional benefit to treatment of acute migraine attacks as compared to routine care only. Many other studies of acupuncture either for tension headache or migraine headache, with a sample size from 50 to 2022 patients, also showed similar results. Another review for chronic tension headache, including 11 trials with 2317 participants, found that acupuncture has statistically significant and clinically relevant short-term (up to 3 months) benefits over control in terms of the number of headache days and pain intensity. Thus acupuncture could be a valuable non-pharmacological tool in patients with frequent episodic or chronic tension-type headaches. Interestingly, the pediatric patient population also benefits from this alternative therapy for headache treatment.

Despite the differences between traditional Chinese medicine and western medicine, the recent Cochrane systematic reviews suggest that acupuncture is an effective and valuable option for patients suffering from migraine or frequent TTH. Moreover, acupuncture seems to be a cost-effective treatment according to international values. There are fewer adverse effects associated with this therapy compared with many standard drug treatment regimes used for headache management.

Other Pain Conditions

Acupuncture has been used to treat many other pain conditions such as postoperative pain or labor pain. Several studies have shown that patients who received acupuncture prior to operation not only had a lower pain level and reduced opioid requirement but also had a lower incidence of postoperative nausea and vomiting and lower sympathoadrenal responses. In a study of acupuncture treatment for labor pain, parturients who received acupuncture during labor significantly reduced the requirement of epidural analgesia with a better degree of relaxation. There was no acupuncture-associated negative effect on labor and delivery as compared with a control group. Osteoarthritis of the knee is another common chronic pain condition that acupuncture can provide some improvement in function and pain relief when compared with sham acupuncture or control groups using education. In addition, the benefit of acupuncture treatment in fibromyalgia and rheumatoid arthritis is supported by several clinical trials. Similarly, chronic lateral epicondylitis (tennis elbow) may benefit from the acupuncture treatment in part due to the effect of acupuncture on the range of motion and reduction in pain on exertion. In some cases, the effects on tennis elbow lasted up to 1 year after ten sessions of acupuncture.

Other Uses of Acupuncture

Besides its analgesic effects, acupuncture has been used for the treatment of many other conditions. For example, a number of clinical trials strongly support a therapeutic role of acupuncture (either needle acupuncture or applying acupressure to the relevant acupoints) in postoperative nausea and vomiting as compared with antiemetics such as droperidol and Zofran. Many cancer patients have used acupuncture for cancer-related fatigue, malaise, and chemotherapy-induced nausea and vomiting. An increasing number of patients are turning to acupuncture either to supplement or replace their conventional treatments for many medical conditions including allergy, asthma, depression, anxiety, obesity, insomnia, premenstrual syndrome, menopause symptoms, assisted conception and infertility, spinal cord injury, smoking cessation, and detoxification from opioids or other drug addiction.

Possible Complications of Acupuncture

NIH consensus panel on acupuncture in 1997 has stated that the documented occurrence of adverse events in practice of acupuncture has been extremely low. The most commonly reported complication is bruising or bleeding at the needle insertion site, followed by the incidence of a transient vasovagal response. Other rare complications include infection, dermatitis, and broken needle fragments. In one prospective large-scale survey with 34,407 acupuncture treatments, no serious adverse events were reported that required hospital admission, prolonged hospital stays, permanently disabling, or death. A total of 43 minor adverse events were reported (0.13%), including severe nausea and actual fainting; unexpected, severe, and prolonged aggravation of symptoms; prolonged and unacceptable pain and bruising; and psychological and emotional reactions. Another survey with a total of 31,822 acupuncture treatments also found only 43 minor adverse events, a rate of 14 per 10,000 treatments (0.14%). Other minor adverse events can be avoided such as patients being left unattended, needles being left in patients, cellulites, and moxa burns. Overall, acupuncture has significantly lower complication rate comparing with many other medical treatments and is a relatively safe treatment modality. However, since acupuncture is an invasive medical intervention, serious complications such as pneumothorax, hemathorax, internal organ puncture, and pericardial effusion could happen if the treatment is not properly administered. Some of these more serious complications generally occur in elderly and more fragile and debilitated patients with complex comorbidities or in the hands of less skilled practitioners. Thus, it is imperative that the acupuncture licensing and regulation mandate the use of standards of acupuncture training through adopting strict requirement for the knowledge of anatomy and sterile techniques.

Perspectives and Future Directions

Alone with the popularity of the CAM and acupuncture in recent years, an increasing number of physicians have combined integrative medicine into their practices. Recommendations for patient who is seeking for physician's opinion about CAM therapy include: first, it is important to know the scientific evidence and effectiveness of CAM therapy that patient is interested. Much information can be found at the National Center for Complementary and Alternative Medicine (NCCAM) and the US Food and Drug Administration (FDA) website. The patient should keep in mind that each individuals may respond differently to treatments, and many factors may contribute to the difference in response, including the person's health condition, comorbidities, application of the therapy, as well as the person's belief in the therapy. Second, safety of the CAM therapy is equally important if not more. A product that is "natural" does not mean it is "safe." Thus, patients should have an in-depth discussion about their medical condition with CAM therapist. Information about particular CAM therapy's benefits and the risks, side effects, and interaction with patient current medical treatment should be covered during the discussion. Third, when choosing a CAM practitioner, one should consider factors such as training background, skill and experience, and licensing. Fourth, whether the therapy will be covered by health insurance is an imperative issue for patient to consider too.

To face the aging population and ever-growing healthcare cost in the United States, more health insurance providers have begun to emphasize preventive and alternative measures. Many CAM therapies may offer good efficacy, safety, and cost-effectiveness, and it is a useful adjunct to conventional treatment to allow us to reach the goal of maintaining health, reducing costs, and improving patient satisfaction.

Reference

1. Barnes PM, Bloom B, Nahin R. CDC National Health Statistics Report #12. Complementary and Alternative Medicine Use Among Adults and Children: United States, 2007. December 10, 2008.

Suggested Reading

1. Berman BM, Langevin HM, Witt CM, Dubner R. Acupuncture for chronic low back pain. N Engl J Med. 2010;363(5):454–61. https://doi.org/10.1056/NEJMct0806114.
2. Eisenberg DM, Davis RB, Ettner SL, et al. Trends in alternative medicine use in the united states, 1990–1997: results of a follow-up national survey. JAMA. 1998;280(18):1569–75.
3. Eisenberg DM, Kessler DC, Foster C, et al. Unconventional medicine in the United States. Prevalence, costs, and patterns of use. N Engl J Med. 1993;328(4):246–52.
4. http://www.mayoclinic.com/health/alternative-medicine.
5. http://en.wikipedia.org/wiki/National. Center for Complementary and Alternative Medicine.
6. Melchart D, Weidenhammer W, Streng A, et al. Prospective investigation of adverse effects of acupuncture in 97,733 patients. Arch Intern Med. 2004;164(1):104–5.
7. National Health statistic report number 18, July 30 2009.
8. nccam.nih.gov/health/whatiscam.
9. NIH consensus conference. Acupuncture. JAMA. 1998;280(17):1518–24.
10. Ulett GA, Han S, Han JS. Electroacupuncture: mechanisms and clinical application. Biol Psychiatry. 1998;44(2):129–38.
11. White A, Hayhoe S, Hart A, Ernst E. BMAS and AACP. British medical acupuncture society and acupuncture Association of Chartered Physiotherapists. Survey of adverse events following acupuncture (SAFA): a prospective study of 32,000 consultations. Acupunct Med. 2001;19(2):84–92.
12. WHO. Acupuncture review and analysis of report on controlled clinical trials. 2002. www.who.int.
13. Zhao ZQ. Neural mechanism underlying acupuncture analgesia. Prog Neurobiol. 2008;85(4):355–75.

12 Palliative Care

Chirag A. Patel and Mellar P. Davis

Key Concepts

- Palliative care is an interdisciplinary care model which addresses physical, emotional, spiritual, functional, and social causes of suffering in patients and families. Palliative care also supports good communication between medical providers and patients/families to assess and focus on achieving the patient's goals of care.
- Palliative care is available to patients/families through all stages of illness and in a variety of health-care settings.
- Patients with life-limiting illnesses from both cancer and noncancer diagnoses commonly experience pain and multiple other bothersome symptoms which affect quality of life.
- The framework of "total pain," which involves physical, psychological, spiritual, and social components of pain, can help guide a more complete assessment of pain in the palliative care patient.
- An interdisciplinary health-care team can help address nonphysical contributors to "total pain."
- Non-opioid analgesics including acetaminophen and nonsteroidal anti-inflammatory drugs (NSAIDs) and adjuvant medications including antidepressants, antiepileptics, and steroids can be useful in addressing pain in the palliative care patient.
- Opioids are commonly used for moderate to severe pain for the palliative care patient. Pain characteristics, administration route limitations, adverse side effects, tolerance, organ failure, variable analgesic response, and medication accessibility are factors to be considered when prescribing and adjusting opioids.

What Is Palliative Care?

The National Consensus Project for Quality Palliative Care (NCP) defines palliative care by stating: "Palliative care means patient and family centered care that optimizes quality of life by anticipating, preventing, and treating suffering. Palliative care throughout the continuum of illness involves addressing physical, intellectual, emotional, social, and spiritual needs and facilitates patient autonomy, access to information, and choice" [1].

The NCP defines key features of the palliative care philosophy to include:

- Interdisciplinary team care coordination
- Communication of care needs between health-care providers and patients/families
- Continuation of services both during and after life-prolonging care
- Family/patient support during the course of the illness, the dying process, and following death [1]

C.A. Patel, MD (✉) • M.P. Davis, MD
Taussig Cancer Institute, Cleveland Clinic,
9500 Euclid Ave/CA-5, Cleveland, OH 44195, USA
e-mail: patelc@ccf.org; mdavis2@geisinger.edu

J. Cheng, R.W. Rosenquist (eds.), *Fundamentals of Pain Medicine*,
https://doi.org/10.1007/978-3-319-64922-1_12

The interdisciplinary team of palliative care can include physicians, mid-level providers, nurses, social workers, case managers, rehabilitation personnel, spiritual providers, and music therapists.

Goals of this interdisciplinary team include addressing:

- Physical symptoms (pain, nausea, dyspnea, delirium, constipation, anorexia, etc.)
- Functional deficits (loss of independence, fatigue, weakness, etc.)
- Psychosocial and spiritual distress (depression, anxiety, existential suffering, caregiver burnout, etc.)
- Advanced care planning issues (establishing goals of care, communicating bad news, discussing withdrawing treatment, etc.)

The terms "hospice care" and "palliative care" are often confused and interchanged inappropriately. Hospice care refers specifically to a subset of palliative care provided to patients during the last months of life through a Medicare benefit.

Palliative care and hospice services can be delivered in multiple forms and settings including:

- Outpatient clinics
- Visits to the patient's place of residence (home, nursing home, etc.)
- Consultations within medical facilities (hospitals, nursing homes, long-term acute care facilities)
- Primary service inpatient care in a palliative medicine unit or hospice unit

Pain in Palliative Care Patients

In patients with advanced illnesses, pain is highly prevalent. The SUPPORT study found that the prevalence of pain in colon cancer patients increased from >25% at 6 months prior to death to >40% at 3 days prior to death [2]. Other studies on advanced cancer patients indicate pain prevalences ranging from about 30 to 90% [3]. In patients with end-stage congestive heart failure, about 75% of patients experience pain [4]. The SUPPORT investigation also found that serious pain was reported by a quarter of COPD patients and one-third of end-stage liver disease patients in the last 6 months of life [5, 6].

In addition to pain, palliative care patients suffer from a wide array of other symptoms. Symptom distress scores in advanced illness patients are similar for cancer and noncancer illnesses. Patients with cancer, AIDS, heart disease, respiratory disease, and renal disease suffer from fatigue, dyspnea, and pain with prevalences above 50% [7]. Other symptoms including depression, anxiety, confusion, nausea, and constipation are also quite common in end-stage diseases. In the palliative care population, depression, anxiety, number of chronic illnesses experienced, social support, and loss of functional ability affect perception and experience of pain [8].

Despite its high prevalence, pain control at the end of life is often suboptimal. Pain at end of life remains either untreated or undertreated very often; about one-third of hospitalized end-of-life patients have severe or significant pain at time of death or discharge to hospice [9]. Some of the challenges with pain control specific to palliative care and hospice patients are listed in Table 12.1. Most pain can be controlled using the World Health Organization's pain relief ladder.

Assessment

Pain assessment has been pushed to the forefront of patient care since the introduction of pain as the "fifth vital sign" in 1996 and the publication of the first clinical guidelines in 1992. The Veterans Administration and Joint Commission on the Accreditation of Hospital Organizations made pain evaluation a top priority shortly thereafter [10]. These steps helped to underscore the need for frequent, proactive monitoring of pain in all patients.

Pain in the palliative care population can be largely physical, or it can involve significant psychosocial or spiritual components. Pain in the palliative care patient population should be

Table 12.1 Challenges with pain control specific to palliative care and hospice patients

Health-care professionals	Lack of pain management training/education	Poor assessment of pain
		Under treatment of pain
	Controlled substance regulations	Use of drug in a lower schedule
		Limiting the number of refills
		Reduced drug dose or quantity
	Worries of adverse effects	Fear of addiction
		Fear of tolerance
Patients	Reluctance in reporting pain	Wanting to be a "good" patient
		Worrying about distracting the treating physician from the primary disease
		Fear that increased pain indicates worsening disease
	Worries of adverse effects	Fear of addiction or being perceived as an addict
		Fear of tolerance or that early pain treatment will preclude effective later pain treatment
		Concerns about side effects such as nausea, confusion, and constipation
	Accessibility of medications	Availability of opioids at a local pharmacies
		Cost of medications

assessed within the framework of "total pain." "Total pain" refers to the multidimensional nature of pain which includes physical, psychological, spiritual, and social aspects of pain. In addition to pain, other concurrent symptoms may contribute to a patient's overall suffering and therefore should be explored and treated.

When assessing the physical component of pain, using a standard assessment scheme can help one avoid overlooking components of importance. The "PQRST" assessment involves asking about:

- Provoking/palliating factors.
- Quality: may help point to a neuropathic, somatic, visceral, or mixed pain etiology.
- Radiation/region.
- Severity: measured using a validated, reproducible scale such as the numeric rating scale or the visual analogue scale. The same scale should be used consistently for each patient, so changes due to treatments can be monitored [11].
- Temporal course: constant versus intermittent; if intermittent, incidental or spontaneous.

Prior use of pain medications, side effects of these medications, and relief of pain with the medications should also be assessed. A patient's prior experiences with pain medications or knowledge of acquaintances who have used pain medications either legally or illicitly can shape compliance to a prescribed treatment plan. In an interview of almost 1000 terminally ill patients, half of patients with moderate to severe pain did not want to change their pain medications, despite their high pain severity rating. In this study, frequently cited reasons for not wanting to change medications included fears of side effects and addiction [12].

Periodic reassessment of the patient's pain control is vital to maintaining adequate analgesia. Pain that worsens after a period of stability can indicate disease progression, tolerance, hyperalgesia from opioid-induced neurotoxicity, increased activity levels, or psychological/spiritual distress.

Cognitive impairment due to delirium can make evaluation of pain more complicated in palliative care and end-of-life patients. Cognitive impairment should be screened for proactively early in the course of an interview with the patient due to the high prevalence of delirium in the palliative care population. Screening methods include the use of the Bedside Confusion Scale, Confusion Assessment Method, or Memorial Delirium Assessment Scale. Patients with mild or moderate cognitive impairment can usually quantify pain severity [13]. If severe cognitive impairment exists, pain can be assessed through the use of nonverbal signs such as grimacing and furrowing of the eyebrows, moaning or groaning, restlessness or combativeness, or changes in activity level [11]. Caregiver assessments are often used in patients with severe cognitive impairment and can be helpful in alerting a clinician to the presence and severity of pain; but clinicians should also use nonverbal cues and treatment trials to assess/treat pain. Heart rate and respiratory rate alterations are poor indicators of chronic pain.

Coexisting symptoms in the palliative care and end-of-life population frequently cause a higher level of distress. Proactive assessment and treatment of these symptoms in addition to pain treatment is crucial in minimizing suffering in patients. In a study of 1000 hospitalized palliative care patients with cancer, the median number of distressing symptoms per patient was 11 [14]. Using a standard symptom screening tool during assessment of a patient will minimize "missed" symptoms. Some commonly used symptom screening scales which take into account physical and nonphysical contributors to suffering include the Edmonton Symptom Assessment Scale, the Palliative Care Outcome Scale, and the Memorial Symptom Assessment Scale.

Obtaining a psychosocial and spiritual history using single-item questions or brief question sets such as the hospital anxiety and depression scale, FICA, or HOPE can help screen for other contributors to "total pain" [15].

Treatment

Treatment of "total pain" within the palliative care population requires simultaneous attention to the multiple factors that can influence the experience of suffering in addition to physical pain.

Psychological, spiritual, and social aspects of total pain benefit from interdisciplinary collaboration between physicians, psychologists, spiritual care services, social workers, and other members of an interdisciplinary health-care team. Cognitive behavioral therapy interventions, which may incorporate relaxation training, controlled breathing, biofeedback, progressive muscle relaxation, imagery, symptom reappraisal, coping strategies, and problem-solving strategies, can produce significant changes in pain experiences, pain behaviors, and social functioning for chronic pain patients [16]. Supportive-expressive group psychotherapy, meaning-centered group psychotherapy, and therapies which address demoralization may also be helpful for patients with advanced illnesses [17].

Treatment of physical pain includes both pharmacologic and non-pharmacologic measures. Pharmacologic options include both non-opioids and opioids as indicated in the WHO ladder. Non-opioids can help minimize the need for higher doses of opioids to control pain but also may result in polypharmacy. Non-pharmacologic measures to address physical pain include cancer-directed therapy, nerve blocks, and neurosurgical techniques.

Pharmacologic Therapy

Non-opioids

Commonly used non-opioid analgesics include NSAIDs and acetaminophen. Both may be useful in relief of mild pain, and NSAIDS especially might be useful in reducing the dose of opioids used for moderate to severe pain [18]. Acetaminophen is appropriate for patients with mild pain from musculoskeletal causes such as osteoarthritis. Its use should be avoided or reduced in patients with liver failure. Use of NSAIDs is especially beneficial for bone pain or inflammatory pain. Caution must be exercised when using NSAIDs in terminally ill patients due to adverse effects including gastrointestinal ulcers/bleeding, coagulations abnormalities, and renal insufficiency. Appropriate dosage for acetaminophen and NSAIDs is determined by patient response and maximum medication dose (while also taking into account comorbidities). If pain relief is not obtained with the maximum dose of one NSAID, switching to a different NSAID may still be of benefit. Acetaminophen and NSAIDs can be given orally or rectally. Ketorolac and acetaminophen are available parenterally also.

Adjuvant pain medications are medications whose primary indication is not analgesia, but have analgesic properties in specific painful conditions. Examples of adjuvants include antidepressants, antiepileptics, steroids, bisphosphonates, N-methyl-D-aspartate (NMDA) receptor antagonists, and muscle relaxants. Anti-inflammatory medications are especially useful in management of pain from bone metastasis, nerve compression, and capsular distension, whereas antidepressants and antiepileptics are particularly useful in management of neuropathic pain states. A recent systematic review found that benefits of antidepressants, anticonvulsants, and other adjuvant analgesics outweighed adverse effects in patients with neuropathic cancer pain [19].

Opioids

Opioids are commonly used in the palliative care population due to their lack of ceiling effect, efficacy in treating moderate to severe pain, and lack of renal and hepatic toxicity. Commonly used opioids in palliative care patients include morphine, hydromorphone, oxycodone, fentanyl, methadone, and buprenorphine.

When beginning an opioid in an opioid-naïve patient, one can start with an intermittent dose every 2–3 h as needed equivalent to 5–10 mg of oral morphine. Fixed schedule or extended-release opioids can be started if frequent dosing is required and/or the pain is continuous in nature. Transdermal fentanyl is not recommended for acute or unstable pain. Around-the-clock dosing can be achieved by using an extended-release formulation, using an immediate-release formulation on a scheduled basis, or using a continuous intravenous (IV) or subcutaneous (SC) infusion. Due to variability of pain severity, a breakthrough dose equal to approximately 10–25% of the daily dose of the scheduled opioid should be made available intermittently. The use of IV or SC patient-controlled analgesia (PCA) is an option that can deliver both a continuous opioid infusion and an intermittent breakthrough dose, but PCA use should be avoided in patients with cognitive impairment (dementia and/or delirium).

If the patient is already on continuous and breakthrough opioids but continues to experience pain, calculate the patient's total opioid use over the past 24 h and determine if the patient is having adverse side effects from the current opioid. If no significant side effects are present, increase the existing opioid dose by either 25–50% of the total daily opioid dose or by the total breakthrough opioids amount used in the past 24 h. Then, either recalculate the breakthrough opioid's dose as equal to 10–25% of the new scheduled dose or titrate it based on efficacy and tolerance of the prior breakthrough opioid dose. If significant side effects are present, opioid rotation or dose reduction is indicated.

Opioid rotation may be required for improvement in the balance between analgesia and side effects [20]. First calculate the total dose used over the prior 24 h. Then, use an equianalgesic table to convert the prior opiate to the 24-h dose of the new opiate. Usually, a decrease in the calculated new opioid dose by 25–50% is performed to account for incomplete cross-tolerance between opioids. Divide the 24-h dose of the new opiate by the number of doses to be given per day and give it on a scheduled basis. Be sure and also order a breakthrough pain dose of 10–25% of the 24-h dose to be given every 2–4 h as needed.

In patients with life-threatening illnesses, it is especially important to note renal and hepatic function changes and to use opioids that will not be affected by the patient's end-organ failure.

Opioid and/or active metabolite accumulation due to organ failure can lead to accentuated analgesic and/or neurotoxic effects. In patients with renal failure, fentanyl, buprenorphine, and methadone are considered relatively safe, and other opioids should be used cautiously [21]. Most opioids undergo some liver metabolism: either oxidation/reduction via the cytochrome P450 enzymes or conjugation/glucuronidation. Hepatic failure can lead to reduced hepatic blood flow and decreased cytochrome P450 enzyme levels, but glucuronidation is less affected. As a result, opioids which are metabolized through glucuronidation are preferred if liver failure is present. In patients with severe liver disease, opioid dosing intervals may need to be longer, and initial doses may need to be reduced; doses can then be titrated based on patient response and tolerance.

Multiple administration routes may need to be considered for palliative care patients. The oral route is the least invasive and is generally preferred due to convenience and cost. Most oral opiates are available in extended-release formulations also. Onset of pain relief usually occurs between 20 and 30 min, with a peak effect at around 1 h. Feeding tubes can accommodate liquid or crushed immediate-release opiates. Most extended-release formulations though cannot be crushed; but liquid (or crushed) methadone or long-acting polymeric morphine beads can be used as long-acting opiates through a feeding tube. Fentanyl and buprenorphine are available as transdermal patches. A lag time of about one-half to three-fourths of a day occurs when a patch is applied or a patch dose is changed. Similarly, the half-life after patch removal is about ½–1 day. Intravenous and subcutaneous routes are also options for morphine, hydromorphone, methadone, fentanyl, and buprenorphine (but not oxycodone in the USA). Medications can be given continuously and/or intermittently. Most extended and immediate release or formulations of opioids can also be absorbed rectally, although morphine and hydromorphone are available in specific rectal formulations [20]. Sublingual or transmucosal administration of opioids is also an option for patients who are unable to swallow and lack parenteral access. Lipophilic medications such as methadone, fentanyl, and buprenorphine are better absorbed sublingually than hydrophilic opioids such as morphine, hydromorphone, and oxycodone. The neuraxial route refers to medication administration at the epidural or intrathecal level. Neuraxial opioids may be an option for refractory pain and/or intolerable side effects. Opioids which can be delivered neuraxially include morphine, diamorphine, hydromorphone, fentanyl, sufentanil, and methadone.

Morphine is widely used and considered to be the first-line opioid for palliative care patients. Its use provides flexibility with dosing (extended- and immediate-release oral formulations are available) and route. Morphine is glucuronidated in the liver to morphine-3-glucuronide (M3G) and morphine-6-glucuronide and eliminated via the kidneys. M3G accumulation can lead to neurotoxicity symptoms such as delirium, myoclonus, and hyperalgesia. Therefore, dosing and frequency must be altered in patients who have renal failure; and its use in patients with fluctuating renal function is not recommended.

Oxycodone is semisynthetic and interacts with both mu and kappa opioid receptors. Oral dosing is similar to that of morphine, with long-acting and short-acting tablets available. Hydromorphone is glucuronidated like morphine, and metabolite accumulation can also lead to neurotoxic side effects. It is five to six times more potent parenterally than morphine. Fentanyl is a synthetic opioid 100 times more potent than morphine. Methadone is inexpensive and has NMDA receptor inhibitor activity. Its potency compared to other opioids varies markedly depending on the patient's current opioid dose, it has multiple drug interactions due to its metabolism via the cytochrome P450 system, and it has relatively complicated pharmacokinetics [22]. Therefore, methadone should only be prescribed by clinicians familiar with its use.

Individuals can be quite variable with respect to analgesic and adverse effects of the different opioids. Dose-limiting side effects may include hallucinations, vivid nightmares, dysphoria, nausea, or cognitive impairment. Therefore, the treating physician must be familiar with multiple opioids and their relative potencies.

Patients and caregivers should be educated about common opioid side effects such as constipation, nausea, drowsiness, and neurotoxicities when opioids are prescribed. Constipation requires a proactive management plan usually involving scheduled laxative use. Both nausea and drowsiness usually resolve after a few days. If they persist, reviewing other potential contributors and treating them appropriately may be of benefit. Other options to address nausea and drowsiness include the use of antiemetics and psychostimulants, respectively, or changing to another opioid [21]. Signs of opioid-induced neurotoxicity include excessive sedation, confusion, delirium, myoclonus, and hyperalgesia. Palliative care patients should be closely monitored for neurotoxicity signs due to concomitant use of multiple psychoactive medications, dehydration, and renal/hepatic impairments.

References

1. National Consensus Project for Quality Palliative Care Task Force M. Clinical Practice Guidelines for Quality Palliative Care 2013 April 15, 2013.
2. McCarthy EP, Phillips RS, Zhong Z, Drews RE, Lynn J. Dying with cancer: patients' function, symptoms, and care preferences as death approaches. J Am Geriatr Soc. 2000;48(5 Suppl):S110–21. PubMed PMID: 10809464.
3. van den Beuken-van Everdingen MH, de Rijke JM, Kessels AG, Schouten HC, van Kleef M, Patijn J. Prevalence of pain in patients with cancer: a systematic review of the past 40 years. Ann Oncol Off J Eur Soc Med Oncol/ESMO. 2007;18(9):1437–49. PubMed PMID: 17355955.
4. Nordgren L, Sorensen S. Symptoms experienced in the last six months of life in patients with end-stage heart failure. Eur J Cardiovasc Nurs/J Work Group Cardiovasc Nurs Eur Soc Cardiol. 2003;2(3):213–7. PubMed PMID: 14622629.
5. Lynn J, Ely EW, Zhong Z, McNiff KL, Dawson NV, Connors A, et al. Living and dying with chronic obstructive pulmonary disease. J Am Geriatr Soc. 2000;48(5 Suppl):S91–100. PubMed PMID: 10809462.
6. Roth K, Lynn J, Zhong Z, Borum M, Dawson NV. Dying with end stage liver disease with cirrhosis: insights from SUPPORT. Study to understand prognoses and preferences for outcomes and risks of treatment. J Am Geriatr Soc. 2000;48(5 Suppl):S122–30. PubMed PMID: 10809465.
7. Solano JP, Gomes B, Higginson IJ. A comparison of symptom prevalence in far advanced cancer, AIDS, heart disease, chronic obstructive pulmonary disease and renal disease. J Pain Symptom Manag. 2006;31(1):58–69. PubMed PMID: 16442483.
8. Lin JI, Wang JJ, Chiu HJ, Lee CY, Cheng SF. Chronic pain and associated factors amongst institutionalized elderly with arthritis. Hu li za zhi J Nurs. 2011;58(1):59–67. PubMed PMID: 21328206.
9. Yao Y, Keenan G, Al-Masalha F, Lopez KD, Khokar A, Johnson A, et al. Current state of pain care for hospitalized patients at end of life. Am J Hosp Palliat Care. 2013;30(2):128–36. PubMed PMID: 22556281. Pubmed Central PMCID: 3681818.
10. National Pharmaceutical Council Inc. In: Council NP, editor. Pain: current understanding of assessment, management, and treatments. Reston: National Pharmaceutical Council; 2001.
11. Persons AGSPoPPiO. The management of persistent pain in older persons. J Am Geriatr Soc. 2002;50(6 Suppl):S205–24. PubMed PMID: 12067390.
12. Weiss SC, Emanuel LL, Fairclough DL, Emanuel EJ. Understanding the experience of pain in terminally ill patients. Lancet. 2001;357(9265):1311–5. PubMed PMID: 11343734.
13. Closs SJ, Barr B, Briggs M, Cash K, Seers K. A comparison of five pain assessment scales for nursing home residents with varying degrees of cognitive impairment. J Pain Symptom Manag. 2004;27(3):196–205. PubMed PMID: 15010098.
14. Walsh D, Donnelly S, Rybicki L. The symptoms of advanced cancer: relationship to age, gender, and performance status in 1,000 patients. Support Care Cancer. 2000;8(3):175–9. PubMed PMID: 10789956.
15. Walsh D. Palliative medicine. Philadelphia: Saunders/Elsevier; 2009. xl, 1475 p.
16. Morley S, Eccleston C, Williams A. Systematic review and meta-analysis of randomized controlled trials of cognitive behaviour therapy and behaviour therapy for chronic pain in adults, excluding headache. Pain. 1999;80(1–2):1–13. PubMed PMID: 10204712.
17. Breitbart W. Spirituality and meaning in supportive care: spirituality- and meaning-centered group psychotherapy interventions in advanced cancer. Support Care Cancer. 2002;10(4):272–80. PubMed PMID: 12029426.
18. Nabal M, Librada S, Redondo MJ, Pigni A, Brunelli C, Caraceni A. The role of paracetamol and nonsteroidal anti-inflammatory drugs in addition to WHO step III opioids in the control of pain in advanced cancer. A systematic review of the literature. Palliat Med. 2012;26(4):305–12. PubMed PMID: 22126843.
19. Jongen JL, Huijsman ML, Jessurun J, Ogenio K, Schipper D, Verkouteren DR, et al. The evidence for pharmacologic treatment of neuropathic cancer pain: beneficial and adverse effects. J Pain Symptom

Manag. 2013;46(4):581–90. e1. PubMed PMID: 23415040.
20. Dalal S, Bruera E. Assessment and management of pain in the terminally ill. Prim Care. 2011;38(2):195–223. vii–viii. PubMed PMID: 21628035.
21. Caraceni A, Hanks G, Kaasa S, Bennett MI, Brunelli C, Cherny N, et al. Use of opioid analgesics in the treatment of cancer pain: evidence-based recommendations from the EAPC. Lancet Oncol. 2012;13(2):e58–68. PubMed PMID: 22300860.
22. Bruera E, Sweeney C. Methadone use in cancer patients with pain: a review. J Palliat Med. 2002;5(1):127–38. PubMed PMID: 11839235.

Suggested Reading

Dalal S, Bruera E. Assessment and management of pain in the terminally ill. Prim Care. 2011;38(2):195–223. vii–viii. PubMed PMID: 21628035.

Davis MP, Srivastava M. Demographics, assessment and management of pain in the elderly. Drugs Aging. 2003;20(1):23–57. PubMed PMID: 12513114.

Walsh D. Palliative medicine. Philadelphia: Saunders/Elsevier; 2009. xl, 1475 p.

Part III

Painful Disease States: Acute Pain

Surgical Pain 13

Ehab Farag, Maria Yared, Wael Ali Sakr Esa, Michael Ritchey, and Loran Mounir Soliman

Key Concepts

- Surgical pain is a complex and difficult problem to fully understand and consequently to manage. In addition to causing patient discomfort, it stimulates the sympathetic nervous system, increases myocardial oxygen demand, delays mobilization, impairs the immune system, and may potentially lead to chronic pain.
- Ineffective management of postoperative surgical pain may increase the risk of developing chronic postoperative surgical pain.
- The use of multimodal analgesia is the best way to manage postoperative pain as it decreases opioid side effects and provides better patient experiences.
- The use of regional analgesia either as single-dose peripheral nerve blocks or continuous peripheral nerve blocks should be utilized whenever possible as they have beneficial effects in improving the quality of postoperative pain management and reducing the incidence of chronic postsurgical pain development.

E. Farag, MD, FRCA (✉)
Cleveland Clinic Lerner College of Medicine, Departments of General Anesthesia and Outcomes Research, Cleveland Clinic, Cleveland, OH, USA
e-mail: FARAGE@ccf.org

M. Yared, MD
Anesthesiology Institute, Cleveland Clinic, Cleveland, OH, USA

W.A.S. Esa, MD, PhD
General Anesthesia and Pain Management, Cleveland Clinic, Cleveland, OH, USA

M. Ritchey, MD
Department of General Anesthesia, Cleveland Clinic, Cleveland, OH, USA

L.M. Soliman, MD
General Anesthesia and Critical Care & Comprehensive Pain Management, Cleveland Clinic, Cleveland, OH, USA

Surgical Pain Anatomy

The experience of pain is the product of a very integrated information-processing network. Nociceptive afferents are usually transmitted by nociceptors, which are specialized peripheral sensory neurons that respond to noxious stimuli. The nociceptors are free, unencapsulated peripheral nerve endings that are found in most tissues of the body including skin, deep somatic tissue, and viscera. C polymodal nociceptors are the most numerous types and respond to a wide range of mechanical, thermal, and chemical noxious stimuli. They are slowly conducting (<3 m/s) and are associated with prolonged burning pain. The more rapidly conducting Aδ fibers (5–30 m/s) are associated with a briefer sharp pain. They are myelinated and respond to mechanical and thermal stimuli. Approximately 15% of C-fibers are silent nociceptors and only become active after

J. Cheng, R.W. Rosenquist (eds.), *Fundamentals of Pain Medicine*,
https://doi.org/10.1007/978-3-319-64922-1_13

tissue injury or inflammation has occurred. After tissue trauma, they respond spontaneously or become sensitized to other sensory stimuli. C and Aδ fibers terminate in the lamina I (marginal zone) and lamina II (substantia gelatinosa) of the spinal gray matter. However, some Aδ fibers also terminate in lamina V which contains wide dynamic range (WDR) cells. Those cells receive input from a diverse range of neurons and have a large receptive field. Excitatory or inhibitory interneurons, which regulate the flow of nociceptive information, are located in laminae V and VI. The spinothalamic tact (STT) is considered the major pain pathway and originates from neurons in laminae V–VII and I. The majority of axons cross locally and ascend contralaterally. Lamina I cells project to the posterior part of the ventromedial nucleus of the thalamus and mediate the autonomic and unpleasant emotional perception of pain. Neurons in the deeper laminae project to the ventral posterolateral nucleus of the thalamus and carry the discriminative aspects of pain. The spinomesencephalic tract terminates in the periaqueductal gray (PAG), activating the descending inhibitory pain networks. The spinoparabrachial–amygdala system originates from lamina I neurons that express neurokinin-1 (NK1) receptors. It is involved in the emotional or affective components of pain (Fig. 13.1).

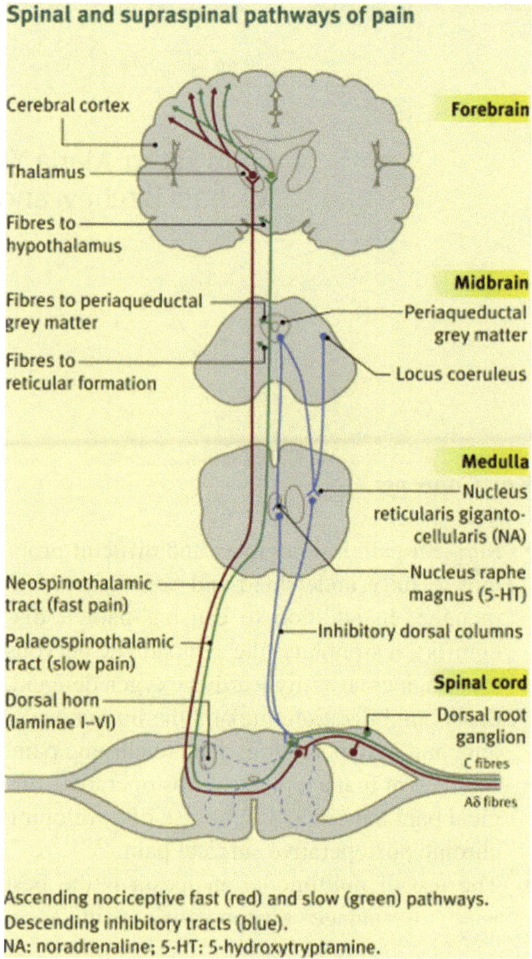

Fig. 13.1 Spinal and supraspinal pathways of pain (Reprinted from Steeds CE. The anatomy and physiology of pain. *Surgery*. 31(2):49–53, Copyright 2013, with permission from Elsevier)

The somatosensory cortex (SS) is located in the postcentral gyrus of the parietal lobe. It is an area that processes inputs related to the sensory system of touch, nociception, temperature, and proprioception. The SS are divided into SI and SII areas, both of them are linked to processing sensory discriminative aspects of pain. However, stimulation of SII results in the reduction of nociceptive behaviors of painful stimuli and the number of c-Fos-positive cells in the spinal horn and trigeminal dorsal horn in conscious rats.

The Role of Glutamate Receptors in Pain Transmission

At the central terminals of primary afferents (C and Aδ fibers), glutamate is the major transmitter that mediates rapid excitatory postsynaptic potentials in the dorsal horn neurons. In the presynaptic terminals, glutamate is taken up into synaptic vesicles in neurons by vesicular glutamate receptor transporters (VGLUTs). VGLUTs mediate the transport of glutamate from the cytoplasm into synaptic vesicles. There are three distinct isoforms of VGLUT 1–3 with similar transport characteristics but with a different pattern of expression in the primary sensory neurons. VGLUT2 is present mainly in lamina I, whereas VGLUT1 is present in deeper laminae. However, some fibers in (laminae III–IV) appeared to contain both transporters. The terminals of thinly myelinated Aδ fibers and unmyelinated C-fibers contain VGLUT2. In contrast, VGLUT3 is mainly present in nonvisceral dorsal root ganglia (DRG). Once glutamate is released, it acts on postsynaptic receptors of second-order neurons in the dorsal horn. There are three main classes of ligand-gated ionotropic glutamate receptors (iGLuRs) – the α-amino-3 hydroxy-5-methyl-4-isoxazolepropionoc acid receptor (AMPAR), the kainate receptor (KAR), and the N-methyl-$_{D-}$ aspartate receptor (NMDAR) – and three groups of the G-protein-coupled metabotropic glutamate receptors (mGluRs), which are involved in initiating and maintaining neuroplasticity. All synaptic transmissions from primary sensory afferents to second-order neurons are excitatory, involving iGluRs and mGluRs, at time scales from milliseconds to tens of seconds. Glutamate, released from primary afferents, binds to receptors localized on second-order neurons to produce fast excitatory postsynaptic potentials (fast EPSPs), mediated by AMPARs and KARs, on the scale of milliseconds.

The contribution of NMDARs during acute pain is limited since those receptors are down-regulated under normal conditions by Mg^{+2}, which blocks the channel pore. Therefore, the recruitment of NMDARs requires disinhibition of the Mg^{+2} block and receptor phosphorylation. Upon sustained, intense noxious stimuli, primary sensory afferents release glutamate along with peptide neuromodulators, such as substance P (SP) and calcitonin gene-related peptide (CGRP). Sustained release of peptides and glutamate results in activation of postsynaptic G-protein-coupled receptors (GPCR) including group I mGluRs. The activation of those receptors results in the inhibition of K^+ channel conductance, which leads to slow EPSPs lasting up to tens of seconds. The slow EPSPs help the temporal summation of fast EPSPs, and the combined depolarized effects of slow EPSPs and fast EPSPs result in the release of Mg^{2+} blockade from the NMDAR channel. The activated NMDARs then allow Ca^{+2} to enter the neurons. This rapid increase in intracellular Ca^{+2} is the initial trigger for activity-dependent plasticity. Of note, the activation of group I mGluRs causes the release of intracellular Ca^{+2} from the endoplasmic reticulum. This step appears to be critical for spreading the stimulation from active synapses to neighboring non-active synapses.

Another pathway involved in pain is the primary sensory afferents' group I mGluRs that are functionally coupled to transient receptor potential vanilloid type 1 (TRPV1) receptors. Inflammation or nerve injury which can occur during surgery leads to the activation of TRPV1 receptors in primary sensory afferents which leads to glutamate release from both peripheral and central terminals. The activation of TRPV1 receptors will further increase the intracellular Ca^{+2} and depolarize primary sensory afferents, leading to increased quantal release of glutamate. On the other hand, the stimulation of metabotropic glutamate 2 (mGluR2) has an analgesic effect as it negatively regulates neurotransmitter release from primary afferent fibers in the dorsal horn of the spinal cord. The analgesic action of L-acetylcarnitine results from upregulation of mGluR2 in the dorsal root ganglia and the dorsal horn of the spinal cord (Fig. 13.2)

The Immune System and Surgical Pain

Surgical pain is unique as it is induced by a combination of tissue injury and inflammation. The molecules released from the damaged cells are recognized by toll-like receptors (TLRs) in immune cells (such as monocytes or macrophages), dendritic cells, and immune-related cells (such as keratinocytes). Binding to TLRs activates nuclear factor -κB (NF-κB) signaling and the release of inflammatory cytokines. The mast cells within immune cells undergo degranulation and release histamine, bradykinin, and other vasodilator mediators. Calcium-dependent cell adhesion molecule called N-cadherin mediates the direct interaction between mast cells and peripheral nerve terminals which ultimately leads to the degranulation of mast cells. N-cadherin is cleaved by metalloproteinase MT5-MMP (MMP-24), which is expressed by neurons. Of interest, it has been shown that mutant mice that are deficient

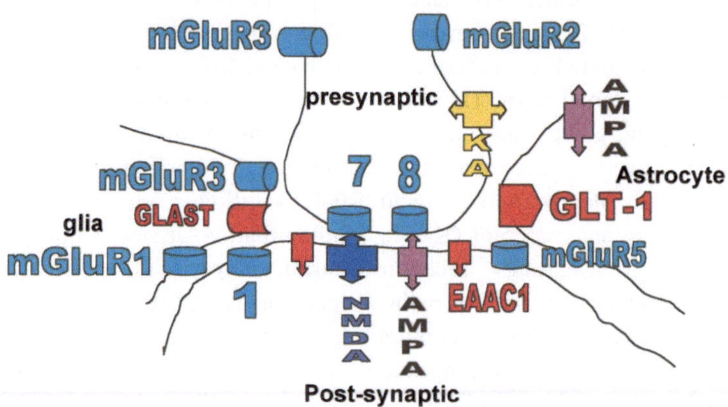

Fig. 13.2 The role of glutamatergic synapses on pain transmission (Reprinted from Meldrum BS. Glutamate as a neurotransmitter in the brain: review of physiology and pathology. *J Nutr*. 130:1007S–15S, Copyright 2000, with permission from The American Society for Nutrition, Inc. The American Society for Nutrition, Inc., does not endorse any commercial enterprise)

in MT5-MMP do not develop inflammatory hyperalgesia. Mast cell degranulation also contributes to the rapid onset of nerve growth factor-induced thermal hyperalgesia.

The release of cytokines as a result of tissue or nerve injury during surgery plays an important role in amplifying pain responses and increasing the recruitment of immune cells, which in turn facilitate neuronal sensitization and pain chronification. Interleukin-1 (IL-1) can bind nerve terminals and induce both substance P release and migration of polymorphonuclear leukocytes. Of note, mast cell degranulation is facilitated by both substance P and CGRP. Another cytokine involved in the pain pathway is TNF-alpha. Schwann cells release TNF-α after nerve injury, which induces MMP-9. In turn, MMP-9 promotes migration of macrophages to the injured site. T-helper type 1 (T_H 1) cells facilitate neuropathic pain by releasing IL-2 and interferon -γ (INFγ), whereas T_H 2 cells counteract this effect by releasing anti-inflammatory cytokines (IL-4, IL-10 and IL-13). It is important to mention that the concentration of IL-17, which is one of the key pro-inflammatory cytokines, is increased in the spinal cord of rats after nerve injury. Interestingly, the cytokines and chemokines act on dorsal root ganglia (DRG) neurons to generate ectopic discharges and enhance primary afferent input to the spinal dorsal horn (Fig. 13.3).

The activation of the immune system does not always enhance the pain response; it has analgesic effect at the same time. The inflammatory process not only evokes leukocyte recruitment but also induces the release of opioid peptides from migrating leukocytes. When neutrophils, vascular endothelium, and other immune cells are activated, they produce lipid mediators such as lipoxins and resolvins. Lipoxins suppress inflammatory pain and promote resolution of inflammation. Resolvins are derived endogenously from omega-3 essential polyunsaturated fatty acids. There are two series of resolvins: the D and E series. Resolvin D1 (RvD1) inhibits IL-1B production in the microglia, and RvD2 attenuates neutrophil migration to the site of inflammation by inhibiting leukocyte–endothelial interactions. Both RvE1 and RvD1 reduce hyperalgesia in animal models of inflammatory pain. RvE1 also inhibits the potentiation of NMDA receptor currents induced by TNF-α.

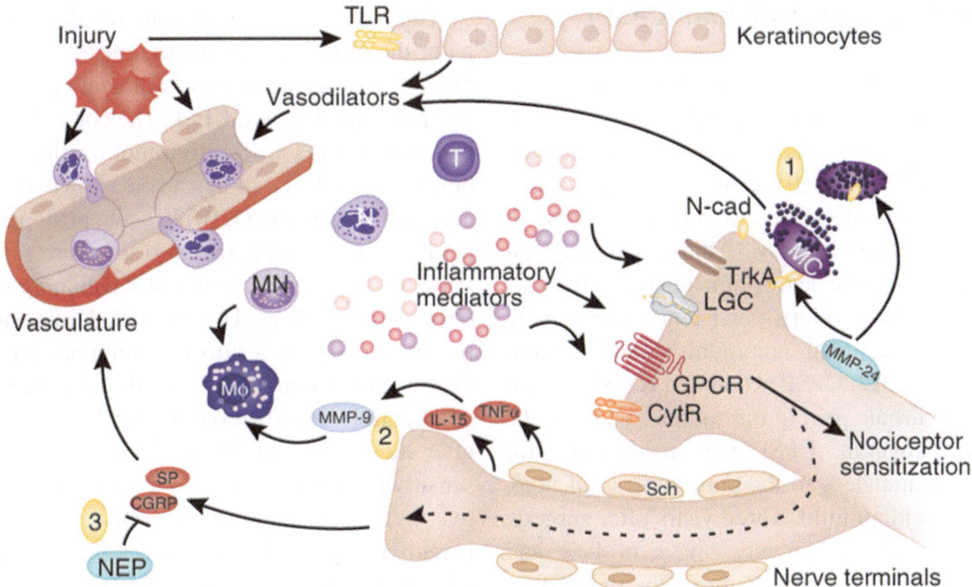

Fig. 13.3 The role of inflammatory mediators on pain transmission (Reprinted with permission from Macmillan Publishers Ltd.: Nature Publishing Group, Ren K, Dubner R. Interactions between the immune and nervous systems in pain. *Nat Med.* 2010;16(11))

Genetic and Epigenetic Predisposition in Surgical Pain

The role of genetics in pain is undeniable. The gene SCN9A encodes a sodium channel (NaV1.7), and if mutated, it can cause either a gain of function resulting in erythermalgia or loss of function resulting in the inability to sense pain. Therefore, the polymorphic SCN9A gene channelopathy is associated with insensitivity to pain. The single nucleotide polymorphism 118G in the human μ-opioid receptor gene (OPRM1) which is present in in up to 17% of the white population and 49% of the Asian population might be associated with a reduction in μ-opioid receptor and expression or signaling. The genetic variants (haplotypes) of the gene that encodes catecholamine-O-methyltransferase (COMT) can determine a person's sensitivity to pain. Individuals with genetic variants that encode for low COMT activity are at higher risk of developing myogenous temporal mandibular joint disorder (TMD), a common musculoskeletal pain condition. The reduction of COMT is also associated with a decrease of enkephalins in certain regions of the CNS which may affect pain and mood. In addition, reduced COMT activity results in elevated levels of catecholamines. Increased levels of catecholamines promote the production of persistent pain states via the stimulation of B_2-adrenergic receptors in the peripheral and central nervous systems.

Epigenetic mechanisms involve changing the likelihood of gene expression by altering the chemical structure or the physical structure of DNA. Histone deacetylase (HDAC) inhibitors are known to modulate gene expression by increasing acetylation of histone proteins, thus remodeling chromatin structure. Therefore, the use of HDAC inhibitors results in analgesia by upregulating the expression of mGluR2 in the dorsal ganglion and dorsal horn. The histone hypoacetylation in the rat brain stem nucleus raphe magnus results in impaired GABA synaptic inhibition, which causes persistent inflammatory and neuropathic pain. The use of HDAC inhibitors is considered potentially new therapeutic targets in an epigenetic approach to the treatment of chronic or inflammatory pain.

Chronic Postsurgical Pain (CPSP)

Chronic postsurgical pain (CPSP) is a major concern of surgeons and perioperative physicians as it significantly worsens quality life of the affected patients. CPSP is defined as chronic persistent pain at the site of surgery, ranging from 1 month to 1 year after surgery. Although nearly all patients have some degree of acute pain after surgery, 30–40% develops persistent chronic pain. In a cross-sectional community sample from Norway in 2012, CPSP accounted for 33% of all cases of chronic pain in the sample, while in the United Kingdom, CPSP was responsible for 22.5% of attendees to the pain clinics. Of note, CPSP is seldom mild. Three years after surgery, pain is usually moderately severe in 12% and severe in 7% of patients diagnosed with CPSP.

The risk factors for developing CPSP include the presence of preoperative pain, severe postoperative acute pain, preoperative anxiety, and the site of the surgery. Female sex and increasing age also appear to be risk factors (Table 13.1).

Table 13.1 Perioperative predictive risk factors for chronic postsurgical pain (CPSP).

Construct	Score
"Capacity overload" in the 6 months prior to surgery (having had more to deal with in the psychological sense than the subject thought (s)he could handle)	1
Preoperative pain in the body part to be operated on	1
Preoperative pain distant from the operative site	1
The presence of two or more indicators suggestive of stress (sleep disorder, exhaustibility/exhaustion, frightening thoughts, dizziness, tachycardia, feeling of being misunderstood, trembling hands, or taking sedatives or sleeping pills)	1
An average pain score >5/10 on days 1–5 postoperatively	1
Points are added to render a score from zero to five. Score correlates with CPSP risk as follows: 0 = 12%, 1 = 30%, 2 = 37%, 3 = 68%, 4 = 82%, 5 = 71%	

Rashiq S, Dick BD. Postsurgical pain syndromes: a review for the non-pain specialist. *Can J Anaesth.* 2014;61(2):123–30. Epub 2013 Nov 2., with kind permission from Springer Science + Business Media

The severity of acute pain predicts chronic pain; therefore the administration of gabapentin prior to surgery decreases both acute postoperative pain intensity and CPSP. The control of postoperative pain is crucial to minimize the risks of developing CPSP. It has been shown that for every unit reduction (1/10) in acute postoperative pain, as measured on a zero-to-ten (zero = worst, ten = best) scale, the odds of developing CPSP decreases by 10%. The increased intensity of postoperative pain results in continuous inputs to the dorsal horn and consequently leads to neuronal central sensitization. Central sensitization after surgery leads to the development of hypersensitivity to pain commonly called postoperative hyperalgesia, a phenomenon that can be paradoxically increased by intraoperative opioid administration. Therefore, the use of regional anesthetic techniques may reduce CPSP not only by decreasing pain sensitization induced by the surgery itself but also by decreasing excessive intraoperative opioid use and the potential for opioid-induced hyperalgesia. Glutamate receptors, like the NMDA receptors, play an important role in the process of central sensitization. Increased intensity of painful stimulation, as seen during and after surgery, activates NMDA receptors on the second sensory neurons. Indeed, subgroup analysis of the gas mixture for anesthesia (ENIGMA) trial showed a 50% decrease in CPSP when 70% nitrous oxide (NMDA antagonist) was used during general anesthesia for noncardiac surgery lasting more than 2 h. However, in the same trial, the use of nitrous oxide for more than 2 h was associated with an increased risk of myocardial infarction.

The surgical site is considered an independent risk factor for CPSP. The top four most frequently affected sites are the chest wall 35%, breast 31%, total joint arthroplasty 20%, and iliac crest bone harvest 19%. Patients contemplating mammoplasty have a greater than 40% risk of CPSP at 3 years, with a 10% chance of this being moderate or severe, and 6% chance of pain being the reason for regretting the operation. Of note, the development of CPSP is not confined to only major procedures, as open inguinal hernia repair carries a 7% risk of developing CPSP. Minimally invasive surgery probably, but not unequivocally, reduces the risk of CPSP, as it was shown that laparoscopic inguinal hernia repair reduces the risk of CPSP by 60% compared with open surgery. Surgical durations greater than 3 h are more likely to be associated with CPSP than shorter ones (Table 13.1).

Chronic pain after thoracic surgery represents a significant problem in 25–60% of patients. The severity of pain in the first 48 postoperative hours is still considered the main indicator for the development of chronic postoperative pain 1.5 years after thoracotomy. The use of regional anesthesia, especially epidural analgesia, is considered the mainstay prophylactic method to reduce the risks developing post-thoracotomy chronic pain. The importance of the severity of postoperative pain has been confirmed after obstetrical delivery as well. It has been shown that the prevalence of persistent pain for 8 weeks in the postpartum period was strongly related to the severity of acute postoperative pain but not to the mode of delivery. Therefore, acute pain services should be available to effectively manage postoperative pain.

Biological Mechanisms for CPSP

Synaptic plasticity is the ability of synapses to strengthen or weaken over time in response to increases or decreases in their activity. The plasticity of the nervous system can be seen in processes, such as peripheral and central sensitization, which increase sensitivity and lower threshold to noxious stimulation.

Peripheral sensitization results mainly from the release of inflammatory mediators due to tissue damage, including prostaglandin E2 (PGE2), bradykinin, and nerve growth factor (NGF). The inflammatory mediators may act on G-protein-coupled receptors (GPCRs) or tyrosine kinase receptors (TKRs) at nociceptor terminals. The binding of PGE2 and bradykinin to the nociceptor nerve terminals leads to the activation of cyclic adenosine monophosphate (cAMP)-dependent protein kinase A (PKA) and the Ca^{2+}/phospholipid-dependent protein kinase C (PKC) which results in phosphorylation of TRPV1. NGF induces activation of p38 mitogen-activated protein kinase (MAPK) in primary sensory neurons. Increased activity of p38 MAPK can lead to an increased expression and transport of TRPV1, resulting in increased sensory hyperalgesia. Other growth factors, such as neuregulin, bind to v-erb-b2-erythrobastic leukemia viral oncogene homolog 2 and 3 receptors (ERBB2 and ERBB3) on Schwann cells. Early ERBB2 activation results in demyelination, while late activation of ERBB2 causes Schwann cell proliferation. Proliferating Schwann cells release NGF as well as the neurotrophin glial-derived neurotrophic factor, prostaglandins, and cytokines like IL-1β and IL-6. The release of IL-6 can trigger sprouting of sympathetic nerve fibers around dorsal root ganglia, which may contribute to chronic neuropathic pain. Thus the nervous and immune systems interact in the periphery and lead to chronic pain development. The released vasoactive mediators such as nitric oxide (NO) result in hyperemia and swelling which have been implicated in the development of neuropathic pain.

Central sensitization results mainly from the action of glutamate on its excitatory inotropic and metabotropic receptors. The activation of mGluRs and neurokinin-1 receptors (NK1Rs) results in the increase of intracellular Ca^{2+} and PKC, which can activate the sarcoma (Src) family kinases, enhance NMDA activity, and produce hyperalgesia.

Brain-derived neurotrophic factor (BDNF) released from microglia plays a key role in the long-term maintenance of central sensitization. BDNF binds to tyrosine receptor kinase B (TrkB) and leads to phosphorylation of extracellular signal-regulated kinase (ERK). The phosphorylated ERK can enter the nucleus to induce transcriptional changes like increased transcription for c-Fos, cyclooxygenase-2, neurokinin (NK), and TrkB genes, which contribute to central pain sensitization and pain.

It has been observed that large-diameter Aβ neurons may begin to express SP under pathological conditions associated with pain hypersensitivity. Since Aβ fibers now express high levels of SP, they now function like C-fibers and can

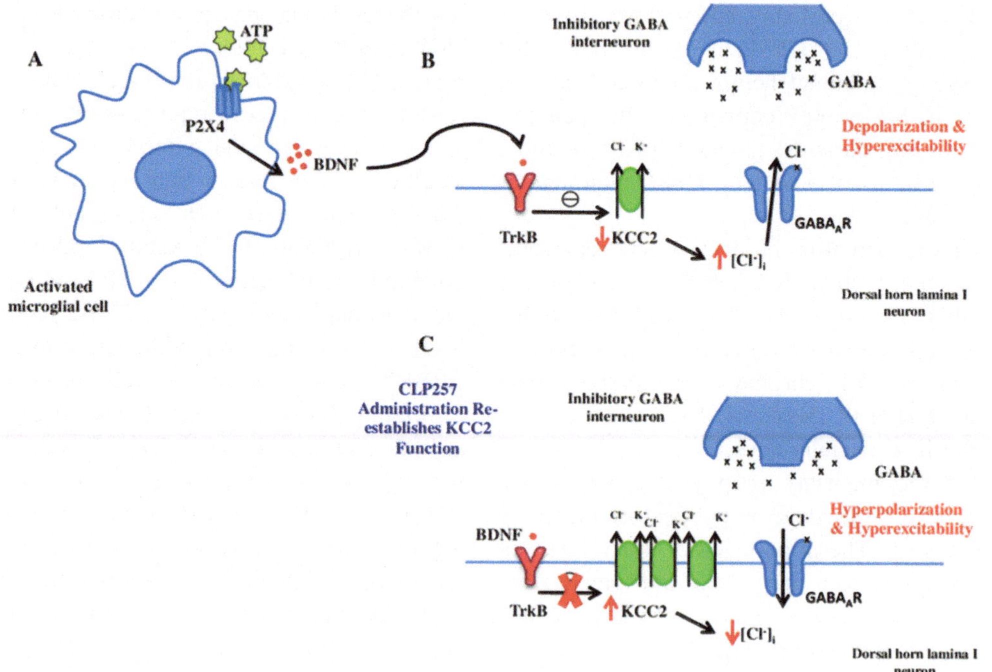

Fig. 13.4 The effect of activated microglia and inhibitory GABA interneurons on transmission of pain at level of spinal cord (With kind permission from Springer Science + Business Media)

increase central excitability. Therefore, this phenotypic switch serves as a key mechanism whereby previously non-nociceptive afferents now have the ability to induce central sensitization and tactile pain hypersensitivity.

Tissue injury during surgery can trigger major changes to the microglia and astrocytes in the dorsal horn. Toll-like receptors 2 (TLR2) expressed on astrocytes and microglia and TLR4 expressed on microglia mediate neuropathic pain processing. TLR2 and TLR4 activation leads to release of pro-inflammatory cytokines like IL-1β, TNFα, and IL-6 and increase in phagocytosis. TNF-α and IL-1β from astrocytes increase the neuronal excitability by enhancing the AMPA/NMDA receptors number and conductivity. Increases in NMDA receptors can initiate a positive feedback loop where increased production of NO increases neuronal excitability. TLR4 enhances pain processing by activating its endogenous ligand fibronectin. Fibronectin in return upregulates the purinergic receptor $P2X_4$ in microglia. The activation of purinergic receptors in the microglia by adenosine triphosphate (ATP) released in the dorsal horn results in mechanical hypersensitivity and the release of BDNF from the microglia. BDNF activates TrkB receptor on the second-order neurons and inverts inhibitory responses medicated by gamma-aminobutyric acid (GABA) to depolarization, thereby facilitating pain transmission. This inversion in GABA function is due to the decreased levels of the potassium–chloride cotransporter KCC2, which results in a decrease in intracellular chloride and a depolarizing shift in lamina I neurons. Therefore, the stimulation of GABA receptors results in extrusion of the chloride from intracellular into the extracellular compartments, thereby inducing depolarization instead of hyperpolarization as in normal conditions. The KCC2-specific activator (CLP257) has been shown to restore chloride transport and normalize sensitized spinal nociceptive pathways. Therefore, restoring chloride homeostasis may prove to be a successful therapeutic target for chronic pain (Fig. 13.4).

Treatment of Surgical Pain

The analgesic ladder introduced for the treatment of cancer pain by the World Health Organization (WHO) ladder has been adapted for the treatment of acute pain. It is made up of three steps. The first step involves the use of non-opioid ± adjuncts like acetaminophen, aspirin, or nonsteroidal anti-inflammatory drugs (NSAIDS). If there is increasing pain intensity, in addition to step 1 medication, weak opioids like codeine or tramadol can be added. In moderate to severe pain or pain persisting or increasing, stronger opioids are considered in addition. All these involve the concept known as multimodal analgesia. The multimodal analgesia realistically can be defined as a combination of an opioid and non-opioid analgesic, with or without regional anesthesia. The use of multimodal analgesia usually results in better quality of analgesia with concurrent reduction of opioid side effects, such as postoperative nausea, vomiting, constipation, and sedation, through an opioid sparing effect.

Suggested Reading

1. Liu XJ, Salter MW. Glutamate receptor phosphorylation and trafficking in pain plasticity in spinal cord dorsal horn. Eur J Neurosci. 2010;32:278–89.
2. Mifflin KA, Kerr BJ. The transition from acute to chronic pain: understanding how different biological systems interact. Can J Anesth. https://doi.org/10.1007/s12630-013-0087-4.
3. Nikolajsen L, Minella CE. Acute postoperative pain as a risk factor for chronic pain after surgery. Eur J Pain Suppl. 2009;3:29–32.
4. Ren K, Bubner R. Interactions between the immune and nervous systems in pain. Nat Med. 2010;16(11):1267–76.

Traumatic Pain

14

Martin J. Carney, Austin L. Weiss, Mark R. Jones, and Alan David Kaye

Key Concepts

- Acute and chronic pain following a traumatic injury bears increasing significance to the United States' healthcare system.
- Complex regional pain syndrome (CRPS) is often initiated by traumatic injuries. A subsequently over-exaggerated immune response produces gross and sustained inflammation that can be devastating to limb function, presenting commonly with continuous and severe pain, hyperalgesia, and allodynia.
- Traumatic brain injury (TBI) afflicts nearly 1.4 million people annually in the United States. The most common sequela of TBI is posttraumatic headache, occurring in 90% of patients. However, up to 43% will experience some form of chronic disability, such as whiplash injuries to the occipital and cervical nerves, and require long-term rehabilitation services.
- Few reliable treatment options exist for spinal cord injury (SCI) patients. A majority of patients (65%) experience chronic pain following SCI, and symptoms can vary greatly. Individual treatment goals and therapies must be implemented under close scrutiny to achieve the best therapeutic effects possible.
- Vertebral fractures are increasing in incidence in the United States, largely owing to the growing aged population. In addition to medical management, several minimally invasive therapies may be indicated for these patients, such as vertebroplasty and kyphoplasty.
- Managing traumatic pain in the acute setting can be challenging and requires knowledge and application of a variety of treatment modalities. Inadequate treatment often results in a common set of negative physiological and psychological outcomes.
- The principles of acute traumatic pain management parallel the multimodal approach to acute pain outlined by the American Society of Anesthesiologists (ASA) Task Force. The guidelines recommend that all surgical patients receive around-the-clock NSAIDs and acetaminophen unless contraindicated

M.J. Carney, BS
Tulane University School of Medicine, New Orleans, LA, USA

A.L. Weiss, MD
Wake Forrest School of Medicine, Department of Anesthesiology, Winston-Salem, NC, USA

M.R. Jones, MD
Brigham and Women's Hospital/Harvard Medical School, Department of Surgery, Boston, MA, USA

A.D. Kaye, MD, PhD, DABA, DABPM, DABIPP (✉)
Department of Anesthesiology, Hospital Director of Anesthesia, Department of Pharmacology, LSU School of Medicine T6M5, Tulane School of Medicine, 1542 Tulane Ave., Room 656, New Orleans, 70112, LA, USA
e-mail: akaye@lsuhsc.edu

J. Cheng, R.W. Rosenquist (eds.), *Fundamentals of Pain Medicine*,
https://doi.org/10.1007/978-3-319-64922-1_14

and that regional anesthesia be considered early on in the pain management process.

Acute Traumatic Pain

Epidemiology and Pathophysiology

Traumatic injury is the leading cause of death for Americans between 1 and 46 years old and the third leading cause of death overall. Of the traumatic injuries reported by the National Trauma Database (NTDB) in 2015, falls were by far the most common mechanism of injury at 44% of cases followed by motor vehicle traffic-related injuries at 26%.

Traumatic injuries often results in a common set of negative physiological and psychological outcomes. From a cardiovascular standpoint, acute pain has been shown to increase heart rate, blood pressure, and myocardial contractility that subsequently lead to increased O2 consumption which can contribute to ischemia. Regarding the respiratory system, poorly managed acute pain in the thorax or upper abdomen can lead to impaired ventilation and to subsequent atelectasis, which potentially can cause decreased vital capacity and increased V-Q mismatch from shunting, and predisposes the patient to the development of pneumonia and respiratory distress.

Release of catecholamines also affects the gastrointestinal tract via sympathetic stimulation, leading to decreased gut motility and the potential for constipation and bowel obstruction. Pain is also a potent cause of nausea and vomiting. Visceral afferent fibers from most organ systems as well as sympathetic afferents have synapses in the vomition centers in the medulla. It is also worth noting that opioids, the cornerstone of acute pain management, share both of these adverse effects on the gastrointestinal system. Pain also causes release of vasopressin (antidiuretic hormone) from the posterior pituitary. This can result in both urinary retention and oliguria. Furthermore, vasopressin is known to increase platelet adhesion, which could induce a prothrombotic state.

Psychologically, pain has many deleterious consequences. It is associated with both acute and chronic anxiety which can in turn increase the fear and psychosomatic perception of future pain. In burn and trauma patients, higher pain scores have been associated with subsequent development of clinical depression and posttraumatic stress disorder (PTSD). There is also evidence that adequate treatment of acute pain may decrease the risk of subsequent PTSD and improve sleep patterns.

Management

Managing traumatic pain in the acute setting can be challenging and requires knowledge and application of a variety of treatment modalities. In 2012, the American Society of Anesthesiologists (ASA) Task Force released a set of acute pain management practice guidelines underscoring the use of multimodal analgesia whenever possible in the perioperative setting. The guidelines recommend that all surgical patients receive around-the-clock NSAIDs and acetaminophen unless contraindicated and that regional anesthesia be considered early on in the pain management process. Anticonvulsants like gabapentin and pregabalin should also be included in the postoperative treatment plans. This type of multimodal analgesia has been developed with the ultimate goal of adequate pain management while reducing the use and/or dose of opioids. All of these aforementioned principles can be applied verbatim to the management of traumatic pain with the addition of some nuances and variation in technique. Ultimately, the goal of the multimodal approach should be to achieve superior pain control while decreasing patients' need for opioid therapy.

Non-opioid Analgesics

With regard to non-opioid analgesics, they are often overlooked or discounted in the trauma setting. In some cases this dismissal denies patients the pain-relieving benefit of these agents and perhaps unnecessarily exposes them to the undesired side effects of high-dose opioids.

Acetaminophen

Acetaminophen is perhaps the most well-known non-opioid analgesic with a modest analgesic potency. It primarily acts upon the central nervous system as an antipyretic and analgesic and lacks any peripheral anti-inflammatory action. Despite its reputation as an "entry-level" pain reliever, acetaminophen can have a profound analgesic benefit without the risks of platelet inhibition, gastritis, and nephrotoxicity that seem to plague NSAID medications. The pain experienced by most trauma patients cannot normally be controlled on acetaminophen alone, but when used in a multimodal regimen, it can effectively reduce the need for opioids and their associated side effects.

The primary risk of acetaminophen is hepatotoxicity. Overdose of acetaminophen can lead to fulminant hepatic necrosis, and it is the leading cause of acute liver failure in the United States. Administration of more than 3000 mg per day should be avoided, and appropriate caution should be exercised when considering the use of acetaminophen in those with pre-existing hepatic disease. Additionally, physicians must take into consideration all other medications by which a patient could receive acetaminophen. Opioid and acetaminophen (e.g., Norco, Percocet) are staples of moderate pain analgesia; however, it is best to prescribe the two classes separately to more accurately monitor acetaminophen intake and decrease the risk of overdose.

Nonsteroidal Anti-inflammatory Drugs (NSAIDs)

NSAIDs exert their analgesic, antipyretic, and anti-inflammatory effects primarily by inhibition of the COX-II enzyme. However, their concomitant inhibition of COX-I increases bleeding risk and therefore limits their use in the trauma setting. NSAIDs also lead to constriction of the afferent arterioles in glomeruli resulting in decreased GFR. Patients in the trauma setting often present in a hypovolemic state, and further decreasing their GFR could certainly cause an acute kidney injury. Additional risks with NSAIDs include bronchospasm in asthmatic patients and gastrointestinal ulceration. Evidence also suggests that there is an increased risk of thromboembolic events (e.g., MI, stroke) in patients who use long-term or high-potency NSAIDs secondary to a relative increase in thromboxane levels that offsets the platelet-inhibiting effects of COX-I blockade.

Ketorolac is perhaps the most commonly used NSAID in the acute pain setting. It is available in IV, IM, and oral formulations and is among the most potent of NSAIDs. Other commonly prescribed NSAIDs in the trauma setting include ibuprofen, diclofenac, naproxen, and the COX-II selective inhibitor celecoxib.

COX-II Selective Inhibitors

The COX-II selective inhibitor celecoxib provides substantial analgesia equal or superior to that of other NSAIDs with the added benefit of less risk for GI and hematologic side effects. It is this quality that makes it a favorable option for the trauma patient. It is worth noting that celecoxib is a sulfa drug and as such can potentially cause sequelae ranging from mild fever to Stevens-Johnson syndrome in allergic patients.

Ketamine

Ketamine is an N-methyl-D-aspartate (NMDA) glutamate receptor antagonist within the phencyclidine family of medications. Producing analgesia at low doses and dissociative anesthesia at high doses, the effects of ketamine are widely variable depending on the administered dose. Notable side effects of ketamine include the possibility of dysphoric or psychotic reactions, indirect sympathetic stimulation leading to tachycardia and hypertension, bronchodilation, increased salivation, and impairment of airway protective reflexes and direct cardiac depression at high doses. Primary benefits of ketamine include its lack of respiratory depression and its intense and persistent analgesic properties.

In the trauma setting, ketamine is usually used as an induction agent due its relative sparing of the cardiovascular system and facilitating hemodynamic stability. It remains underutilized, however, as an analgesic and may be particularly useful in opioid-intolerant patients, those with a history of chronic pain, or those currently receiving naloxone or buprenorphine. In this regard, ketamine has been shown to be very effective in trauma-related settings where moderate and even deep sedation is required. As an example, a child requiring stitches in the tongue can be effectively and safely managed with titration of ketamine. As part of a multimodal regimen in the trauma setting, ketamine can be safely administered as a low-dose infusion (e.g., 0.1–0.4 mg/kg/h) or added to a PCA at an even lower dose (e.g., 0.01 mg/kg) with 5–10-min lockout intervals.

Although rather uncommon, dysphoria can occur even at low doses (e.g., <0.5 mg). Therefore, any patient who receives ketamine should be monitored for hallucinations and any alterations in affect. Co-administration of benzodiazepines (e.g., midazolam) has been shown to decrease these dysphonic reactions in the emergency department and trauma settings.

Practitioners are historically weary of using ketamine in patients with significant mental health history; however, recent literature suggests that ketamine may be beneficial in patients suffering from major depressive disorder or those with risk factors for PTSD.

Analgesic Adjuncts

In addition to the analgesics above, multiple adjunct medications may contribute to pain relief and can be considered as part of an analgesic regimen in the trauma patient. These include anticonvulsants such as gabapentin or pregabalin, antidepressants such as tricyclics, selective serotonin reuptake inhibitors or selective norepinephrine reuptake inhibitors, and alpha-2 agonists such as clonidine or dexmedetomidine. Evidence of analgesic benefit for each of these exists, but does not yet place them in the category of routine pain medications. They are not frequently included in the routine management of pain in the trauma population. They may be useful, however, for patients with pain that is difficult to manage despite the first-line treatment with opioids, non-opioid analgesics, or regional analgesia techniques. Limiting side effects for anticonvulsants typically include sedation and for alpha-2 agonists include hypotension, bradycardia, and sedation.

Opioids

Opioid therapy is often considered the cornerstone of managing moderate to severe pain. Acting mainly on mu, kappa, delta, and sigma receptors, they exert their strongest effects in the areas of analgesia, sedation, cough suppression, and euphoria. Their primary sites of action include the dorsal horns, brain stem, cortex, and portions of the peripheral nervous system. The side effect profile for opioids is long and dependent on the class but for most includes respiratory depression, nausea and vomiting, urinary retention, constipation, and itching. Effectively balancing the desired properties of opioids with their undesired effects is a learned skill and to some degree dependent on the individual patient and the extent of their injury.

The classification and characteristics of separate opioids is an extremely large topic that, by itself, could fill the pages of this text and will therefore not be discussed in this chapter. The following section will instead focus on the principles of opioid administration as they pertain to the trauma setting.

Opioids do not possess any anti-inflammatory properties. Instead, their application lies within their ability to increase the threshold and modify the perception of pain. Characteristically dull, continuous pain is more effectively quelled by opioids than is more sharp, intermittent pain. Furthermore, it should be noted that opioid analgesia reaches maximal pain reduction when administered prior to the painful stimulus.

The most commonly used opioids in the management of acute pain in the trauma setting include morphine, hydromorphone, fentanyl, oxycodone, and hydrocodone. Alternative methods of delivery such as intramuscular, transdermal, and transmucosal are available as well. Moderate to severe pain following acute trauma is best controlled initially with IV agents secondary to their reliable and rapid onset of action and their utility in those who are unable to tolerate oral agents such as in the settings of thoracic or abdominal trauma. Patient-controlled analgesia (PCA) with IV opioids should be considered for any patient who is able to participate. PCA has been shown to improve both patient pain control and satisfaction, and although higher total doses of opioids might be given, there is no associated increased risk of respiratory depression. Of the various opioids prescribed for use in PCA, hydromorphone may have the most suitable pharmacologic profile with an onset comparable to morphine but with lower incidence of itching and nausea and the lack of clinically significant active metabolites.

Regional Anesthesia in the Trauma Setting

Trauma is inherently unpredictable. Therefore, approach to traumatic pain management requires an arsenal of various treatment methods and a physician who is well versed in each of them. While opioid-based intervention is almost a given in the trauma setting, the application of regional and/or neuraxial anesthesia is much more dependent on the type and location of injuries. Regional or neuraxial techniques can be used as the primary form of pain control for injuries limited to the extremities, and it can also serve as an adjunct to general anesthesia and postoperative pain control in patients with more extensive injuries including those to the thorax and abdomen. Clinical evidence has shown that pain control with the use of regional and neuraxial techniques leads to a decreased physiologic stress response to trauma and surgery, improved return of bowel and bladder function after laparotomy, decreased incidence of chronic pain, and perhaps most importantly, increased patient satisfaction.

There are, however, many common issues and concerns that prevent the widespread utilization of regional and neuraxial anesthesia in the trauma setting. First and foremost are the relative and absolute contraindications. Neuraxial techniques can be contraindicated in trauma patients secondary to:

- Infection at the injection site
- Hemodynamic instability/hypovolemia
- Coagulopathy/thrombocytopenia/anticoagulation
- Ventricular outflow obstruction
- Increased intracranial pressure
- Spinal trauma
- Patients at risk of compartment syndrome (e.g., crush injuries)
- Patient refusal/inability to obtain consent

However, with peripheral nerve blocks, the contraindications are fewer as they can safely be performed in hypovolemic patients and those receiving LMWH. Although most studies thus far have been equivocal, compartment syndrome still remains a fairly common relative contraindication for both modalities. Finally, exparalel is a lipid emulsion bupivacaine preparation with durations of action of 3–4 days. The Food and Drug Administration is expected to consider the use of Exparel, for peripheral nerve blocks in the coming year.

Both neuraxial and regional anesthesia are thought to potentially mask the pain, paresthesias, and paralysis cardinally associated with compartment syndrome of the extremities. This lack of symptoms could then lead a delay in diagnosis, contributing further to limb ischemia and tissue necrosis. It is therefore important to recognize patients at risk of compartment syndrome including those with fractures to the distal radius and ulna, tibial plateau fractures, crush injuries, and those with recent prolonged ischemia of an extremity. Furthermore, if the use of regional anesthesia is an option for at-risk patients, it should be thoroughly discussed, closely monitored, and clearly documented with the surgical team.

Thoracic Trauma

Thoracic trauma is most frequently encountered after motor vehicle collisions and accounts for approximately 21% of trauma incidents in the United States annually. Of those chest injuries, rib fractures are by far the most common.

Rib Fractures

Treatment of injuries to the bony thorax (i.e., rib fractures) generally consists of chest physiotherapy and pain control, with great emphasis on the latter. Patients with fewer than three fractured ribs and no other injuries can typically be discharged home on oral pain medications without the need for further intervention. In contrast, multiple rib fractures (MRFs) often inflict severe pain that cannot be adequately or safely controlled with oral or IV analgesics alone. The pain from MRFs limits a patient's ability to take full breaths, which can lead to atelectasis and a decrease in functional residual capacity (FRC). These factors can then cause a restrictive ventilation pattern, V-Q mismatch, and acute respiratory distress. The prevention of these sequelae is the main indication of neuraxial and regional anesthesia in this setting.

Regional pain management of rib fractures is typically achieved through the application of thoracic epidural anesthesia (TEA), paravertebral blocks (PVBs), and intercostal nerve blocks. All of these approaches tend to provide superior pain relief compared to NSAIDs or opioids alone, but they are all inherently invasive and therefore carry certain risks. Another option is a Lidoderm patch.

TEA, much like lumbar epidurals, delivers bilateral segmental analgesia that can be maintained for days via an epidural catheter. TEA using a long-acting local anesthetic in conjunction with opioid medication is currently regarded to be the best method of pain control in patients with MRFs. In order to obtain optimal results, the epidural catheter should be placed in the spinal cord segment that corresponds to the approximate middle of the multiple ribs involved. As with lumbar epidural anesthesia, complications of TEA include bradycardia and hypotension from sympathetic blockade, systemic anesthetic toxicity, headache, dural puncture, direct spinal cord injury, meningitis, epidural abscess, and hematoma.

PVBs and ICBs are a reasonable second-line option for MRFs in patients who either refuse epidural anesthesia or in those whom epidural anesthesia is contraindicated. Unlike epidural anesthesia, PVBs and ICBs provide unilateral analgesia that is typically limited to one segmental dermatome. While PVBs may achieve some degree of cephalocaudal spread in one to two adjacent segments, ICBs are strictly limited to a single rib and dermatome. As a result, multiple injections are often required to achieve adequate coverage in the setting of MRFs. The average effective duration of a single-shot PVB or ICB ranges from 12 to 16 h depending on the anesthetic used, and the use of catheters to provide continuous administration is possible albeit complicated by the lack of segmental spread of anesthetic. Therefore, multiple catheters may be required especially in patients with bilateral or multi-segmental rib fractures.

Notable complications associated with PVBs and ICBs include pneumothorax, local site infection, local anesthetic toxicity, and unintentional neuraxial spread of anesthetic leading to epidural or intrathecal anesthesia. Furthermore, it is important to note that these risks may be compounded by the need for serial injections or multiple-site injections with catheters.

VATS/Thoracotomy

It is well known among surgeons, anesthesiologists, respiratory therapists, and post-op patients that thoracotomies and video-assisted thoracoscopic surgeries (VATS) are accompanied by rather significant postoperative pain. Postoperative pain associated with chest wall surgery can impede recovery and increase time spent intubated on mechanical ventilation. It can also lead to atelectasis, pneumonia, delayed ambulation, and high cost from the prolonged hospital admission. On a larger timescale, both VATS and thoracotomies have been shown to carry a high risk of developing chronic pain.

Much like the management of multiple rib fractures, TEA is the gold-standard management post-thoracotomy and is associated with improved analgesia and a decreased side effect profile compared to opioids. Though not yet studied in the trauma setting, TEA has also been shown to possibly decrease the risk of chronic pain post-VATS and post-thoracotomy. It should also be noted that infusion of a local anesthetic in combination with an epidural opioid, such as fentanyl, results in greater analgesia than either alone. Adjunctive neuraxial opioids are usually well tolerated; however significant respiratory depression remains a risk that requires careful consideration and close monitoring. For patients whose pain is incompletely controlled with epidural local anesthetic and opioids, a wise strategy may be to continue the epidural with local anesthetic alone and provide them with opioids via an alternative method as necessary.

The technique of performing a thoracic epidural should be a skill mastered by every anesthesiologist, but it is beyond the scope of this chapter and will not be discussed herein. More detailed information can be found in the suggested reading or within other chapters of this text.

Abdominal Trauma

In 2015, 11% of all trauma incidents in the United States involved some degree of abdominal injury. This significant proportion of a prevalent pathology necessitates review of common presentations and therapies.

Laparotomy

Abdominal trauma is similar to thoracic trauma in the fact that the nature of the injury in patients requiring surgery typically prohibits any preoperative placement of neuraxial or regional anesthesia. In the postoperative setting, however, low thoracic epidural anesthesia (LTEA) and high lumbar epidural anesthesia (HLEA) are invaluable. Epidural anesthesia post-laparotomy can provide optimal pain control, improved pulmonary function, and possibly an earlier return to ambulation and normal bowel function. Care must be taken when placing an epidural catheter in the post-laparotomy setting, however, as upright positioning is not recommended with a fresh abdominal incision. Instead, placement with the patient in the lateral position is recommended. LTEA at the T10 level provides analgesia to almost the entire abdomen while avoiding any significant impairment of the lower extremities.

Unlike neuraxial approaches, transversus abdominal plane (TAP) and rectus sheath blocks do not exert any visceral analgesia, and they only provide unilateral blockade. Nonetheless, these approaches do possess qualities that make them potentially invaluable in the trauma setting. Their lack of effects on the sympathetic nervous system allows them to be more widely used postoperatively as there is less concern for hypotension or bradycardia. From a technical standpoint, TAP and rectus sheath block are also more easily performed than LTEAs and PVBs in patients with fresh abdominal incisions, because the patient lies supine for the former two and must be upright or lateral for the latter. TAP and rectus sheath blocks should be considered for any patient in whom neuraxial analgesia is contraindicated.

The TAP block is typically performed to provide unilateral analgesia to the anterior abdomen below the umbilicus but can also be administered bilaterally for low midline incisions or horizontal incisions that cross the midline. In a proper TAP block, the needle is inserted along the lateral abdominal wall between the iliac crest and the 12th rib. Local anesthetic is then injected just deep to the internal oblique within the plane of the transversus abdominis; therefore, accurate and methodical identification of each muscle layer via ultrasound is imperative and helps to avoid peritoneal perforation.

Adequate analgesia of the midline for patients undergoing laparotomy can also be achieved locally via the rectus sheath block. This method utilizes a similar ultrasound-guided approach as the TAP block; however, since it is performed deep to the rectus abdominis muscle, extra care must be taken not to advance the needle through the peritoneum.

Trauma in the Extremities

Upper Extremity

Neuraxial and peripheral anesthesia for extremity trauma can provide a multitude of benefits to the patient including superior pain control and decreased requirement for opioids and, if administered preoperatively, can forego the need for general anesthesia. Unfortunately the use of these methods has been limited by the concerns for potentially masking the symptoms of compartment syndrome. Its use is also limited by the need for some patients to have their nerve function closely monitored postoperatively or after a closed reduction of a fracture. Sometimes it may be the nature of the injury itself that makes administering a peripheral nerve blockade unfeasible and impractical.

Brachial Plexus Block

Regional anesthesia for upper extremity trauma more commonly involves brachial plexus blockade but can sometimes require selective blockade of terminal nerves, namely, the median, radial, and ulnar nerves. Brachial plexus blocks can be done through a variety of approaches including the interscalene, supraclavicular, infraclavicular, and axillary approaches. The techniques involved in each of these approaches are critical skills for an anesthesiologist to master but are out of scope for this chapter.

Risks associated with each approach include injury to the great vessels, systemic anesthetic toxicity, unintentional neuraxial spread, phrenic block, and pneumothorax. It should be noted that many of these complications have seen a decrease in incidence following the advent of ultrasound-guided techniques. Some unique limitations to certain approaches also exist in the trauma setting. For example, interscalene blocks are near impossible in patients wearing a C-collar. Most of these approaches, except the axillary approach, are also contraindicated in any patient with baseline respiratory insufficiency, as an accidental phrenic blockade could prove disastrous in this scenario.

Lower Extremity Trauma

Lower extremity trauma is often encountered in the same settings as chest trauma and encompasses a large portion of sport-related trauma. Management of these injuries can range from a simple closed reduction to a full amputation, and the approach to regional pain management equally diverse.

Peripheral regional anesthesia for the lower extremity can be performed via lumbar plexus block; femoral nerve block; saphenous nerve block; proximal sciatic nerve block; distal i.e., popliteal, sciatic nerve block; and ankle block. Unfortunately, the innervation of the lower extremity does not provide as convenient a distribution of anesthesia as the upper extremity. In other works, there is no single block that provides anesthesia to the entire lower extremity.

Femoral Nerve/"Three-in-One" Block

The femoral nerve block is one of the most commonly performed lower extremity blocks especially in the non-trauma setting such as routine knee arthroplasty. In the trauma patient however, it can be used in any procedure requiring anesthesia to the anterior thigh and lower leg. Ideal scenarios include patellar fractures, large anterior thigh lacerations, isolated burns, and as an adjunct for below-knee amputations.

It is important to remember that the femoral block does not provide anesthesia to the region of the medial thigh covered by the obturator nerve nor to the lateral thigh covered by the lateral femoral cutaneous nerve. Therefore, in scenarios requiring anesthesia to the entire thigh, the use of the "three-in-one" block, a modified femoral block, should be considered. This block attempts to cover all three distributions by administering a large volume of anesthetic underneath the iliac fascia in a rostral direction to achieve retrograde spread to the lumbar plexus.

The primary risk of femoral nerve blockade is that of direct vascular injection and subsequent anesthetic toxicity. If catheters are placed, patients are also at increased risk of infection due to the catheter's proximity to the groin.

Lumbar Plexus Block

Formed by the L2-L4 nerve roots, the lumbar plexus is the origin for crucial lower extremity nerves including the femoral, genitofemoral, lateral femoral cutaneous, and obturator nerves. Altogether the lumbar plexus supplies innervation to the anterior, medial, and lateral portions of the thigh as well as the anteromedial portion of the lower leg. Lumbar plexus blocks are widely used in orthopedics for postoperative analgesia in hip and femur surgery but also have applications in the trauma setting. Because the block only anesthetizes the aforementioned portions of the thigh and lower leg, it is insufficient as a sole anesthetic and must often be complemented with a sciatic nerve block to provide complete anesthesia to the leg.

While the lumbar plexus block covers a larger distribution than the more commonly administered femoral block, it also bears the burden of additional risks. Retroperitoneal bleeding secondary to needle trauma is an uncommon but potentially severe complication especially in patients with coagulopathies and those on anticoagulation. Bowel, bladder, and vascular injury are well-documented risks as well. As with other blocks, there is a risk of neuraxial spread and anesthetic toxicity.

Sciatic and Popliteal Blocks

Derived from the L4 to S3 nerve roots and originating at the lumbosacral plexus, the sciatic nerve provides sensation to the posterior portion of the upper leg and the entire lower leg minus the medial saphenous distribution anteromedially. The sciatic nerve block is indicated in a variety of trauma scenarios especially those precipitated by falls and motor vehicle injuries. The length of the sciatic nerve offers a unique advantage in that it can be blocked at various sites along its course from a variety of approaches depending on the size and location of the trauma.

Sciatic blocks placed in the proximal leg are typically used in conjunction with femoral or lumbar plexus blocks for full-leg anesthesia after extensive trauma to the knee or in the case of amputation. Distal sciatic blocks (i.e., popliteal blocks) provide anesthesia to the remainder of the lower leg minus the anteromedial portion covered by the femoral distribution. A block placed here is ideal in isolated distal tibial fractures and in extensive foot or ankle trauma. Full anesthesia to the lower leg is achieved by blocking both the popliteal nerve as well as the saphenous (femoral nerve origin).

Risks associated with sciatic blocks include temporary foot drop secondary to loss of peroneal motor innervation; however, inadvertent damage to the nerve during injection could lead to a permanent inability to dorsiflex the foot. Preoperative sciatic blocks should be avoided in cases where there is a significant risk of surgical damage to the sciatic nerve that could lead to foot drop. Foregoing the block until after the surgery in this case allows for a neurological exam of function to take place prior to block placement.

Certain sciatic approaches also carry specific risks. Popliteal blocks carry a high risk of vascular injury to the popliteal artery, while parasacral sciatic blocks carry similar risks to previously mentioned paravertebral block such as neuraxial spread. Finally, it is worth re-mentioning that sciatic blocks are absolutely contraindicated in the setting of tibial plateau fractures.

Chronic Traumatic Pain

Epidemiology

Chronic pain following traumatic injury has grown increasing relevance in clinical practice throughout the United States. A 2008 estimate suggested that nearly 100 million Americans suffer with chronic pain. This undeniable burden suggests a variety of practitioners will inevitably deal with complaints of pain throughout their future career. Nearly one fifth of chronic pain patients identify traumatic injury as the direct cause. Improved survival of trauma patients has occurred due to protocol adjustments within the prehospital and operating suites, as well as the increased availability of level I trauma centers.

Pathophysiology

Injury type and mechanism dictates the physiologic foundation of chronic pain in trauma patients. Altercations of nerve plexus following crush or other injuries to the periphery can lead to a rewiring and general disability of the limb involved. Central injuries on areas such as the brain or spinal cord can have wide-ranging disturbances depending on the structures affected. Paresthesias to complete loss of function compose the spectrum of possibility. With limb salvage not always a possibility, phantom limb pain will also frequently follow a loss of an extremity.

Types and Clinical Evaluation

Complex Regional Pain Syndrome (CRPS)

CRPS is often initiated by a traumatic injury. The initial trauma, however, leads to an immunologic cascade resulting in gross and sustained inflammation. The results of this disease progression can be devastating to limb function and quality of life. The classic presentation is continuous pain, hyperalgesia, and allodynia in the setting of autonomic dysregulation. Acutely, this presents as edema, redness, and increased temperature. Symptoms progress over time, and the effected limb develops trophic changes: contracture, loss of function, bone density loss, and decreased nail and hair growth. The majority of cases resolve, but outcomes can be severe. Progressive disability is common and some patients require amputation. Orthopedic procedures are those most commonly plagued by this complication. Figure 14.1 demonstrates the severity and potential complication issues with CRPS.

Traumatic Brain Injury (TBI)

TBI prevention and management permeates a variety of acute care settings and practice types. Clinical estimates demonstrate that nearly 1.4 million people in the United States are sustaining this injury type each year. The most common sequelae of a TBI are posttraumatic headache, with up to 90% of patients at risk following this breed of trauma. Most importantly, of patients hospitalized with a TBI, nearly 43% will progress to some form of chronic disability. This high rate of complication severely affects quality of life and places a considerable burden on rehabilitation services. Most commonly in the United States, this variety of head trauma is sustained from falls, motor vehicle accidents, and assault.

A variety of intra- and extracranial structures can be disturbed upon injury, leading to diverse symptomatology and necessitating individual care and treatment plans. Aside from this conglomerate of pain syndromes, post-TBI headache remains a near universal symptom and should be addressed. An exact etiology remains a topic of debate, but theories suggest aberrance in cerebral blood flow, trigeminal nerve damage, or a combination of both to be likely possibilities. Tension and migraine headaches are most common in the setting of TBI and should be treated with NSAIDs and triptans or ergot derivatives, respectively.

Trauma to structures in the head other than the brain may also result in head and neck pain. For example, whiplash can result in trauma to the temporomandibular joint (TMJ), occipital nerves, and cervical joints and nerves. Whiplash injuries frequently occur after rear-end automobile

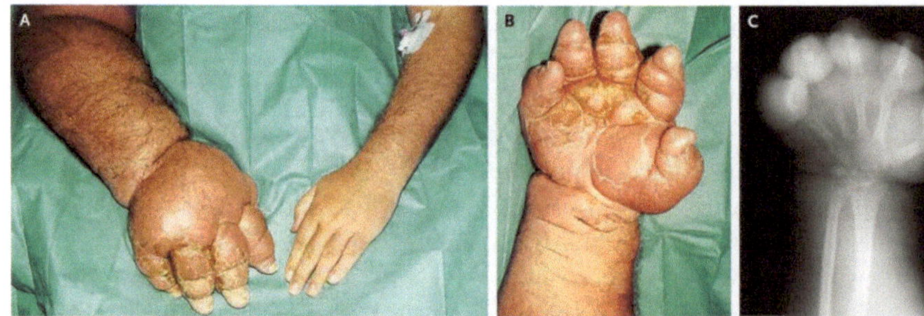

Fig. 14.1 CRPS after metacarpal fracture and ultimately requiring amputation (With permission from: Guttmann O, Wykes V. Complex regional pain syndrome type 1. *N Engl J Med.* 2008;359:508)

collisions, and the mechanism of injury is an abrupt backward then forward motion of the head. Figure 14.2 depicts the mechanism of whiplash injury. Medical treatment in this instance must be tailored to the structures injured and type of pain elicited. A carefully formed plan agreed upon by both patient and physician is necessary to move forward with pain management.

Spinal Cord Injury (SCI)

Very few reliable treatments exist in the realm of spinal cord injury, while nearly 65% of SCI patients report chronic pain following trauma. Because of this lack of standardization, treatment protocols vary greatly and are tailored to individual symptomology and pain relief. Table 14.1 outlines potential treatment modalities and side effects. Both nociceptive and neuropathic pain can be seen in this injury population. These broad classifications of trauma-induced SCI pain demonstrate the inherent variability of treatment regimens. The large subset of patients suffering from SCI complications requires closer attention and treatment rubric for current and future patients.

Phantom Limb Pain

While phantom sensation is always described after amputation, up to 80% of these are described as painful. Generally the distal portion of the missing limb comprises a burning, cramping, or tingling sensation. Phantom limb pain results in a chronic issue and is thought to be due to severed nerve fibers at the exact site of amputation. Treatment includes emphasis on prevention of pain through re-afferentiation through mirror therapy. Aggressive pain control postoperatively may also decrease the likelihood and severity of phantom pain symptomology.

Posttraumatic Abdominal Pain

Postsurgical abdominal pain occurs in the days to weeks following surgical manipulation and can manifest as a chronic syndrome. Neuropathic entrapment syndrome can happen when direct pressure exists on a nerve. This application of pressure causes sharp, tingling pain in the distribution of that nerve body. Similarly, visceral abdominal pain suggests a stimulation and sensitization of nociceptors generally occurring following direct trauma. Conservative medical treatment, steroid injections, regional anesthetic blocks, abdominal massage, radiofrequency ablations, and cryotherapy are all options to alleviate posttraumatic abdominal pain.

Vertebral Fracture

Posttraumatic vertebral fracture is increasing in incidence in the United States, with the elderly population being most at risk. This age stratification is due to older individuals having decreased

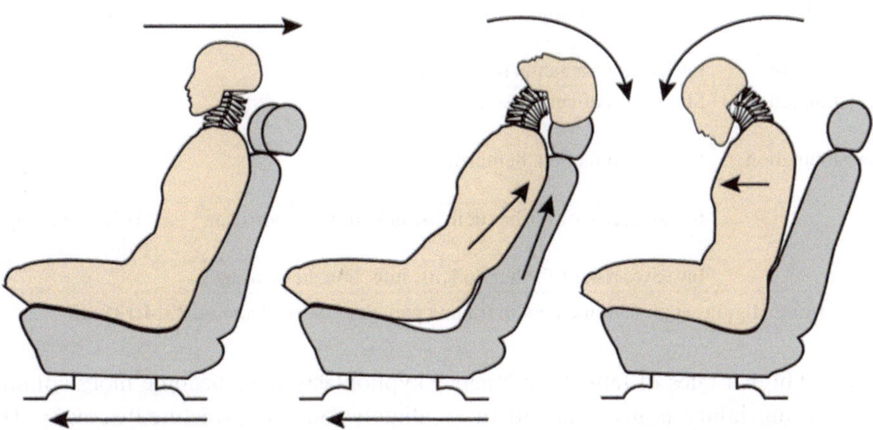

Fig. 14.2 Injury mechanism following whiplash. Rear-end collision – a common mechanism of injury. Note the ineffectiveness of an improperly adjusted head restraint (With permission from: IIHS (1997): "Special Issue: Head Restraints" (PDF, 575 KB), Status Report Vol.32, No.4. Website: http://www.iihs.org/externaldata/srdata/docs/sr3204.pdf)

Table 14.1 SCI medication options and side effects

Treatment	Disadvantages or side effects	Special considerations
Pregabalin/gabapentin/ gabapentinoid agents	Somnolence, dizziness, asthenia, dry mouth, edema, constipation	
Opioids	Constipation, drowsiness, tolerance, dependence, respiratory depression	
Mixed serotonin/ noradrenaline reuptake inhibitors	Hypertensive effects, gastrointestinal disturbance, dry mouth, reduced appetite, sweating, drug-drug interactions, including serotonin syndrome	
Mexiletine	Gastrointestinal upset, cardiovascular, hematological disturbance, skin reactions	
Topiramate	Drowsiness, dizziness, ataxia, anorexia, fatigue, gastrointestinal upset, ocular issues, kidney stones	
Lamotrigine	Potentially life-threatening skin rash, hepatic effects, diplopia, blurred vision, dizziness	
Dronabinol	Dizziness, drowsiness, irritability	
Older anticonvulsants	Drowsiness, dizziness, liver dysfunction, hematological effects	
Acupuncture	Invasive, vagal reactions	Effectiveness for below-level neuropathic pain uncertain
Ketamine	Dysphoria, increased secretions, increased intracranial pressure	
Propofol	Hypotension, arrhythmias, bradycardia, respiratory failure	
Alfentanil	Short-term duration, invasive, respiratory depression, bradycardia, sedation, hypotension, nausea, vomiting	
Morphine	Respiratory depression, sedation, hypotension, nausea, vomiting, constipation	Effectiveness demonstrated for mechanical allodynia
Baclofen	Reports of increased or "unmasked" neuropathic pain, sedation, rash	Stronger evidence for spasm-related pain
Intrathecal morphine and clonidine	Invasive, tolerance, hypotension, respiratory depression, drowsiness	
Subarachnoid lignocaine	Invasive, central nervous system disturbance	
Spinal cord stimulation	Invasive, infection	At-level neuropathic pain, incomplete injuries
Deep brain stimulation	Invasive, intracranial hemorrhage, infection	
Motor cortex stimulation (transcranial)	Short-term effect, infection, hemorrhage	
Motor cortex stimulation (epidural)	Invasive, infection, hemorrhage	
DREZ	Invasive, risk of further deficits, infection, hemorrhage	At-level neuropathic pain
Cordotomy	Invasive, risk of further deficits, infection, hemorrhage	

With permission from: Higgins et al. Chronic pain in trauma patients. *Anesth Trauma*. 2014:131–43

bone density and higher rates of falls. Immediate imagining following injury is necessary to rule out spinal damage and surgical intervention. Aside from bed rest and a spine brace, minimally invasive procedures such as vertebroplasty and kyphoplasty have become more common immediately following fracture discovery. These interventions are percutaneous procedures that involve intraosseous injection of cement into vertebral bodies under fluoroscopic guidance.

Suggested Reading

1. Apfelbaum JL, Ashburn MA, Connis RT, Gan TJ, Nickinovich DG. Practice guidelines for acute pain management in the perioperative setting. Anesthesiology. 2012;116:248–73.
2. de Mos M, Huygen FJ, van der Hoeven-Borgman M, et al. Outcome of the complex regional pain syndrome. Clin J Pain. 2009;25:590–7.
3. Joshi GP, Ogunnaike BO. Consequences of inadequate postoperative pain relief and chronic persistent postoperative pain. Anesthesiol Clin North Am. 2005;23(1):21–36.
4. Karanikolas M, Aretha D, Tsolakis I, et al. Optimized perioperative analgesia reduces chronic phantom limb pain intensity, prevalence, and frequency: a prospective, randomized, clinical trial. Anesthesiology. 2011;114:1144–54.
5. McGirt M, Parker S, Wolinsky J, Witham T, Bydon A, Gokaslan Z. Vertebroplasty and kyphoplasty for the treatment of vertebral compression fractures: an evidenced-based review of the literature. Spine J. 2009;9(6):501–8.
6. Merritt CK, Salinas OJ, Kaye AD. Pain control in acute trauma. In: Scher CS, editor. Anesthesia for trauma. 1st ed. New York: Springer Science and Business Media; 2014.
7. Nampiaparampil DE. Prevalence of chronic pain after traumatic brain injury. JAMA. 2008;300(6):711–9.
8. Simon BJ, et al. Pain management guidelines for blunt thoracic trauma. J Trauma. 2005;59:1256–67.

Mechanisms of Labor Analgesia 15

Beth H. Minzter and Jagan Devarajan

Key Concepts

- Labor pain is a severe acute pain perceived by women during the birthing process. This pain can be associated with visible tissue deformation and injury.
- Each stage of labor produces a different type of pain which is transmitted by specific neural pathways. These pathways may overlap.
- Pain during the first stage of labor is predominantly visceral and transmitted by the sympathetic fibers from T10 to L1. Second-stage labor pain is predominantly somatic pain and transmitted by the S2- S4 fibers of the pudendal nerve.
- Untreated labor pain is associated with cardiorespiratory stimulation and can occasionally have psychological consequences including depression.
- Regional analgesia is the most effective and most commonly used analgesic modality for labor pain. Regional analgesia techniques can be converted to provide anesthesia for operative deliveries, thereby helping to avoid general anesthesia.
- Epidural analgesia is the most commonly utilized method of regional analgesia for labor pain. Epidural analgesia is associated with delayed onset and can require a large amount of local anesthetic to block the sacral segments. Combined spinal–epidural analgesia provides more rapid-onset analgesia.
- Bupivacaine and fentanyl are the medications most commonly employed for neuraxial analgesia, although ropivacaine is used in some centers instead of bupivacaine.
- The addition of fentanyl to the local anesthetic improves the quality of neuraxial analgesia and can decrease the amount of local anesthetic and the incidence of motor block and hypotension.
- More often than not, supplemental administration of local anesthetic is required to provide analgesia during the second stage of labor in addition to the continuous infusion of epidural medication.
- Hypotension and motor block are the side effects most associated with local anesthetic use and pruritus is the side effect most commonly encountered with opioids.
- Patient-controlled analgesia using remifentanil intravenously is an option available for laboring mothers who request analgesia and

B.H. Minzter, MD, MS (✉)
Department of Pain Management, Cleveland Clinic, Cleveland, OH, USA
e-mail: MINZTEB@ccf.org

J. Devarajan, MD
Department of Anesthesiology, Cleveland Clinic Medina Hospital, Westlake, OH, USA

J. Cheng, R.W. Rosenquist (eds.), *Fundamentals of Pain Medicine*,
https://doi.org/10.1007/978-3-319-64922-1_15

have contraindications to or do not want neuraxial analgesia.

- Paracervical and lumbar sympathetic plexus blocks can be used for the first stage of analgesia although they are infrequently used. Pudendal nerve block and perineal infiltration can be utilized to supplement epidural analgesia during the second stage of labor.

Labor Pain

Pain during labor and delivery is one of the most severe pains perceived by women, referred to as the *poena magna* – the "great pain" or "great punishment" by the Romans. The degree of pain falls somewhere between low back pain and digit amputation without anesthesia. The intensity of labor pain varies between individuals. Pain scores are lower in multiparous women compared to those in nulliparous women. Though education during the antenatal period about childbirth and knowledge about labor and labor pain do help in reducing pain scores, they do not eliminate the need for analgesics. During progression of labor, pain scores soar with cervical dilation and the intensity of uterine contractions. The vast majority of parturients request some type of analgesia during childbirth.

Pathophysiology

First Stage of Labor

- Pain during the first stage of labor arises from distention of the lower uterine segment and cervix as a result of uterine contractions. C fibers from the receptors pass through the paracervical ganglia, the hypogastric nerve and plexus, and the lumbar sympathetic chain and terminate between T10 and L1 levels in the spinal cord (Fig. 15.1).
- Pain during the first stage of labor is of visceral origin and is diffuse and poorly localized.
- The pain impulses are transmitted along the contralateral ventral spinothalamic tract, relayed in the thalamus, and terminated in the post central gyrus of the somatosensory cortex.
- The above anatomical course illustrates that pain during the first stage of labor can be blocked at paracervical, hypogastric, paravertebral, lumbar sympathetic, epidural, or spinal levels.

Second Stage of Labor

- During the second stage of labor, in addition to first-stage pain related to uterine contractions, afferent fibers are activated from the cervix, vagina, and perineum.
- These afferents pass through the pudendal nerve with cell bodies at the dorsal root ganglia located between S2 and S4. These afferents are mostly A-delta fibers and the somatic pain is relatively well-localized.
- The anatomical basis of the second-stage labor pain reflects that analgesia during the second stage of labor is obtained either by blockade of receptors at the perineum, pudendal nerve block, or by conduction block of S2, S3, and S4 roots via caudal, epidural, or spinal drugs.

Effects of Labor Pain on Parturient

- Increased activity of sympathetic nervous system and catecholamines which can cause tocolysis.
- Increased maternal peripheral vascular resistance and decreased uteroplacental perfusion.
- Hyperventilation causing respiratory alkalosis, leading to further uterine artery vasoconstriction and leftward shift of oxyhemoglobin dissociation curve leading to decreased fetal oxygen delivery.
- Pain-induced psychological and psychosocial consequences, including depression and negative thoughts about sexual relationships and childbirth.
- Effective regional analgesia helps prevent these negative effects and can help make the

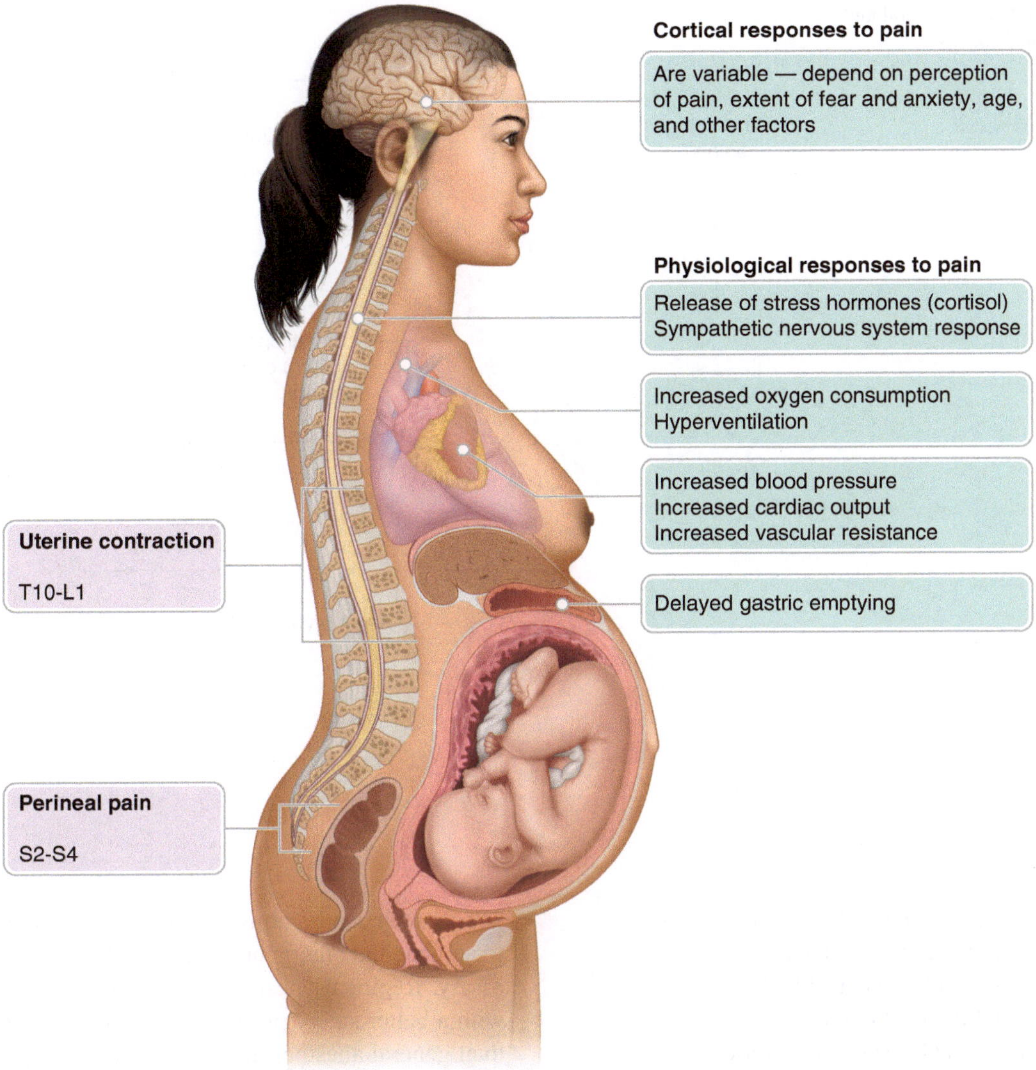

Fig. 15.1 Components of labor pain and involved nerve roots and physiologic responses if untreated

labor experience a memorable and pleasant one.

Treatment

Analgesic Options

Nonpharmacologic

1. Emotional support
2. Touch and massage
3. Positioning
4. Biofeedback
5. TENS
6. Acupuncture

Pharmacologic

1. Systemic analgesia
   (a) Parenteral opioid analgesia
   (b) Inhalational analgesia
2. Regional analgesia (Fig. 15.2)
   (a) Continuous epidural (CEA)
   (b) Combined spinal–epidural (CSE)
   (c) Continuous spinal analgesia

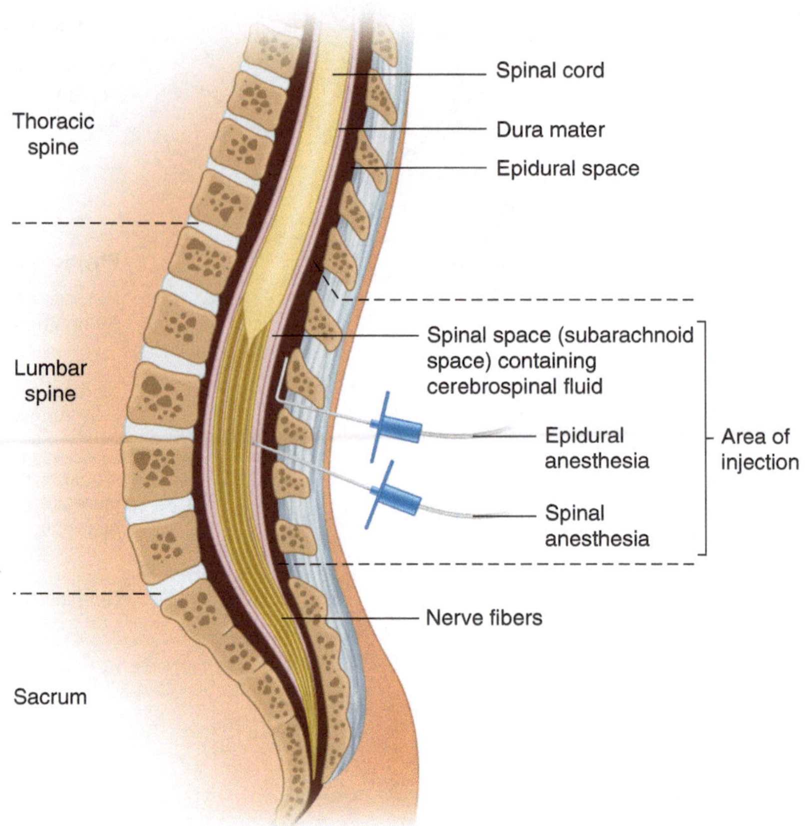

Fig. 15.2 Epidural and spinal spaces

3. Peripheral nerve blocks (Fig. 15.3)
   (a) Paracervical block
   (b) Lumbar plexus block
   (c) Pudendal nerve block
   (d) Local perineal infiltration

We will discuss in detail regional analgesia, currently the most common modality of labor analgesia and utilized approximately 60–84% of the time. Use of parenteral and inhalational analgesics is beyond the scope of this chapter.

Neuraxial Analgesia

Neuraxial analgesia is the most effective analgesic modality for labor in today's practice, which tremendously improves the parturient's obstetric experience and satisfaction scores. In addition to minimizing the adverse effects of pain on mother and fetus, it can be utilized to provide anesthesia for urgent and emergent cesarean delivery if necessary. Regional anesthesia has been associated with a better safety profile for operative delivery than general anesthesia. It can also provide postoperative analgesia following repair of perineal tear and surgical delivery.

Contraindications

- Maternal refusal.
- Infection at the epidural placement site.
- Coagulopathy–thrombocytopenia is more common among pregnancy (6–10%). However, severe thrombocytopenia (less than 100,000/ml) limiting regional analgesia is very rare. Risk and benefits should be weighed for individual patients and decisions made in coordination with patient and obstetrician.

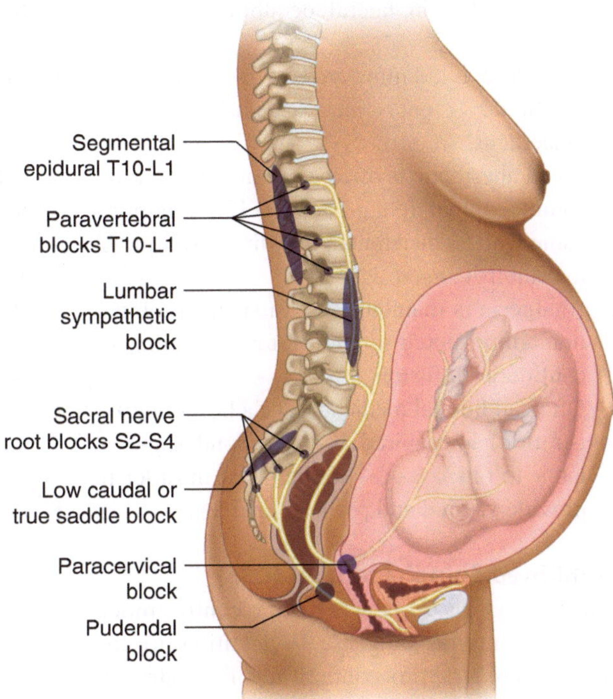

Fig. 15.3 Different peripheral nerve blocks for labor analgesia

Objectives of Epidural Analgesia

- Versatility and flexibility with ability to titrate in accordance with changing labor conditions
- Safety of drugs and techniques for mother and baby
- Minimal to no effect on the progress of labor and delivery
- Provision of reliably high-quality pain relief with minimal breakthrough pain
- Minimal motor block in order to retain parturient's ability to push during the second stage of labor

Types of Neuraxial Analgesia

Epidural Analgesia

Establishment of analgesia by placing an epidural catheter is the most commonly utilized modality of labor analgesia.

Advantages

- Presence of an epidural catheter allows provision of continuous peripartum analgesia.
- No dural puncture.
- Tested working epidural catheter allows conversion to epidural anesthesia for cesarean delivery.

Disadvantages

- Slow onset of analgesia particularly when performed in the late stages of labor
- Requirement of large volume of local anesthetic to provide sacral analgesia with resultant potential for systemic local anesthetic toxicity

Procedure

- Epidural catheter is placed in lumbar intervertebral space usually between L2-L3 and

L3-L4 either in lateral decubitus or sitting position.

- Test dose is administered to recognize subarachnoid or intravascular catheter placement.
- Local anesthetic is often combined with lipid-soluble opioid (e.g., 10 ml 0.125% bupivacaine with 50 mcg fentanyl in divided aliquots) to establish analgesia.
- Analgesia is maintained with same combination administered as intermittent injections or continuous infusion.
- Often additional medication (via bolus administration) is required in the second stage of labor to block S2-S4 dermatomes in order to provide vaginal and perineal analgesia.

Combined Spinal–Epidural (CSE)

This method has become popular recently among obstetric anesthesiologists. In addition to the standard epidural procedure, it involves intrathecal (subarachnoid) administration of either low-dose local anesthetic or opioid or a combination of both drugs. The intrathecal space is accessed via a needle-through-needle technique (e.g., 27 g BD™ Whitacre needle through 18 g epidural needle).

Advantages

- Rapid establishment of high quality of analgesia – particularly useful when analgesia is requested late in the first stage or during the second stage of labor.
- Faster onset of sacral analgesia with lower dose of drug particularly when analgesia is requested late in the labor process. In this circumstance, it also decreases the incidence of fetal drug exposure and maternal systemic toxicity.
- Opioid administration alone can establish sufficient first-stage analgesia – this may be helpful in patients with preload-dependent critical cardiac illness
- Decreased incidence of motor block and hypotension.

Disadvantages

- The epidural catheter is left untested until the spinal effect wears off after approximately 1–2 h. Hence this technique is not advised for patients with difficult airway and abnormal fetal heart tracings given the potential need for urgent or emergent delivery.
- Very low risk of postdural puncture headache; studies have shown little to no increased risk of headache after dural puncture with a 27 G pencil point needle.
- Higher incidence of pruritus associated with intrathecal versus epidural opioid administration.
- Occasionally fetal bradycardia can develop following CSE – presumably due to tonic uterine contraction secondary to abrupt reduction of catecholamines following rapid establishment of spinal analgesia.

Continuous Spinal Analgesia

This technique is not often used today. Sometimes a continuous subarachnoid catheter is utilized in a patient after an unintentional dural puncture or in whom there is anticipated difficulty identifying the epidural space.

Microcatheters were being developed to provide continuous spinal analgesia; As a result of the increased incidence of cauda equina syndrome associated with the microcatheters, they are not used anymore. Cauda equina syndrome with these smaller-gauge catheters is presumed to be due to maldistribution of local anesthetic, with pooling of high concentration of local anesthetic at the cauda equina.

Another disadvantage of the use of spinal catheters is the potential error in dosing. If the catheter is mistakenly thought to be in the epidural space and a large dose of local anesthetic is administered, unanticipated and/or high subarachnoid block can occur with potential hemodynamic instability and cardiorespiratory arrest. Therefore when an anesthesiologist decides to use this technique, the catheter has to be labeled clearly and all anesthesia providers and labor and delivery nurses should be well-informed about the presence of the subarachnoid (i.e., spinal) catheter.

Side Effects and Potential Complications

- Postdural puncture headache
- Central nervous system infection due to dural puncture and presence of the catheter

Caudal Analgesia

Caudal analgesia is very infrequently used. It may be considered in a patient who has had lumbar spine surgery, now rendering the lumbar epidural space inaccessible or nonexistent. In general, a large amount of local anesthetic is required via caudal administration to block the higher lumbar segments. Absorption into the systemic circulation of this large volume of local anesthetic can lead to high maternal and fetal plasma levels. Additionally there is potential for fetal or uterine injury when accessing the caudal canal.

Dural Puncture Epidural (DPE)

This method involves making a dural puncture with either a 27 or 25 G pencil point spinal needle without administration of any subarachnoid medications during performance of the epidural procedure. This facilitates better analgesia during labor in terms of a lower incidence of unilateral, asymmetrical or incomplete analgesia compared to epidural analgesia alone without a dural puncture. Dural puncture epidural also compares better than combined spinal epidural analgesia with respect to a lower incidence of side effects such as maternal pruritus, hypotension, and combined uterine tachysystole and hypertonus. In both of the above instances, some studies indicate that this newer modality has resulted in fewer physician "top up" interventions and improved maternal satisfaction.

Monitoring During Neuraxial Analgesia

- Maternal hemodynamics (heart rate and blood pressure). Blood pressure should be measured at 1–3-min intervals during injection of the test dose and bolus epidural administration of local anesthetic. After analgesia is established and hemodynamics are stable, blood pressure can be measured at 15–30-min intervals
- Oxygenation using continuous pulse oximetry.
- Extent of sensory and motor block. The adequacy and extent of sensory and motor block should be assessed following test dose and initial bolus dose. Subsequently the block should be measured every few hours and also every time that analgesia is felt to be inadequate or when there is unexplained hypotension.
- Continuous fetal heart rate monitoring. Though it would be ideal to continue fetal heart rate monitoring during the entire placement of the epidural catheter, practically it is not possible. General practice is to check FHR before and after the procedure by trained personnel.

Intravenous Hydration

Regional analgesia causes peripheral vasodilatation and a decrease in preload sometimes results in hypotension. Uteroplacental perfusion, a primary determinant of fetal well-being, is critically dependent on blood pressure. Untreated hypotension can cause alterations in fetal heart rate and may lead to fetal bradycardia. Preloading the patient with 500–1000 ml of lactated Ringer's solution before institution of the block can decrease the incidence of hypotension. Fluids should be administered with caution in patients with preeclampsia and cardiac conditions to prevent development of pulmonary edema.

Maternal Positioning

All pregnant patients should avoid flat supine position in order to prevent aortocaval compression. This is particularly true in patients receiving regional analgesia which prevents compensatory vasoconstriction. All patients should be tilted 30° to the left. Epidural can be performed in either lateral decubitus or sitting position.

Lateral Decubitus Position

- Allows continuous fetal monitoring and reduces the incidence of orthostatic hypotension
- May be more comfortable for some patients, particularly those who are in late labor
- Aortocaval compression with extreme lumbar flexion
- May be technically challenging to perform epidural procedure in the lateral position, particularly in obese patients

Sitting Position

- Helps to identify the midline and also provides better respiratory mechanics and comfort.
- Though lateral position decreases the incidence of epidural venous puncture and cannulation, dural puncture is unlikely influenced by positioning.

Epidural Test Dose

- Epidural catheter can be unintentionally placed in the intrathecal space or in a blood vessel. If unrecognized, serious complications can occur with dosing. A test dose is administered to identify catheter misplacement.
- Intravascular and intrathecal test doses are usually administered as one injection though they can be administered separately.
- Lidocaine 45–60 mg or bupivacaine 7.5 mg combined with epinephrine 15 mcg (3 ml of 1:200,000 solution) is commonly used as test dose.
- An increase of heart rate of 20 beats per minute within 45 s of injection is considered positive (intravascular injection). An increase in systolic blood pressure of 15–25 mmHg can also be considered positive.
- Although 15 mcg epinephrine is highly sensitive for an intravascular catheter tip, it is also associated with false-positive results as uterine contractions are commonly associated with increase in heart rate. Therefore the test dose should be administered between contractions.
- Metallic taste, tinnitus, and dizziness may also be observed with intravenous lidocaine to help identify intravascular administration of local anesthetic.
- Sensation of warmth within a minute of injection and rapid sensory loss and inability raise a straight leg at the hip within 4 min of injection is considered positive for subarachnoid placement of the catheter.
- Administration of combined local anesthetic and epinephrine can enhance motor blockade.
- Of note, the test dose neither completely guarantees placement of epidural catheter in the epidural space nor completely rules out intravascular or intravenous placement. Hence it is always advisable that every dose should be considered as a test dose and local anesthetic should be administered in 3–5 ml increments with observation of the patient's response after each injection.
- Catheters should always be aspirated before administration of medications.
- Sensory and motor blockade should be checked regularly during CEA.

Choice of Drugs

Combination of bupivacaine and fentanyl is most commonly employed for labor analgesia.

- Both are highly protein bound and associated with minimal transplacental transfer and fetal effect.
- These two drugs are inexpensive and have a proven safety record. A typical initial bolus dose is bupivacaine in the epidural space 6.25 or 12.5 mg (10–20 mL of a 0.0625% solution or 5–10 mL of a 0.125% solution) in combination with a fentanyl dose of 15–25 micrograms.
- Lower doses of local anesthetic in combination with opioid spares motor blockade. Maintenance of motor power is essential for maternal expulsive efforts. Moreover, pelvic floor muscle relaxation can cause abnormal rotation of the fetal head and can cause dysfunctional labor. Onset of effect is usually 10 min and peak action occurs at 20 min.

- Bupivacaine can also be combined with sufentanil instead of fentanyl.
- For maintenance of analgesia either 0.125% or 0.0625% bupivacaine combined with 2 mcg/ml of fentanyl is commonly used.
- Some advocate adding epinephrine to the mixture to improve the quality of analgesia. Epinephrine enhances analgesia by alpha-2 adrenoceptor agonist action. However, addition of epinephrine can potentiate motor blockade.
- Ropivacaine and levobupivacaine are other local anesthetics used for labor analgesia. They are approximately 40% less potent than bupivacaine.
- Though initial studies showed less motor block with ropivacaine, there was no difference in motor block between the two drugs when they were administered inequipotent doses.
- It is usually administered at 8–12 ml/h of 0.08–0.2% solution.

CSE

In combined spinal–epidural analgesia, fentanyl is commonly administered with or without bupivacaine as initial intrathecal dose.

- High lipid solubility of fentanyl facilitates rapid transfer into the spinal cord and decreases onset of action.
- It also improves the quality of analgesia and prolongs the duration of action of subsequently-administered epidural medications. Fentanyl is delivered at a dose of 15–25 mcg combined with 2.5 mg of bupivacaine. Sufentanil can also be used instead of fentanyl at a dose of 2.5–5 mcg. Neonatal outcomes are equally good with both choices of drugs.
- Epinephrine, clonidine, and neostigmine are adjuvants that have been used for provision of labor analgesia. Among them, epinephrine is most commonly used. It is administered at 25–50 mcg/h as infusion combined with bupivacaine and fentanyl.
- Epinephrine decreases the local anesthetic absorption from epidural blood vessels and decreases plasma concentration. It also augments analgesia by additional alpha-2 adrenoceptor agonist activity. At this dose, the epinephrine administration and absorption do not affect uteroplacental perfusion nor fetal outcomes. Though it enhances motor block, it does not affect obstetric outcomes.
- Clonidine is not widely used as it causes bradycardia, hypotension, and sedation. Neostigmine causes increased incidence of nausea and vomiting and hence is not used.

Mode of Administration

Epidural medication can be administered as intermittent boluses, continuous infusion, or patient-controlled epidural infusion.

Intermittent Bolus Administration

- It consists of injecting 8–12 ml of combination of local anesthetic and opioid whenever the epidural effect starts to wane.
- This is a labor intensive practice and is associated with breakthrough pain and decreased overall satisfaction.

Continuous Infusion

- It is the most common mode of analgesia.
- It is administered at the rate of 8–12 ml/h of combination of local anesthetic and opioid.
- The advantage of this technique is maintenance of stable analgesia and hemodynamics with less breakthrough pain and decreased incidence of potential systemic local anesthetic toxicity.
- It also enhances satisfaction scores and safety profile.
- Intravascular migration of the catheter can be determined by regression of analgesia; intrathecal migration of the catheter can be detected by rapid ascent of sensory and motor blocks.

Patient-Controlled Epidural Analgesia (PCEA)

- It involves patient-activated bolus with or without background infusion of local anesthetic and opioid.
- PCEA has been shown to result in decreased amount of local anesthetic with a lower degree of motor blockade.
- Patient satisfaction scores are better than other methods with equivalent outcomes.
- Typical PCEA prescription is a patient-activated bolus of 4–8 ml every 15–30 min along with background infusion of 4–10 ml/h.

Ambulatory Labor Analgesia

- Low-dose opioid-based spinal analgesia with CSE technique followed by maintenance of epidural with low-dose infusion is termed "walking epidural."
- The intention of this technique is analgesia with preservation of motor power and ambulatory capability.
- The ability to ambulate does not affect maternal and fetal outcomes. Epidural test dose of lidocaine with epinephrine can impair the ability to walk.
- The addition of epinephrine to maintenance epidural infusion augments motor block and hence can affect maternal mobility.
- Before ambulating, patient should be checked for orthostatic hypotension and FHR should be monitored.
- Patient should not be allowed to ambulate alone.

Analgesia for the Second Stage of Labor

- Blockade of somatic impulses between S2 and S4 requires a larger amount of more concentrated local anesthetic.
- Usually continuous epidural analgesia during the first stage of labor results in blockade of sacral segments.
- If additional analgesia is required, it is often supplemented by 1–2% lidocaine 5–10 ml.
- This supplemental injection will also provide analgesia for outlet forceps and episiotomy suturing if necessary.

Adverse Effects of Regional Analgesia

Hypotension

- Sympathetic blockade as a result of regional anesthesia causes peripheral vasodilatation, decreased venous return and cardiac output, often leading to hypotension.
- Occasionally blood pressure decreases due to decreased sympathetic tone associated with pain relief.
- Hypotension is considered significant if it is greater than 20% decreased from baseline or if it is associated with maternal symptoms of dizziness or nausea or if it is associated with non-reassuring fetal heart rate patterns.
- Since uteroplacental perfusion is dependent on maternal blood pressure and is incapable of autoregulation, blood flow to the fetus may decrease with a fall in blood pressure.
- Decreased fetal perfusion if prolonged may lead to fetal acidosis.
- Incidence of hypotension is lower with low-dose epidural dosing and usually corrected with 500 ml of crystalloid administration.
- Aortocaval compression should be avoided by either lateral positioning or supine placement with left lateral tilt.
- If hypotension persists or non-reassuring FHR develops, ephedrine (5–10 mg) or phenylephrine (50–100 mcg) may be administered.

Nausea and Vomiting

- Nausea and vomiting during labor can be related either to the process of labor or to hypotension due to regional analgesia or sometimes to neuraxial opioids.
- It is difficult to estimate the contribution of each toward nausea and vomiting.

- Opioids act on the receptors at the area postrema at the chemoreceptor trigger zone or at the nucleus tractus solitarius and induce vomiting.
- If nausea and vomiting are persistent or bothersome, ondansetron or metoclopramide can be used to treat it.

Pruritus

- Pruritus is related to neuraxial opioid administration and is more common with intrathecal opioid than epidural opioid.
- It is related to actions of opioid on the central opioid receptors at the trigeminal nucleus in the medulla and is not associated with histamine release.
- Coadministration of bupivacaine with the opioid decreases the incidence of pruritus and that of epinephrine worsens the pruritus.
- Pruritus is often self-limited and disappears in 30–45 min of intrathecal opioid administration. However, if it is bothersome, it can be treated intravenously with the partial agonist–antagonist nalbuphine 2.5–5 mg.

Fever

- There is a small but finite (less than 1 °C) rise in core body temperature (max 38 °C) associated with epidural analgesia.
- This occurs more commonly in women who deliver in warm rooms and is more commonly associated with nulliparous women and dysfunctional labor.
- The increase in temperature was thought to be related to sympathectomy which prevents sweating and heat loss from the lower half of the body.
- Growing evidence indicates that the fever is often due to maternal inflammation
- If the temperature goes beyond 38 °C, it should be treated with tepid sponges or acetaminophen as higher temperatures can affect the fetal brain.

Urinary Retention

- Urinary retention during neuraxial analgesia is due to inhibition of S2-S4 sacral segments.
- This decreases parasympathetic outflow to detrusor muscles and internal and external anal sphincters causing decreased urge to urinate.
- If bladder distension occurs and patient is unable to urinate, catheterization should be performed.

Inadequate Analgesia

Incidence – 5–13%

Causes

- Progression of labor
- Inadequate coverage of sacral segments
- Migration of epidural catheter into blood vessel or paravertebral space
- Unilateral analgesia
- Malpositioned fetal head
- Occipitoposterior position (usually with significant back discomfort)
- Bladder distension

Management

- Assessment of progress of labor.
- Rule out bladder distension.
- Check sensory level and extent of sacral blockade.
- Site of epidural catheter should be checked to rule out accidental displacement.
- Epidural catheter should be aspirated.
- Treatment starts with injection of 5–10 ml dilute concentration of local anesthetic with opioid and observation of the response.
- If the pain is from the perineum or vagina, a larger amount of more concentrated local anesthetic may be required ("perineal dose"). This is usually injected with patients in the sitting position though evidence of greater efficacy this way is not clear.
- If there is no relief and the provider cannot determine sensory level, the epidural catheter needs to be replaced.

- If the block is asymmetric or unilateral, some providers prefer to place the patient with the unblocked side in the dependent position to see if analgesia can be improved.
- Occasionally withdrawing the epidural catheter by a cm or two may be helpful to address the unilateral block and effectuate bilateral analgesia.

Effects of Regional Analgesia on Labor

- Labor analgesia is associated statistically with prolonged labor.
- Controversy exists whether there is an associated increase in instrumental operative deliveries associated with labor analgesia.
- It is difficult to research the impact of epidural analgesia on delivery as there are many conflicting factors involved.
- Randomized studies and impact studies illustrate that labor analgesia is associated with mild prolongation of the second stage of labor, which does not affect maternal and fetal outcomes.
- Similarly, the incidence of operative and cesarean delivery is not increased by epidural analgesia.
- There is also no difference in incidence of operative deliveries or duration of labor between women who received epidural analgesia either in early or late stages of labor. Therefore epidural analgesia can be administered whenever the mother is in labor and becomes uncomfortable and requires analgesia.

Postdural Puncture Headache

- Incidence is 1–2% and depends on the experience of the anesthesia provider and the relative difficulty in accessing the epidural space.
- Due to the large bore size of the Tuohy needle, the incidence of PDPH is high after accidental dural puncture (60–70%) with an epidural needle and is greater in thin versus obese patients.
- If dural puncture is recognized at the time of procedure, the catheter can be replaced at a different interspace. However, if there is difficulty in finding epidural space, then the catheter can be threaded into the intrathecal space and used as a spinal catheter.
- Insertion of the spinal catheter after accidental dural puncture decreases the incidence of PDPH theoretically due to fibrotic reaction around the spinal catheter. The thought is that this minimizes leakage of CSF.
- If it is recognized that the epidural catheter is in the subarachnoid space, then it can be used as an intrathecal catheter for labor analgesia.

Total Spinal Anesthesia

- Subarachnoid block is often due to unrecognized migration of the epidural catheter into the intrathecal space.
- Total spinal anesthesia happens more commonly during cesarean delivery and is less likely to occur during labor due to use of low-dose local anesthetic.
- It is determined by high level of sensory blockade, heaviness or inability to move the arms, dyspnea, and – if true "total spinal" – apnea.
- Severe hypotension and cardiovascular collapse can occur.
- Agitation, restlessness, and confusion are followed by loss of consciousness.
- Administration of 100% oxygen, airway management with ventilation, avoidance of aortocaval compression, and administration of fluids and vasopressors are required to maintain oxygenation and circulation.
- Endotracheal intubation is often required to facilitate ventilation and prevention of aspiration of gastric contents.

Subdural Block

It is recognized by an uneven, patchy block which tends to ascend while sparing lower and sacral segments and is associated with poor pain relief. The epidural catheter needs to be replaced.

Back Pain

- Backache is common after labor and delivery and about 50% of patients suffer backache.
- Epidural does increase incidence of immediate postpartum backache but the difference disappears in 48 h.
- The immediate postpartum backache related to epidural is presumed to be due to tissue trauma related to needle insertion and responds well to NSAIDs.

Nerve Injury

- Nerve injury and epidural hematoma following labor epidural are rare given that pregnancy itself produces a hypercoagulable state.
- Nerve injury due to obstetric causes, such as prolonged and dysfunctional labor, is more common than that due to epidural-related causes.
- When prolonged sensory or motor block occurs, it should be evaluated immediately.
- Prolonged nerve block after epidural may occasionally be due to the use of high doses of local anesthetic for provision of analgesia for the second stage of labor or for anesthesia for cesarean delivery or with the use of epinephrine.
- However, if prolonged block occurs in conjunction with severe backache and uneven and/or bilateral progression of sensory and motor block, the patient should be evaluated emergently for a space-occupying lesion (epidural hematoma or abscess) using suitable imaging technique (such as MRI with gadolinium).
- Prompt recognition and immediate treatment will improve outcomes and can prevent devastating neural complications.

Alternative Regional Analgesia Techniques

Paracervical Block

It consists of blockade of paracervical ganglia (*Frankenhäuser's ganglion)* located posterolaterally to cervicouterine junction. It provides mild to moderate analgesia in 50–75% of parturients during the first stage of labor.

- Neither sensory nor motor block is observed.
- It does not delay progress of labor.
- 2-Chloroprocaine is the choice of local anesthetic for paracervical block; however, the effect is short lived and usually lasts about 40 min. One percent lidocaine can also be used. Bupivacaine is not advised for paracervical block as it may cause severe prolonged fetal bradycardia.
- Fetal bradycardia (15–25% incidence) and hence this technique is not used widely

Rare Complications

- Laceration of vaginal mucosa
- Parametrial hematoma
- Nerve injury to sacral plexus
- Retropsoas or subgluteal abscess

Lumbar Sympathetic Plexus Block

- As pain impulses during the first stage of labor travel along the lumbar sympathetic chain before they enter between T10 and L1 segments, lumbar sympathetic plexus can provide analgesia for the first stage of labor.
- It is not commonly used as it can be a painful invasive procedure with minimal benefits and is not always easy to perform or successfully performed without fluoroscopic guidance.
- The major complication of lumbar plexus block is hypotension. The other procedure-related complications include local anesthetic systemic toxicity, total spinal or epidural anesthesia, and retroperitoneal hematoma.

Pudendal Nerve Lock and Perineal Infiltration

- Both are used together to provide analgesia for the second stage of labor as pudendal nerve block alone has a high failure rate.
- Local anesthetic is injected behind the posterior fourchette of the vagina. It provides modest pain relief.
- Complications are rare though high levels of maternal and fetal plasma concentration of

local anesthetic are observed. Hence it is advisable to use short-acting and less cardio-toxic local anesthetics such as lidocaine or 2-chloroprocaine. Fetal scalp injury is possible but rare.

Suggested Reading

1. American Society of Anesthesiologists Task Force on Obstetric Anesthesia. Practice guidelines for obstetric anesthesia: an updated report by the American society of anesthesiologists task force on obstetric anesthesia. Anesthesiology. 2007;106(4):843–63.
2. Capogna G, Stirparo S. Techniques for the maintenance of epidural labor analgesia. Curr Opin Anaesthesiol. 2013;26(3):261–7.
3. Chestnut D, Polley L, Tsen L, Wong C. Chestnut's obstetric anesthesia: principles and practice. 4th ed. Philadelphia: Saunders an imprint of Elsevier Inc; 2009.
4. Datta S, Kodali B, Segal S. Obstetric anesthesia handbook. 5th ed. New York: Springer; 2010.
5. Gomar C, Fernandez C. Epidural analgesia-anaesthesia in obstetrics. Eur J Anaesthesiol. 2000;17(9):542–58.
6. Loubert C, Hinova A, Fernando R. Update on modern neuraxial analgesia in labour: a review of the literature of the last 5 years. Anaesthesia. 2011;66(3):191–212.

16 Ischemic Pain

Magdalena Anitescu

Key Concepts

- Ischemic pain is caused by tissue hypoxia and acidosis.
- Various receptors and neurohumoral substances are implicated in the transmission of acid nociception. A special class of receptors, called acid-sensing ion channels (ASIC), on peripheral and central neurons facilitates the transmission of ischemic pain.
- Critical limb ischemia is an advanced type of vaso-occlusive disease associated with severe pain at rest for more than 2 weeks, ulcers, and skin breakage.
- Opioids have limited efficacy for the pain of critical limb ischemia typically because of their side effects. Methadone may be beneficial because of its anti-neuropathic properties through NMDA receptor antagonism.
- Besides vascularization, lumbar sympathetic blocks and neurolysis, regional anesthesia, and spinal cord stimulation can offer pain relief to patients with advanced peripheral arterial disease and chronic pain.
- Mesenteric ischemia, a special type of ischemic pain, is caused by atherosclerosis of the mesenteric artery; median arcuate ligament syndrome (MALS) is a condition associated with abdominal pain due to decrease blood flow in celiac artery distribution by fibrous compression of this arterial bed.
- Sympathectomy by celiac ganglionectomy during surgery or local anesthetic blockade can offer pain relief; spinal cord stimulation may lessen pain in patients with ischemia in the mesenteric arterial bed.

Ischemic Pain

Among the common pain syndromes, ischemic pain holds a unique place. Although other pain syndromes are generally associated with direct injury to peripheral receptors, ischemic pain is caused by tissue hypoxia [1]. One classic example of ischemic pain is myocardial infarction. An imbalance between oxygen supply and demand in a heart with limited oxygen reserves may predispose a patient to serious comorbidities. Cardiac pain is primarily acute pain. Although the receptors for sensing ischemic pain may be the same in acute and chronic conditions, the focus of this chapter is on the diagnosis and treatment of chronic ischemic conditions associated with refractory pain.

M. Anitescu, MD, PhD (✉)
Department of Anesthesia and Critical Care, University of Chicago Medicine, 5841 S. Maryland Ave, MC 4028, Chicago, IL 60637, USA
e-mail: manitescu@dacc.uchicago.edu

J. Cheng, R.W. Rosenquist (eds.), *Fundamentals of Pain Medicine*,
https://doi.org/10.1007/978-3-319-64922-1_16

Pathophysiology

Altered tissue perfusion from reduced arterial blood flow predisposes an organ to hypoxia. A chronic limited oxygen supply leads to continuous hypoxia, accumulation of lactic acid, and unrelenting ischemic pain [1, 2]. The association between local acidosis and pain was recognized more than 80 years ago. Severe muscle aches during strenuous exercise were recognized as a consequence of anaerobic metabolism and accumulation of lactic acid. Severe ischemic pain was produced by blocking arm blood flow with a tourniquet during a mild forearm exercise [3]. Similar sensations are experienced when running or swimming at a sprint for 40–50 s. The muscle pain experienced with direct physical stress under anaerobic conditions is, in fact, a type of ischemic pain [2] and confirms that lactic acid is a potential mediator. Other agents have also been identified as mediators for ischemic pain (Table 16.1).

Ion channels on sensory neurons react to the local presence of acid [4]. Those structures called acid-sensing ion channels (ASIC) were confirmed in the peripheral and central nervous system [5]. ASICs are expressed in peripheral sensory neurons and in nociceptive pathways of the spinal cord dorsal horn [6]. ASICs belong to the voltage-insensitive, amiloride-sensitive epithelial Na channels/degenerin family (Fig. 16.1). Through their position in the body, ASICs are well equipped to detect, differentiate, and react to pH variations within physiologic and pathophysiological ranges [7]. Inhibition of ASICs has relieved pain in human and animal models of ischemic pain, and ASICs act as membrane-bound H-gated nociceptors [8]. From the many subtypes, ASIC3 channels are predominantly expressed in peripheral sensory neurons and seem to be markedly involved in multiple nociceptive mechanisms including mechano- and chemosensation [9].

Table 16.1 Mediators of ischemic pain

Mediators	Year first described
Bradykinin	1980
Serotonin	1988
Adenosine	1993
Substance P	1996
Oxygen radicals	1995
Histamine	1981
Protons, lactate	1968

Data from Naves and McCleskey [2]

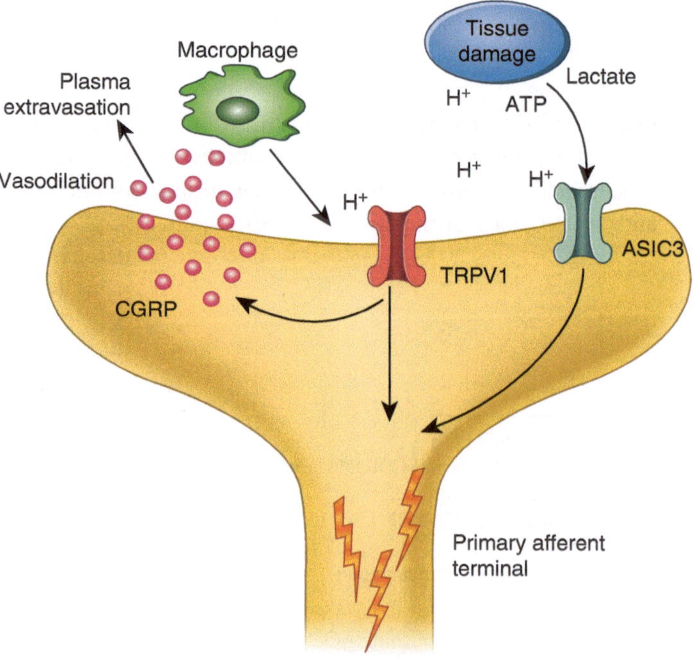

Fig. 16.1 Acid sensing ion channel type 3 and acid-induced nociception

Table 16.2 Signs and symptoms of conditions associated with ischemic pain

Types of conditions	Examples	Symptoms and diagnosis
Degenerative, inflammatory vascular conditions: arterial and venous ischemic diseases, microangiopathies, lymphatic vessels disease	Arterial insufficiency	Claudication (pain with walking)
	Atherosclerosis obliterans	Critical limb ischemia (pain at rest or the presence of ulcer or gangrene on feet); pain often worse at night
	Buerger's disease (thromboangiitis obliterans)	Ischemic signs and symptoms in toes and/or fingers: coldness, pain
	Raynaud's phenomenon	Ischemia of fingers and toes and sometimes of the ears and nose, marked by severe pallor and pain
	Deep venous thrombosis	Pain in affected leg, tenderness along the course of major veins Leg pain on foot dorsiflexion (Hoffman sign) Massive edema with cyanosis and ischemia (phlegmasia cerulea dolens)
	Polyarteritis nodosa	Polymorphic skin rashes, persistent livedo reticularis, ischemia or gangrene
Conditions affecting the bone	Sickle cell disease	Bone pain caused by pressure in marrow and vascular occlusion Visceral pain caused by ischemia (cholecystitis, spleen infarction/rupture, appendicitis, pancreatitis, bowel ischemia)
	Avascular necrosis of joints, especially shoulder, hip, or knee (joint "angina")	Limping Pain at rest, night pain (bone "migraines")
Conditions affecting the muscles	Compartment syndrome, crush injury	Pain with passive extension of fingers Irreversible changes after 6–8 h. of ischemia
Ophthalmologic conditions	Painful ophthalmoplegia	Pain, restriction of extraocular eye movement, proptosis, chemosis, and eyelid edema
	Mucomycosis	Slowly progressive, ischemic infarctions that cause necrosis of the skin, nasal mucosa or palate
Neuronal ischemia	Carpal tunnel syndrome	
Skin conditions associated with ischemia	Erythromelalgia	Ischemic ulcers may be present and could lead to infection and gangrene
	Vascular ulcers	Pain may vary from nonexistent to extreme Venous ulcers are most common around the middle of the ankle above the malleolus and may extend all the way around the leg

Several types of acute pain from ischemic events have been described: acute coronary syndrome, arterial embolism with acute arterial occlusion, compartment syndrome, ischemic bowel, and acute deep venous thrombosis [1]. Chronic ischemic pain has been characterized best in peripheral vascular disease where the main cause is arterial insufficiency. Other conditions that lead to tissue ischemia and chronic pain are described in Table 16.2. In addition, decrease blood flow in the mesenteric artery distribution by either atherosclerotic process or fibrous bands over the celiac artery has been associated with a special type of ischemic pain whose main symptom is postprandial abdominal pain.

Peripheral Arterial Insufficiency

Peripheral artery insufficiency happens with progressive occlusion of the peripheral arteries. Pain progresses in parallel to the degree of occlusion. When pain is severe, lasts for more than 2 weeks at rest, and is associated with ulcers and tissue loss, the condition is called critical limb ischemia (CLL). The patient may lose a limb as a result [9].

Epidemiology

Ischemic pain from peripheral arterial insufficiency is found in 5–15% of adults aged 55 years or older. Chronic critical limb ischemia (CLL) is present in 1–2% of the adult population with peripheral arterial disease [1, 9]. Mortality is 50% in 5 years and 70% in 10 years after diagnosis if CLL [9]. Overall the annual incidence of critical ischemic vascular disease is 0.25–0.45 patients per 1000 people [10].

Pathophysiology

Obstructive atherosclerotic or thromboembolic processes lead to chronic arterial insufficiency with ultimate progression to critical limb ischemia (CLL). The initial response to ischemic events is angiogenesis and capillary sprouting to increase blood flow to the critically ischemic limb; eventually, arterioles become maximally vasodilated. The proliferation of neo-vessels, friable structures with decreased wall thickness, predisposes patients to edema. Patients alleviate their pain by keeping their limbs in a dependent position. This position further aggravates the edema when hydrostatic pressure increases and compresses the already compromised capillaries. As a consequence, perfusion lessens with decreases in oxygen and nutrients to the cells thus worsening the ischemia and pain [9, 10].

Clinical Features and Diagnosis

The first symptom of vascular insufficiency is claudication. Patients complain of pain when walking and pain disappears at rest. Intermittent claudication progresses over years and becomes more severe with fewer pain-free intervals. When critical limb ischemia (CLL) is achieved, pain is constant, even at rest, and is accompanied by slow-healing ulcers [10]. The affected extremity discolors with ischemic pain. In time, the color becomes dark blue, while the pain from intermittent claudication becomes constant pain at rest. The limb is usually cold, and, in advanced stages of critical limb ischemia, skin lesions appear, which heal poorly. The low blood supply in some distal areas may progress to tissue necrosis [11].

Treatment

Chronic critical limb ischemia is difficult to treat. The main treatment goals are to restore function and to maintain skin integrity while relieving pain [12]. Revascularization surgery may be performed in patients with painful arterial occlusive disease; however, a tenth of patients with intermittent claudication may not be surgical candidates, and their condition may progress within 5 year to critical limb ischemia. Twenty to thirty three percent of those patients, considered to have unsalvageable limbs, will require amputations [12, 13].

Medical Management

Medical treatment of ischemic limb pain is directed to symptom management. Among the various treatment modalities are medications and infusion therapies. Recently gene and cell therapy have emerged as possible solutions to relieve pain in patients with ischemic, arterial vaso-occlusive pain.

Table 16.3 Practical approach to symptom management in chronic ischemic pain

Agent	Comments
Opioids	Remain the cornerstone of the management of severe pain
	Consider methadone for the dual action opioid and neuropathic agent
	Opioid doses need to be titrated to effect
	There are two types of pain treated with opioids: breakthrough and incident pain; incident-related pain requires strong short-acting opioids
Membrane stabilizers	Various agents: gabapentin, pregabalin
	Add early to the pain management regimen
	Require a period of titration
Antidepressant	Various agents with different mechanisms of action: serotonin and norepinephrine reuptake inhibitors, tricyclic antidepressants (low dose)
	Add early when depression is suspected
	Effective as anti-neuropathic agents

Data from Woelk [12]

Medications

Opioids are still the mainstay of medications in patients with arterial occlusive disease. Effective up-titration of opioids, however, is limited by side effects in a patient population with comorbidities such as chronic renal insufficiency and ischemic cardiac disease. Ischemic pain has a neuropathic component. Among the opioids, methadone acts as an anti-neuropathic agent through its antagonist properties at the NMDA receptor. Other agents to treat neuropathic pain may be used to treat symptoms of critical limb ischemia [12]. Gabapentin in doses up to 1200–4800 mg daily reduced pain from 9 to 5 on numerical rating scale at rest and with activity in patients with critical limb ischemia [14]. Depression also can worsen arterial vasoconstriction and increase platelet activation. Adding antidepressants to the pain regimen has been a benefit for patients with arterial vaso-occlusive disease [15]. Table 16.3 offers a practical approach to symptom management.

Infusion Therapies

Infusion therapies are emerging as adjuvant modalities for chronic pain syndromes. Sub-anesthetic doses of ketamine as well as lidocaine infusions have mitigated pain and improved quality of life in refractory chronic pain syndromes [16–18].

Ketamine

A known and potent NMDA receptor antagonist, ketamine is an effective agent when administered intravenously for chronic regional pain syndrome [19]. Since neuropathic and chronic ischemic pain share clinical manifestations, it has been suggested that a single ketamine infusion be administered at sub-anesthetic doses in an outpatient setting. In a double-blind randomized, controlled trial, 0.6 mg/kg delivered over 4 h added to an opioid regimen improved pain significantly and decreased allodynia, hyperalgesia, and hyperpathia when compared to placebo [20].

Our current protocol of sub-anesthetic doses of a ketamine infusion for outpatients is reserved for patients with severe chronic pain unresponsive to multiple pain management modalities. A ketamine dose of 0.3 mg/kg is administered over 30–40 min, and vital signs are monitored every 5 min. Table 16.4 describes the protocol in detail.

Lidocaine

A potent local anesthetic widely used in regional analgesia and anesthesia, intravenous lidocaine is a potent analgesic for chronic neuropathic pain syndromes [21, 22]. Short infusions of lidocaine decreased ischemic pain ratings [23]. We use lidocaine infusions in refractory pain states, including chronic ischemic pain unresponsive to multiple treatment modalities. A protocol for 1 mg/kg bolus followed by 4 iv administered over 30–40 min is described in Table 16.5.

Table 16.4 University of Chicago protocol for ketamine infusion

Consultation
Obtain baseline EKG and cardiac history
Evaluate the patient for arrhythmias before scheduling procedure
Day of procedure
Assess the patient for fasting and alertness
Determine effects of previous infusion, if any on:
Pain reduction
Duration of effects
Patient function after infusion
Decrease in use of pain medication since infusion
Verify that patient has companion to accompany patient home
Obtain signed consent on the consent form
Procedure
Apply standard monitors: blood pressure, EKG, pulse oximeter, capnography
Start iv. Access and pretreat with:
Midazolam 2 mg iv
Ondansetron 4 mg iv
Begin ketamine infusion with 0.3 mg/kg in 100 ml bag for 30–45 min
Record at 1, 5, 10, 15, 20, 25, and 30 min the following:
Time of administration
Blood pressure
Heart rate
Pulse oximetry
Pain score
Depending on the patient's vital signs and pain scores, the infusion may be extended to 60 min
Stop the infusion in the event of the following adverse effects:
Hallucinations
Blood pressure increase >20% of baseline
Severe anxiety
Nausea
Unmanageable, symptomatic nystagmus:
Most adverse effects disappear when infusion is stopped
Assess the patient for urgent management
Recovery
Patients recover within 30–60 min after the procedure
Vital signs are monitored every 5–15 min during recovery
At the end of the recovery period, the patient is discharged from the clinic to the accompanying caregiver
Follow-up
In 4 weeks patient returns for evaluation of treatment or repeat infusion
Infusion doses may be increased to 0.6 mg/kg – 1 mg/kg, depending on the effect of the infusion on pain scores and patient function or satisfaction with pain relief

Table 16.5 University of Chicago protocol for lidocaine infusion

Consultation
Obtain baseline EKG and cardiac history
Evaluate the patient for arrhythmias before scheduling procedure
Day of procedure
Assess the patient for fasting and alertness
Determine effects of previous infusion, if any on:
Pain reduction
Duration of effects
Patient function after infusion
Decrease in use of pain medication since infusion
Verify that patient has companion to accompany the patient home
Obtain signed consent on the consent form
Procedure
Apply standard monitors: blood pressure, EKG, pulse oximeter, capnography
Start iv. Access and administer 1 mg/kg lidocaine bolus over 3–5 min
Follow with 4 mg/kg lidocaine (or 2–4 mg) administered slowly over 30 min (or 20–30 min)
Record at 1, 5, 10, 15, 20, 25, and 30 min the following:
Time of administration
Blood pressure
Heart rate
Pulse oximetry
Pain score
Stop the infusion in the event of seizure activity or cardiac instability
Recovery
Patients recover within 30–60 min after the procedure
Vital signs are monitored over 15 min during recovery
At the end of the recovery period, the patient is discharged from the clinic to the accompanying caregiver
Follow-up
In 4 weeks the patient returns for evaluation of treatment or repeat infusion
The dose of lidocaine is not increased if the initial infusion was performed with 4 mg/kg over 20 min

Other Therapeutic Agents

A number of noninterventional therapies recently emerged as possible treatments for pain from critical limb ischemia. Regenerative medicine has shown promise in experimental models of critical limb ischemia [24]. The positive results from small pilot studies using gene therapy were not confirmed in larger follow-up studies such as the TAMARIS trial using non-viral fibroblast growth factor for revascularization. More studies are needed to identify the role for gene therapy in treating pain and arterial occlusion in peripheral arterial disease [25].

Therapeutic angiogenesis using stem cells has also been tried in patients with critical limb ischemia when endovascular or surgical revascularization is not recommended [26]. A recent meta-analysis of small, nonrandomized, clinical studies using cell-based therapies in patients with arterial vascular disease showed improvement in both objective and subjective endpoints [27].

Interventional Therapies

A number of interventional therapies have been used to treat severe ischemic pain in patients that are not surgical candidates and have severe side effects from the analgesic medication.

Sympathetic Chain Blocks and Neurolysis

As ischemic pain has a strong neuropathic component, many interventions for neuropathic pain can be used to treat unrelenting chronic, vaso-occlusive pain. Among the various interventions sympathetic chain blocks have been performed in patients who are not candidates for revascularization [24]. Although it had no effect on limb salvage or mortality rate in patients with severe critical ischemic pain, lumbar sympathetic block gave patients relief from pain at rest in multiple cohort studies [28, 29]. Therefore, chemical or surgical neurolysis can be considered one option for patients with pain at rest who are not candidates for surgery [30]. Thermal radiofrequency ablation of thoracic sympathetic ganglia was efficacious in the treatment of upper extremity limb ischemia [31]. After two cycles of 60 s at a temperature of 80 °C, at T2 and T3 sympathetic chain levels, peripheral perfusion of the upper limb improved, pain was reduced, and quality of life increased with only minimal side effects [32].

Table 16.6 Literature review of ischemic pain and regional anesthesia

Case report authors and year	Regional anesthetic	Drug	Ischemic pain	Regional analgesia masking ischemia
Hyder et al. 1996 [35]	Single shot Femoral 3-in-1 block	0.5% bupivacaine	Yes	Yes
Noorpuri et al. 2000 [36]	Single injection Ankle block	0.25% bupivacaine	Yes	No
Uzel and Steinman 2009 [37]	Single injection Femoral block	0.75% ropivacaine	Yes	No
Cometa et al. 2011 [38]	Continuous catheters Femoral and sciatic	0.75% ropivacaine bolus 0.2% ropivacaine infusion	Yes	No
Nair et al. 2013 [39]	Continuous catheter Supraclavicular	0.75% ropivacaine bolus 0.2% ropivacaine infusion	Yes	No
Walker et al. 2012 [34]	Continuous Popliteal catheter Single shot Saphenous nerve	0.5% bupivacaine bolus, 0.2% ropivacaine infusion	Yes	No

Data from Kucera and Boezaart [33]

Regional Anesthesia

Pain relief in response to blockade of the sympathetic chain raised the possibility of a sympathetic component for ischemic pain. Sympathectomy, chemical or surgical, has proved advantageous in controlling pain in patients with critical limb ischemia [32]. Regional anesthesia, administered through peripheral nerve catheters, has controlled pain in patients with peripheral ischemic disease, especially when acute compartment syndrome is anticipated [33]. Local anesthetic blockade of the sciatic nerve through peripheral nerve catheters placed in the popliteal fossa increased blood flow and treated pain in patients with ischemic pain [34]. Several case reports in the literature support the use of regional anesthesia to treat severe ischemic pain primarily because the signs and symptoms of a developing compartment syndrome are not masked [33]. Table 16.6 summarizes the case reports.

Spinal Cord Stimulators

Used initially for patients with severe pain from complex regional pain syndromes, spinal cord stimulators have been applied for pain from refractory angina and peripheral vascular disease [40–42]. Epidural electrodes placed either percutaneously or through mini-laminectomy modulated central signals to decrease pain. Stimulation of sensory unmyelinated c-fibers and myelinated A-delta fibers by the epidural electrodes activates a cascade of receptors: extracellular signal-regulated kinase (ERK), protein kinase B (PKB), and transient receptor potential vanilloid 1 (TRPV1). Nerve terminals then release potent microvascular vasodilator agents, calcitonin gene-related peptide (CGRP), and endothelial nitric oxide (NO) to relax smooth muscle. Another mechanism is through inhibition of sympathetic nicotine transmission, ganglionic and postganglionic, to suppress sympathetic vasoconstriction [40].

A variety of studies have advocated spinal cord stimulators for patients with peripheral vascular disease who are not candidates for revascularization. In a 20-year retrospective analysis of the use of stimulators for peripheral vascular disease [43], the modulating therapy was effective for pain relief in 88% of the patients. Of 260 patients followed longitudinally, the method was particularly efficient in patients with ulcers and severe vascular pain. Spinal cord stimulators may improve local microcirculation and skin perfusion, thus contributing to wound healing and limb preservation. Fewer patients with non-reconstructible critical limb ischemia and intermediate skin perfusion (measured by capillary microscopy, laser Doppler perfusion, or transcutaneous oxygen measurement in the foot) needed amputation when treated with stimulators compared with standard medical management [44].

In patients with critical limb ischemia 12 months after stimulator implantation, limb salvage was superior and pain relief improved even though fewer analgesics were needed [45]. A trial period with external leads may be conducted to identify patients who would benefit from stimulator implant [40].

Mesenteric Ischemia

Two conditions are associated with the persistent pain of mesenteric ischemia: chronic mesenteric ischemia and median arcuate ligament syndrome.

Clinical Features and Diagnosis

Chronic mesenteric artery ischemia is a condition present in some patients with atherosclerotic disease. Described as early as the mid-1400s, it has been renamed in the twentieth century "intestinal angina" [46]. The name stems from the characteristic clinical features of the condition. Pain begins after a big meal and progresses over time to pain after small meals or even at rest in advanced cases [47]. Patients who are usually between 50 and 60 years of age have other comorbidities such as peripheral vascular disease, cardiac disease, stroke, or claudications. Diarrhea because of malabsorption is another common symptom. Weight loss in advanced cases makes patients cachectic because they fear eating and excruciating postprandial pain.

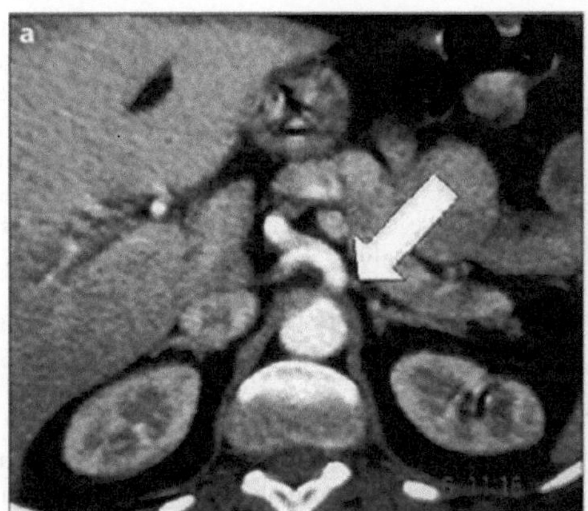

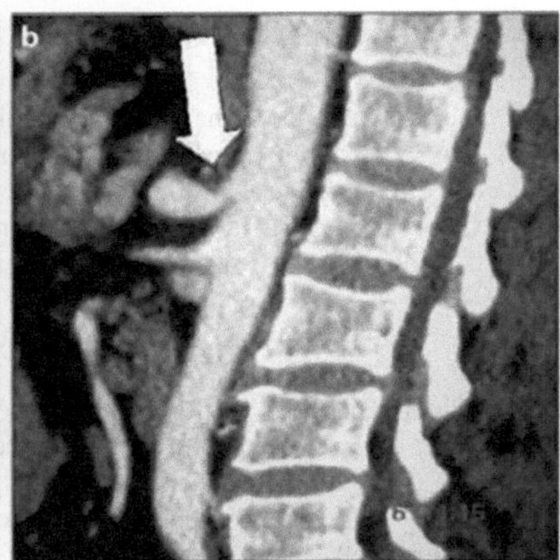

Fig. 16.2 Celiac artery compression syndrome; axial (**a**) and sagittal (**b**) CT image show hypertrophied median arcuate ligament causing severe stenosis (*hooked* appearance) of the celiac axis at the anterior margin of abdominal aorta with poststenotic dilatation (From Karahan et al. [48]; with permission)

Median arcuate ligament syndrome (MALS) results from compression at the celiac artery by fibrous bands. Patients with MALS are younger than patients with mesenteric artery ischemia. In MALS abdominal pain may or may not be associated with eating. Patients do not experience weight loss or diarrhea.

Diagnosis of the two syndromes is difficult to establish in the early stages of the disease. Abdominal pain, diarrhea, and weight loss are associated with many other conditions. Frequently time is spent on upper or lower endoscopies before a vascular component is suspected. Angiography is the best diagnostic test to identify the mesenteric vessels, especially the lateral views. The presence of collaterals and narrowed native vessels suggests a diagnosis of chronic mesenteric ischemia [47]. A computed tomography angiogram is the test of choice to diagnose MALS (Fig. 16.2). A typical "hook sign" is revealed in the lateral views [49].

Treatment

Because the superior mesenteric and celiac arteries are the main blood supply to the bowel, they are vital for adequate intestinal perfusion. Symptomatic ischemia in these vascular beds requires revascularization. Left untreated, severe bowel ischemia may progress to bowel infarction, peritonitis, or death. Prophylactic revascularization has been proposed in cases of noncritical mesenteric ischemia, but results were inconclusive [50].

Patients diagnosed with MALS may undergo decompression procedures as well. Celiac ganglionectomy is sometimes associated with postoperative diarrhea [51]. In inconclusive cases, celiac plexus blocks can be of benefit. Performed preoperatively, pain relief in response to the local anesthetic may provide information on the results of decompressive surgery. Patients with persistent symptoms in the postoperative period, primarily from incomplete ganglionectomy, may also benefit from celiac plexus block. A combination of local anesthetic and corticosteroids may relieve pain through anti-inflammatory properties and direct blockade of the sympathetic nerve terminal.

Although not the main indication for the treatment of pain associated with mesenteric and celiac artery ischemia, spinal cord stimulators (SCS) have been used in several cases as an analgesic modality in visceral pain [52]. Modulation of pain signals in the spinal cord and brain and increase blood flow in visceral ischemic areas are the proposed mechanisms by which SCS may provide pain relief in patients with abdominal pain due to chronic ischemic arterial disease.

References

1. Romero R, Souzdalnitski D, Banack, T. Ischemic and visceral pain. Essentials of pain management. Vadivelu N, New York: Springer, 2011; 545–556.
2. Naves L, McCleskey E. An acid-sensing ion channel that detects ischemic pain. Braz J Med Biol Res. 2005;38:1561–9.
3. Lewis T. Pain in muscular ischemia. Arch Intern Med. 1932;49:713–27.
4. Krishtal OA, Pidoplichko VI. A receptor for protons in the nerve cell membrane. Neuroscience. 1980;5:2325–7.
5. Akaike N, Ueno S. Proton-induced current in neuronal cells. Prog Neurobiol. 1994;43:73–83.
6. Gu Q, Lee L-Y. Acid-sensing ion channels and pain. Pharmaceuticals. 2010;3:1411–25.
7. Dubé GR, Elagoz A, Mangat H. Acid sensing ion channels and acid nociception. Curr Pharm Des. 2009;15:1750–66.
8. Wemmie JA, Price MP, Welsh MJ. Acid-sensing ion channels: advances, questions and therapeutic opportunities. Trends Neurosci. 2006;29:578–86.
9. Li W-G, Xu T-L. ASIC3 channels in multimodal sensory perception. ACS Chem Neurosci. 2010;2:26–37.
10. Coats P, Wadsworth R. Marriage of resistance and conduit arteries breeds critical limb ischemia. Am J Phys Heart Circ Phys. 2005;288:H1044–50.
11. Devulder J, van Suijlekom H, van Dongen R, Diwan S, Mekhail N, van Kleef M, Huygen F. Ischemic pain in the extremities and Raynaud's phenomenon. Pain Pract. 2011;11:483–91.
12. Woelk CJ. Management of critical limb ischemia. Palliative care files. Can Fam Physician. 2012;58:960–3.
13. Slovut DP, Sullivan TM. Critical limb ischemia: medical and surgical management. Vasc Med. 2008;13(3):281–9.
14. Morris-Stiff G, Lewis MH. Gabapentin improves pain scores of patients with critical limb ischaemia: an observational study. Int J Surg. 2010;8(3):212–5.
15. Heartsill LG, Brown TM. Use of gabapentic for rest pain in chronic critical limb ischemia. Ann Pharmacother. 2005;39(6):1136.
16. Patil SK, Anitescu M. Efficacy of outpatient ketamine infusions in refractory chronic pain syndromes: a 5-year retrospective analysis. Pain Med. 2012;13(2):263–9.
17. Niesters M, Martini C, Dahan A. Ketamine for chronic pain: risks and benefits. Br J Clin Pharmacol. 2013;77(2):357–67.
18. McCleane G. Intravenous lidocaine: an outdated or underutilized treatment for pain? J Palliat Med. 2007;10:798–805.
19. Sigtermans MJ, Van Hilten JJ, Bauer MCR, et al. Ketamine produces effective and long-term pain relief in patients with complex regional pain syndrome type 1. Pain. 2009;145:304–11.
20. Mitchell AC, Fallon MT. A single infusion of intravenous ketamine improves pain relief in patients with critical limb ischaemia: results of a double blind randomized controlled trial. Pain. 2002;97:275–81.
21. Tremont-Lukatsetall IW, Challapalli V, McNicol ED, et al. Systemic administration of local anesthetics to relieve neuropathic pain: a systematic review and meta-analysis. Anesth Analg. 2005;101:1738–49.
22. Rosen N, Marmyra M, Abbas M, Silberstein S. Intravenous lidocaine in the treatment of refractory headache: a retrospective case series. Headache. 2009;49:286–91.
23. Frolich MA, McKeown JL, Worrell MJ, Ness TJ. Intravenous lidocaine reduces ischemic pain in healthy volunteers. Reg Anesth Pain Med. 2010;35(3):249–54.
24. Golap O, Yilik L, Yurekli I, Gur S, Gurbutz A. Postoperative treatment of critical limb ischaemia. Eur J Vas Endovasc Surg. 2012;43:729.
25. Belch J, Hiatt WR, Baumgartner I, et al. TAMARIS committees and investigators. Effect of fibroblast growth factor NV1FGF on amputation and death: a randomized placebo-controlled trial of gene therapy in critical limb ischaemia. Lancet. 2011;377:1929–37.
26. Slovut DP, Sullivan TM. Critical limb ischemia: medical and surgical management. Vasc Med. 2008;13:281–91.
27. Fadini GP, Agostini C, Avogaro A. Autologous stem cell therapy for peripheral arterial disease meta-analysis and systematic review of the literature. Atherosclerosis. 2010;209:10–7.
28. Ruiz-Aragon J, Marquez CS. Effectiveness of lumbar sympathectomy in the treatment of occlusive peripheral vascular disease in lower limbs: systematic review. Med Clin (Barc). 2010;134:477–82.
29. Boisers M, Peeters P, D'Archambeau O, et al. AMS INSIGHT-absorbable metal stent implantation for treatment of below-the-knee critical limb ischemia: 6 month analysis. Cardiovasc Intervent Radiol. 2009;32:424–35.
30. Sanni A, Hamid A, Dunning J. Is sympathectomy of benefit in critical leg ischaemia not amenable to revascularization? Interact Cardiovasc Thorac Surg. 2005;4:478–83.
31. Gabrhelik T, Stehlik B, Adamus M, Zalesak B, Michalek P. Radiofrequency upper thoracic sympathectomy in the treatment of critical upper limb ischemia – a case series. Biomed Pap Med Fac Univ Palacky Olomouc Czech Repub. 2012;156:1–7.
32. Chuang KS, Liu JC. Long-term assessment of percutaneous stereotactic thermocoagulation of upper thoracic ganglionectomy and sympathectomy for palmar and craniofacial hyperhidrosis in 1742 cases. Neurosurgery. 2002;51:963–70.
33. Kucera TJ, Boezaart AP. Regional anesthesia does not consistently block ischemic pain: two further cases and a review of the literature. Pain Med. 15.2 (2014); 316–319.

34. Walker BJ, Noonan KJ, Bosenberg AT. Evolving compartment syndrome not masked by a continuous peripheral nerve block: evidence-based case management. Reg Anesth Pain Med. 2012;37:393–7.
35. Hyder N, Kessler S, Jennings A, et al. Compartment syndrome in tibial shaft fracture missed because of a local nerve block. J Bone Joint Surg Br. 1996;78:499–500.
36. Noorpuri B, Shahane S, Getty C. Acute compartment syndrome following revisional arthroplasty of the forefoot: the dangers of ankle block. Foot Ankle Int. 2000;21:680–2.
37. Uzel A, Steinman G. Thigh compartment syndrome after intramedularry femoral nailing: possible femoral nerve block influence on diagnosis timing. Rev Chir Orthop Traumatol. 2009;95:309–31.
38. Cometa MA, Esch AT, Boezaart AP. Did continuous femoral and sciatic nerve block obscure the diagnosis or delay treatment of acute lower leg compartment syndrome? A case report. Pain Med. 2011;12:823–8.
39. Nair GS, Soliman LM, Maheshwani K, et al. Importance of vigilant monitoring after continuous nerve block: lessons from a case report. Ochsner J. 2013;13(2):267–9.
40. Naoum JJ, Arbid EJ. Spinal cord stimulation for chronic limb ischemia. Methodist Debakey Cardiovasc J. 2013;9:99–102.
41. Deer TR, Raso LJ. Spinal cord stimulation for refractory angina pectoris and peripheral vascular disease. Pain Phys. 2006;9(4):347–52.
42. Reig E, Abejon D, del Pozo C, et al. Spinal cord stimulation in peripheral vascular disease: a retrospective analysis of 95 cases. Pain Pract. 2001;1(4):324–31.
43. Reig E, Abejon D. Spinal cord stimulation: a 20 year retrospective analysis in 260 patients. Neuromodulation. 2009;12(3):232–9.
44. Ubbink DT, Spincemaille GH, Prins MH, et al. Microcirculatory investigations to determine the effect of spinal cord stimulation for critical leg ischemia: the Dutch multicenter randomized controlled trial. J Vasc Surg. 1999;30(2):236–44.
45. Ubbink DT, Vermeulen H. Spinal cord stimulation for non-reconstructable chronic critical leg ischemia (review). Cochrane Database Syst Rev. 2009;1:1–7.
46. Mikkelsen WP. Intestinal angina. Am J Surg. 1957;94:262.
47. Glebova NO, Freischlag JA. In: Asher E, editor. Management of acute and chronic mesenteric ischemia. Haimovici's vascular surgery. 6th ed. Malden: Blackwell; 2012. p. 639–52.
48. Karahan OI, Kahnman G, Yikilmaz A, et al. Celiac artery compression syndrome: diagnosis with multislice CT. Diag Interv Radiol. 2007;13:90–3.
49. Sultan S, Hynes N, Elsafty N, et al. Eight years experience in the management of median arcuate ligament syndrome by decompression, celiac ganglion sympathectomy and selective revascularization. Vasc Endovasc Surg. 2013;47(8):614–9.
50. Valentine RJ, Martin JD, et al. Asymptomatic celiac and superior mesenteric artery stenosis are more prevalent among patients with unsuspected renal artery stenosis. J Vasc Surg. 1991;14:195.
51. Tulloch AW, Jimenez JC, Lawrence PF, et al. Laparoscopic versus open celiac ganglionectomy in patients with median arcuate ligament syndrome. J Vasc Surg. 2010;52(1):1283–9.
52. Caruso C, Lo Sapio D, Ragosa V, et al. Abdominal angina due to obstruction of mesenteric artery treated with spinal cord stimulation: a clinical case. Neuromodulation. 2011;14:146–50.

Part IV

Painful Disease States: Chronic Musculoskeletal Pain

Spine Pain

17

Michael B. Jacobs and Steven P. Cohen

Key Concepts

- Spine pain is an extremely common condition, with annual costs in the USA totaling more than $140 billion per year.
- Acute and subacute spine pain commonly resolves without interventions within several months. However, chronic pain is a more challenging clinical condition and often requires an interdisciplinary approach to treatment.
- Mechanical spine pain results from injury to muscles, fascia, discs, bones, or joints. Neuropathic spine pain results from injury to nerve roots, and central sensitization can ensue following prolonged symptoms from a mechanical injury.
- A focused differential diagnosis of spine pain can be made using history and physical exam, but a definitive diagnosis may require diagnostic interventions and/or imaging.
- Treatment of chronic spine pain should be individualized with an interdisciplinary approach that includes medications, physical therapy, psychological therapy, complementary and alternative medicine therapies, interventional pain treatments, and/or surgery.

M.B. Jacobs, MD, MPH
Physical Medicine & Rehabilitation, Walter Reed National Military Medical Center, Bethesda, MD, USA

S.P. Cohen, MD (✉)
Anesthesiology, Neurology, and Physical Medicine & Rehabilitation, Johns Hopkins School of Medicine and Walter Reed National Military Medical Center, Baltimore, MD, USA
e-mail: scohen40@jhmi.edu

Epidemiology

Spine pain is extremely common and poses an economic burden for individuals, families, and communities. Approximately half of all working Americans report an episode of low back pain (LBP) in the last year, and it represents the most frequent cause of disability in those younger than 45 years of age. Males and females have a similar risk of developing LBP, with individuals who have a first-degree relative with LBP being at increased risk. Approximately two-thirds of people will experience a significant episode of neck pain during their lives, with the annual prevalence rate exceeding 30%. Outcomes associated with neck pain are related to the status of pending litigation. Spine pain costs the USA an estimated $140 billion annually, with more than half being due to lost productivity.

J. Cheng, R.W. Rosenquist (eds.), *Fundamentals of Pain Medicine*,
https://doi.org/10.1007/978-3-319-64922-1_17

Categorization

Spine pain includes neck pain, which occurs from the occiput to the superior scapular region; mid-back pain, which is located from the superior scapular region to the costal margin; and low back pain, which includes pain between the costal margin and gluteal folds.

Spine pain can be categorized as acute (lasting less than 6 weeks), subacute (lasting 6 to 12 weeks), or chronic (lasting more than 12 weeks). Most cases of spine pain will resolve in the acute or subacute phase. Chronic spine pain is associated with poorer treatment outcomes.

Spine pain can also be categorized as mechanical or neuropathic. Mechanical pain implies pain originating from the vertebral column, such as that emanating from the facet or sacroiliac joints, vertebral bodies, muscles, ligaments, or discs. Neuropathic pain is caused by injury or dysfunction involving the somatosensory system, such as pain that develops as a consequence of nerve compression from a herniated disc or spinal stenosis. Neuropathic pain involves 37–59% of cases of LBP. In addition, some patients have both mechanical and neuropathic pain. For example, hypertrophy of the facet joints can cause mechanical LBP but also compress an exiting nerve root, resulting in neuropathic pain, and degenerative discs, which are a frequent cause of mechanical LBP, are more likely to herniate, and cause nerve root impingement than non-degenerative discs.

Pathophysiology

The most common etiologies of spine pain include injury or degenerative changes in vertebral or adjacent paraspinal structures. Mechanical pain is caused by activation of nociceptors from a painful stimulus, such as injury to muscles, soft tissues, bones, joints, or skin. The injury may be caused by a seemingly innocuous event, like a cough or change in position, from a traumatic event like a fall or motor vehicle crash, or from a repetitive activity like running or lifting. Neuropathic pain can also be caused by the activation of nociceptors from a painful stimulus, but the injury occurs directly in tissues of the nervous system, such as peripheral nerves, nerve roots, or the spinal cord, which can result in myelopathy. In essence, two things separate neuropathic from nociceptive pain. First, neuropathic pain directly affects nervous tissue, thereby bypassing the stage of transduction. Second, injury to a major nerve is more likely to lead to chronic pain than injury to a nonnervous somatic structure. In addition, repetitive activation of nociceptors from any cause can result in peripheral and central sensitization.

Clinical Features and Diagnosis

Important historical features to annotate include how and when the pain began. The examiner should obtain a detailed history that includes pain pattern, intensity, duration, location, exacerbating and alleviating factors, and associated symptoms such as weakness, numbness, or paresthesias. "Red flag" symptoms should be investigated, such as fever, unexplained weight loss, or bowel or bladder dysfunction, which may indicate an urgent pathological process. A comprehensive review of systems should include a history of psychiatric disease or current symptoms of psychological involvement, pending litigation, and other potential forms of secondary gain. These factors are sometimes referred to as "yellow flags" and may help determine a risk for chronicity as part of a biopsychosocial model of pain.

Myofascial Pain

Up to 80% of LBP has no clear etiology and is usually attributed to injury of muscles and soft tissues. Increased muscle fiber activity has been found in LBP patients irrespective of the cause, so myofascial involvement will be either a primary or secondary feature in most cases. Spasms and tender points are common features on exam. The presence of trigger points, which are taut bands of muscle with "contraction knots" that reproduce a patient's typical symptoms when palpated, may be a source of peripheral/central sensitization and identify a target for multimodal treatment.

Cervical strains and sprains usually follow a traumatic event such as a fall, motor vehicle accident, or sports injury. Pain may be associated with posterior headaches and demonstrate a somatic referral pattern. Mechanical neck pain is often aggravated by cervical motion and improves with rest. Physical examination may demonstrate decreased range of motion, muscle spasm, and tenderness in the cervical paraspinal region. Neurological exam is generally normal with "give-way or pain-induced" weakness. X-rays may demonstrate a fracture, show loss of cervical lordosis, and indicate spondylolisthesis or stenosis, but unlike MRI, plain films are incapable of demonstrating disc pathology.

Facet Arthropathy

Facet joint (or zygapophyseal joint)-mediated pain may account for 10–15% of mechanical LBP, with the prevalence increasing with age. The prevalence of cervical facet-mediated pain is between 27% and 63% of individuals with chronic neck pain, being frequently associated with a history of whiplash injury. The prevalence of thoracic facet-mediated pain is estimated to be approximately 42–48% in patients with chronic mid-back pain.

Patients with facetogenic pain typically report unilateral or bilateral paraspinal pain, with or without sclerotomal referral. Referral patterns often extend into the proximal extremity, but there is significant overlap between different spinal levels (e.g., between L4-L5 and L5-S1 facet joint pain) and between different structures (i.e., facetogenic and discogenic pain from L5 to S1). In addition, greater stimulus intensity may result in more distal pain radiation. Paraspinal tenderness may be the only reliable finding consistent with facet-mediated pain, but a thorough exam will help to rule out other etiologies. Other exam maneuvers typically performed, such as "facet loading" (i.e., pain worsened by extension-rotation), do not correlate well with diagnosis. Currently, the most reliable method of diagnosis is to inject local anesthetic into the facet joint or to block the nerves that innervate the joint (i.e., medial branch or posterior primary ramus block). In general, imaging is not very useful in selecting patients for facet interventions, though patients with normal imaging are less likely to have facetogenic pain.

Sacroiliac Joint Pain

Sacroiliac joint-mediated pain may account for 15–25% of cases of mechanical LBP, with highest prevalence found in young adults and elderly. The source of pain can include intra- and extra-articular pathology. Extra-articular pathology is more common in younger individuals, while intra-articular pain is more likely to present as bilateral symptoms and occur in the elderly. Pain is often described in the sacral region of the back, with occasional radiation into the posterior thighs or groin. The extension in the distal extremity is noted in less than 30% of individuals. No individual examination maneuver correlates well with diagnosis, but a combination (≥3) of positive provocative tests (e.g., Patrick's and Gaenslen's tests) has been shown to be associated with ≥75% sensitivity and specificity in identifying individuals with a painful sacroiliac joint. The most accurate diagnostic test is a low-volume anesthetic injection (Fig. 17.1).

Internal Disc Disruption (IDD)

IDD, also known as discogenic pain, may account for between 20% and 45% of cases of mechanical LBP and is more common in younger and middle-aged adults. Pain is often reported to be midline in the low back and is worsened with sitting or bending. The pain may radiate into the legs in a non-dermatomal pattern. There is generally more midline and less paraspinal tenderness compared with facet- or sacroiliac-mediated pain. Diagnosis is usually made based on a combination of

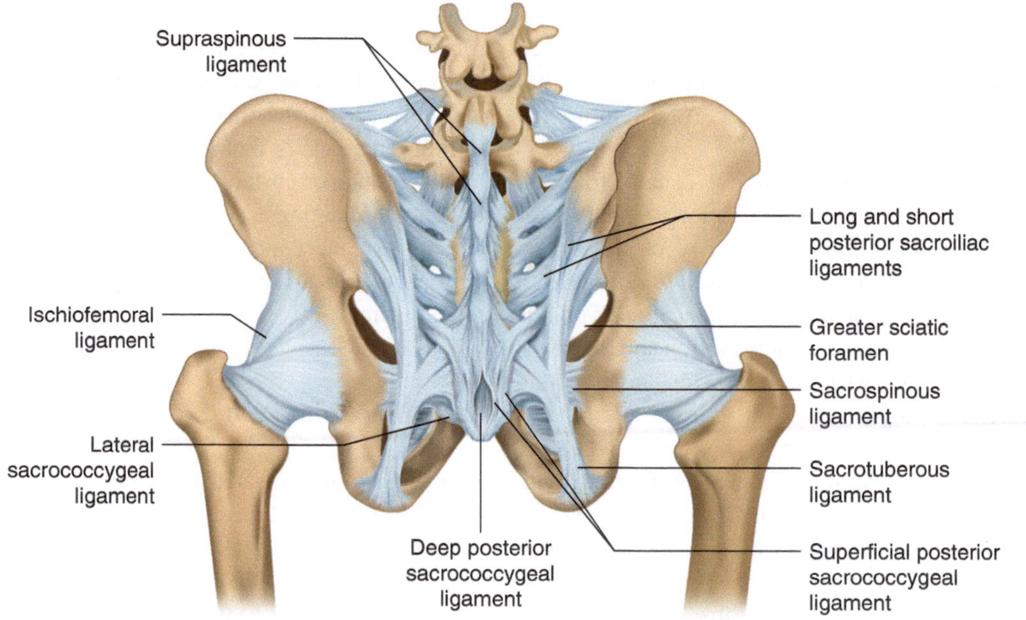

Fig. 17.1 Posterior view of the articulations and associated ligaments of the sacroiliac joint and surrounding structures. Injury to any of the surrounding ligaments or joint can result in sacroiliac joint pain

symptoms, degenerative changes of the discs on imaging, and a lack of response to facet or sacroiliac joint injections. Provocative discography is sometimes considered to be the "gold standard" for identifying a painful disc but is characterized by a high false-positive rate in some patients (e.g., those with somatization and other forms of psychopathology and individuals with previous back surgery), and there is some evidence that piercing the annulus with a needle may accelerate future disc degeneration and increase the risk for herniation.

Approximately 30% of people with chronic neck pain report a history of trauma. In patients with neck pain and a history of trauma, 20% of patients may have IDD alone, and another 40% may have combined IDD and facet pathology. In video-radiographic studies performed in restrained cadavers in the 1970s, motor vehicle accidents resulted in injury to the intervertebral discs in 90% of cases and the anterior longitudinal ligament in 80%. Axial pain usually predominates in those with IDD, but patients may also report a variety of symptoms such as occipital headaches, nonradicular arm pain, facial pain, anterior chest wall pain, dysphagia, ocular dysfunction, and tinnitus. Symptoms may be aggravated by coughing, sneezing, or lifting and improve when the head is supported. Physical exam may demonstrate tenderness to palpation along the spinous processes but is otherwise nonspecific. MRI is noninvasive and usually reveals loss of disc height, signal intensity, and disc bulging but is inherently nonspecific. The only technique that purports to correlate symptoms with pathology is discography, but the procedure is invasive, carries significant risk, and has not been definitively shown to improve surgical outcomes in the MRI era.

Herniated Disc

Herniated disc is a common cause of lumbar radiculopathy, particularly in younger people, with the peak prevalence occurring between 35 and 50 years of age. Patients will commonly report intermittent radiation of neuropathic pain in a unilateral dermatomal distribution, with leg pain often more significant than back pain. Exam may reveal sensory changes, motor weakness, or abnormal deep tendon reflexes corresponding to the affected nerve root. A positive straight leg raising test is over 80% sensitive for detecting L5 or S1 nerve root involvement, while a positive crossed straight leg raise test is highly specific for lumbar radiculopathy but carries low sensitivity. Electrodiagnostic studies can be helpful in challenging diagnostic cases and is a very specific test for lumbar radiculopathy. MRI is usually not required and many patients with herniated discs experience no symptoms. When present, the location of the herniation strongly influences the symptoms, with the most common scenario being a posterolateral herniation causing symptoms in the subjacent traversing nerve root (i.e., L4-L5 affecting the L5 nerve root; Fig. 17.2).

Cervical radiculopathy is associated with an annual prevalence rate ranging between 83 and 350 per 100,000 people, with a peak incidence occurring in the 50–55-year age range. Patients with cervical radiculopathy due to disc herniation often report the acute onset of limb pain, whereas radicular pain due to degenerative changes occurs more gradually. Pain usually follows a dermatomal distribution (though in many cases there is multiple nerve root involvement) and is exacerbated by activities that increase subarachnoid pressure, such as coughing or sneezing. Physical exam may demonstrate atrophy, weakness, and changes in sensation and reflexes in the areas innervated by the affected nerve root(s). A Spurling's maneuver may exacerbate symptoms but has a sensitivity rate of around 50%, and the shoulder abduction test may relieve symptoms. A Hoffman's sign should be assessed for possible myelopathy. MRI is the best imaging modality to identify and assess cervical radiculopathy, but because of the low specificity, findings must be correlated with signs and symptoms for accurate diagnosis. Electrodiagnostic exam is highly specific for cervical radiculopathy, can rule out other etiologies for limb pain, and may assist in surgical planning.

Spinal Stenosis

Spinal stenosis is both a clinical and radiological diagnosis, occurring more commonly in people

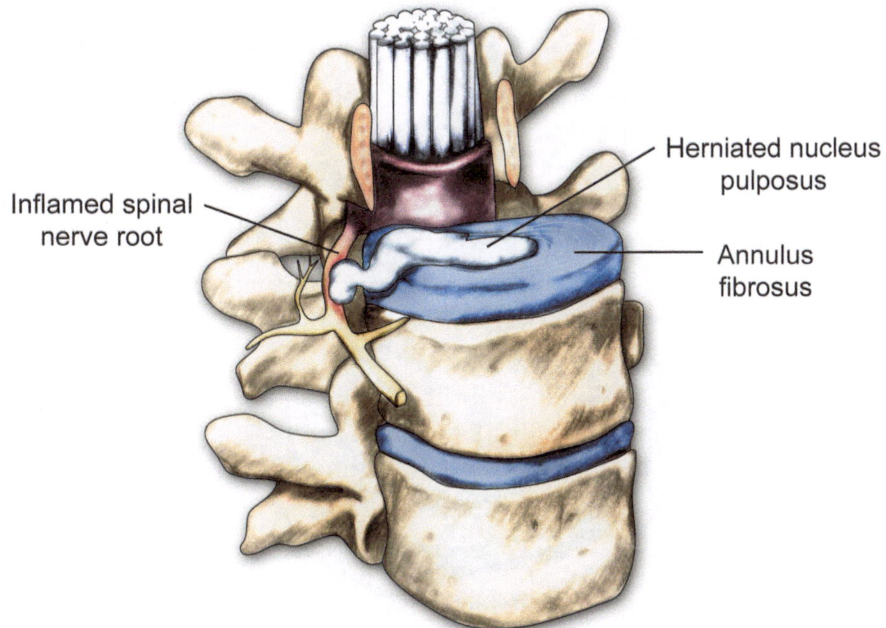

Fig. 17.2 Herniated nucleus pulposus causing nerve root impingement. Radicular symptoms may result from either chemical mediators released from degenerated discs or mechanical irritation

over the age of 60 years. It is characterized by narrowing of the spinal canal resulting in unilateral or bilateral neuropathic leg symptoms. Classically, patients present with neurogenic claudication, which is calf or foot pain that improves with forward bending (e.g., when leaning over to push a shopping cart, known as the "shopping cart sign") or rest. Specific etiologies may include disc bulge, ligamentum flavum hypertrophy, facet hypertrophy, osteophyte formation, and spondylolisthesis, which are most apparent on MRI. Electrodiagnostic studies may also help distinguish spinal stenosis from radiculopathy or other causes of leg pain, such as plexopathy, peripheral neuropathy, or polyneuropathy (Figs. 17.3 and 17.4).

Visceral/Other

Visceral pain may be referred to the low back and accounts for less than 2% of LBP cases. Causes may include gastrointestinal disease (e.g., inflammatory bowel disease or diverticulitis), renal disease (e.g., nephrolithiasis), vascular disease (e.g., abdominal aortic aneurysm), and pelvic visceral disease (e.g., endometriosis or prostatitis).

Psychogenic Pain

Chronic pain and psychological distress are often closely associated. Patients with concurrent psychiatric illness are more likely to develop chronic pain after an acute pain episode, and those with chronic pain are more likely to develop active psychiatric symptoms. A thorough psychological assessment of patients with chronic pain may help to identify those most likely to benefit from psychological interventions such as cognitive-behavioral therapy and procedural interventions.

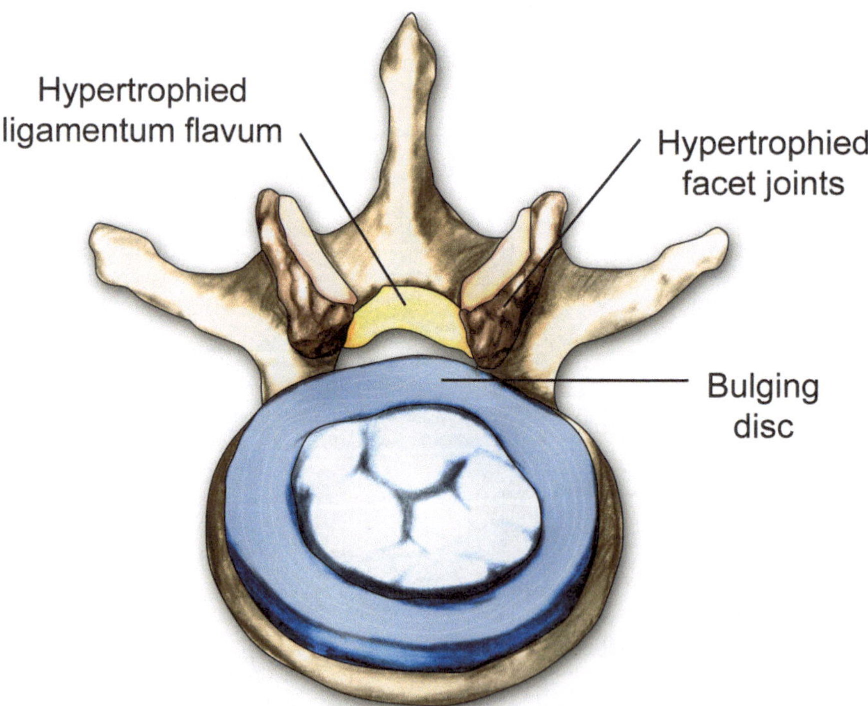

Fig. 17.3 Axial view of a vertebral body demonstrating central spinal stenosis. In addition to the illustrated pathologies, other causes of spinal stenosis include foraminal narrowing, osteophyte formation, spondylolisthesis, postsurgical changes, and congenitally short pedicles

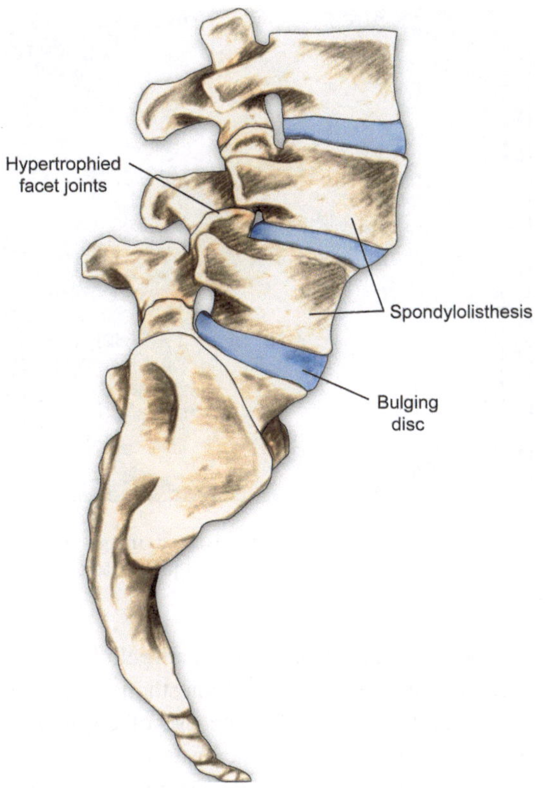

Fig. 17.4 Sagittal view of a lumbar spine demonstrating and foraminal spinal stenosis at L4-L5 and L5-S1

Treatment

Most cases of acute low back pain without red flag symptoms will resolve spontaneously within 4–6 weeks, and over 70% improve by 12 weeks. Bed rest should be avoided after 24 h, with a slow but steady return to activities and exercise as tolerated. Heat or cold modalities and over-the-counter medications, such as acetaminophen or ibuprofen, are often sufficient to control symptoms. For more severe acute pain or pain not improving with home-based therapies, additional treatment options should be considered.

Pharmacotherapy

Acetaminophen and nonsteroidal anti-inflammatory drugs (NSAIDs) are first-line treatments for nociceptive pain. Acetaminophen is considered the safest medication for spine pain but may have lesser efficacy than NSAIDs. NSAIDs are clearly helpful but contain a ceiling effect, potential for side effects with prolonged use, and are not considered very helpful for neuropathic pain.

Muscle relaxants may be beneficial for acute and chronic spine pain, but they are not effective for neuropathic pain. Benzodiazepines are effective for muscle spasm but should be used with caution due to a high risk of side effects.

Opioids are a reasonable option for the treatment of acute moderate to severe pain not relieved with NSAIDs, acetaminophen, or muscle relaxants. Opioids should be avoided or used with caution in chronic pain and should only be considered when other medications and nonpharmacologic interventions have failed. Long-term opioid use requires regular monitoring for analgesia, side effects, functional gains, and aberrant behaviors.

Tricyclic antidepressants (TCAs) are effective for chronic spine pain. In addition, TCAs, anticonvulsants, (e.g., gabapentin and pregabalin), and serotonin-norepinephrine reuptake inhibitors (e.g., duloxetine) may be beneficial for the treatment of radicular or neuropathic pain. The choice of medication is often based on the side effect profile. Particularly in the elderly, the use of these medications should be monitored for cognitive and psychomotor effects.

Complementary and Alternative Medicine (CAM)

CAM therapies have become more commonly utilized for treatment of pain over the past few decades. Many CAM treatments are recommended for back pain because they are relatively noninvasive and unlikely to cause harm for most patients. Massage therapy, spinal manipulation, and to a lesser extent transcutaneous electrical nerve stimulation (TENS) may be useful for short-term benefit of acute and chronic non-neuropathic spine pain, although there is less evidence for long-term benefit. Acupuncture is more effective than no treatment for both axial and radicular pain, but there is conflicting evidence for benefit compared to sham acupuncture, and questions regarding whether "sham" acupuncture constitutes a true placebo. Herbal medications may provide short-term benefit in nonspecific LBP. There is no evidence that lumbar or cervical traction is helpful for axial or radicular low back or neck pain.

Exercise

Exercise has not been proven to be effective in acute spine pain, but studies support its effectiveness in the treatment of chronic spine pain. It is likely that many combinations of strengthening, flexibility, and aerobic exercises produce similar benefits. Specific strategies recommended include postural retraining, lumbar stabilization/core strengthening, and scapular stabilization, depending on the pain location and deficits identified on exam. For those who cannot tolerate land-based activities, aquatic exercise may provide benefits such as reduced gravitational stress, pain reduction, and decreased fear avoidance.

Interventional Procedures

Various interventional procedures are available for the treatment of spine pain in either the acute or chronic stage. Epidural steroid injections (ESIs) may be used as a first-line treatment for radicular pain or when other treatment strategies are not successful. ESIs have been shown in some studies to reduce the need for surgery and tend to work best in patients with intermittent symptoms, limb pain greater than axial pain, and for shorter duration of symptoms (less than 6 months). They are also used to reduce pain associated with spinal stenosis, although the effects tend to be short-lived for this indication.

Both intra- and extra-articular corticosteroid injections may be helpful for sacroiliac joint-mediated pain but are less helpful for the treatment of facet-mediated pain and ineffective for discogenic pain (Fig. 17.5).

Trigger point injections are helpful to reduce pain associated with myofascial trigger points. Dry needling is as effective as needling with local anesthetic, but post-procedure pain relief may be greater with the use of local anesthetic. There is insufficient evidence that the use of corticosteroids or botulinum toxin increases effectiveness, though botulinum toxin appears to be effective for cervical dystonia.

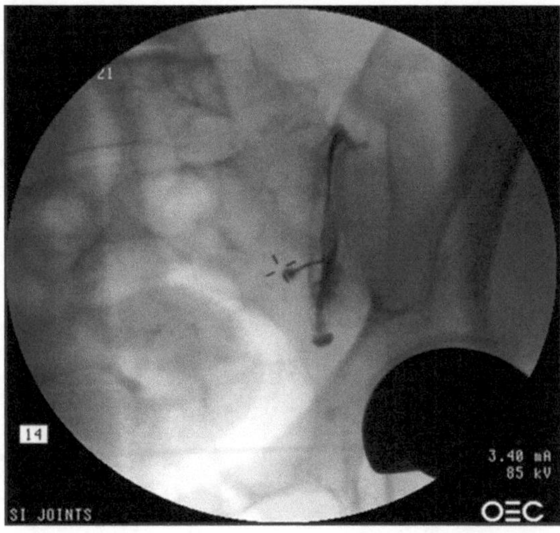

Fig. 17.5 Anteroposterior fluoroscopic image demonstrating a right-sided intra-articular SI joint block

Radiofrequency denervation, which generates heat to lesion nerves innervating painful joints, has been shown in randomized controlled studies as being a useful treatment in lumbar and cervical facet and SIJ-mediated pain. Variations in radiofrequency technique (e.g., cooled radiofrequency and fluid modulation) are available to enhance lesion size and may be particularly beneficial for the treatment of SI joint pain, whereby the number and location of the lateral branches that innervate the joint vary from patient to patient, side to side, and level to level (Figs. 17.6 and 17.7).

Vertebral augmentation procedures, including kyphoplasty or vertebroplasty, may be considered for the treatment of acute or subacute vertebral compression fractures that do not respond to medications. Although non-placebo-controlled randomized trials support kyphoplasty for osteoporotic compression fractures, two placebo-controlled studies evaluating vertebroplasty failed to demonstrate a statistical difference in either pain or function. It is important to note that in patients with vertebral fractures, increased

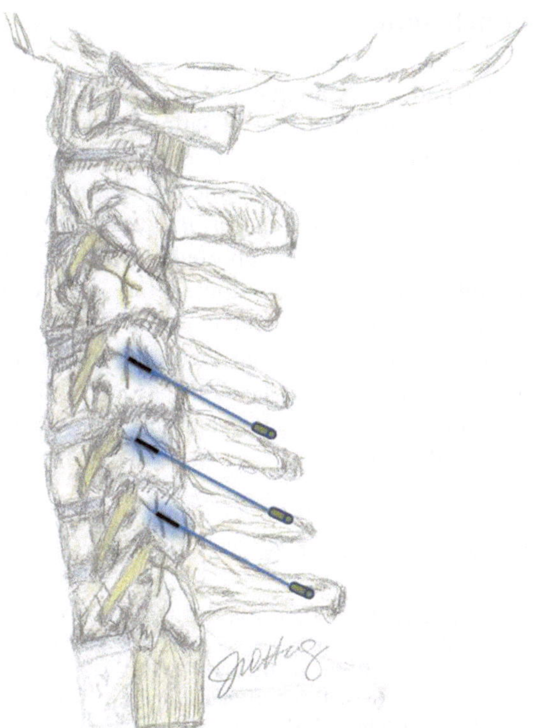

Fig. 17.6 Lateral view of radiofrequency denervation of the C4-C6 cervical facet joints (From Brummett CB, Cohen SP. Pathogenesis, diagnosis, and treatment of zygapophyseal (facet) joint pain. In: Benzon HT, Rathmell JP, Wu CL, Turk DC, Argoff CE, Hurley RW, editors. *Raj's Practical Management of Pain*. 5th ed. London: Mosby Elsevier; 2013. p. 816–45; with permission. Drawing by Julie H.Y. Huang, MD, MBA)

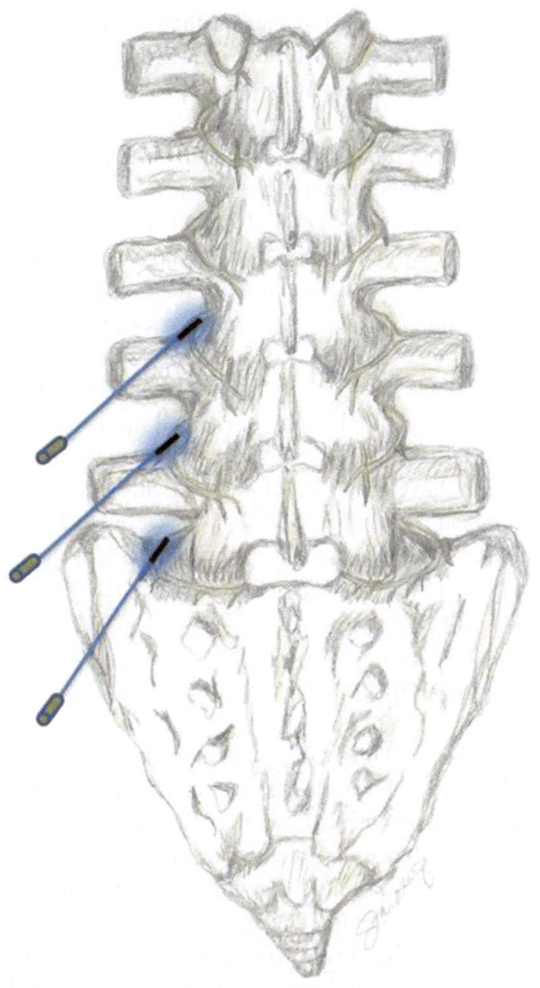

Fig. 17.7 Posterior view of radiofrequency denervation of the L3-L4 medial branches and L5 dorsal ramus, innervating the L4-S1 facet joints (From Brummett CB, Cohen SP. Pathogenesis, diagnosis, and treatment of zygapophyseal (facet) joint pain. In: Benzon HT, Rathmell JP, Wu CL, Turk DC, Argoff CE, Hurley RW, editors. *Raj's Practical Management of Pain*. 5th ed. London: Mosby Elsevier; 2013. p. 816–45; with permission. Drawing by Julie H.Y. Huang, MD, MBA)

stress on the affected facet joints may play a significant role in pain generation.

Percutaneous disc decompression is an alternative to surgery for radicular pain, which may provide at least a year of significant pain improvement in well-selected individuals with small (<6 mm), contained herniated discs confirmed by discography or advanced imaging.

Spinal cord stimulation is a neuromodulatory treatment which has demonstrated effectiveness compared to conventional management and repeat surgery in the treatment of failed back surgery syndrome associated with radicular symptoms. The best candidates for spinal cord stimulation are those with extremity pain greater than axial pain of neuropathic origin. In addition to post-laminectomy syndrome, spinal cord stimulation has been shown in uncontrolled studies to be an effective treatment for radicular pain in select patients who have not undergone surgery and to a lesser extent axial spinal pain.

Surgery

In general, the outcomes of surgery are best when it is performed acutely for progressive nerve root injury due to a herniated disc. Patients should be referred early for "red flag" symptoms or if they display motor or reflex deficits on exam. Decompressive surgery may improve symptoms for up to 6 months in patients with lumbar radiculopathy, but most studies have shown that there is no significant difference in outcomes after 2 years compared to those individuals treated conservatively. In patients with spinal stenosis or significant spondylolisthesis, benefits from surgery can last for up to 2 years. For chronic axial LBP due to degenerative processes, studies have shown that only about 15–40% of patients will experience significant pain relief and functional improvement from surgery. For neck pain, recent systematic reviews have failed to demonstrate any long-term significant differences for surgery compared to conservative treatment for mechanical neck pain, cervical radiculopathy, or myelopathy.

Prevention

Primary prevention of spinal pain is difficult to achieve for a variety of reasons, including the early age of onset of the first-time episode, the high prevalence and recurrence rates, and a lack of known modifiable risk factors. As a result, most efforts are aimed at secondary prevention.

Exercise has been proven to reduce the incidence of LBP and neck pain development and recurrence. Unfortunately, there is insufficient evidence for many other strategies used by patients and recommended by practitioners, including stress management, back supports, shoe inserts, and back schools/educational programs. Workplace training (e.g., material handling) has not been clearly proven to reduce the incidence of LBP or disability.

Conclusions

Spinal pain is a leading cause of disability in all age groups in industrialized nations. In addition to the personal and social consequences, it exacts an enormous economic toll. Despite the increasing expenditures for the treatment of back and neck pain, the reported prevalence and disability rates have continued to grow. The ideal management of spinal pain involves an interdisciplinary approach incorporating pharmacotherapy, structured exercise programs, and psychological and interventional therapies when indicated.

Suggested Reading

1. Balague F, Mannion AF, Pellise F, Cedraschi C. Non-specific low back pain. Lancet. 2012;379:482–91.
2. Benzon HT, Rathmell JP, Wu CL, Turk DC, Argoff CE, Hurley RW. Practical management of pain. 5th ed. Philadelphia: Mosby; 2014.
3. Bicket MC, Gupta A, Brown CH, Cohen SP. Epidural injections for spinal pain. A systematic review and meta-analysis evaluating the 'control' injections in randomized control trials. Anesthesiology. 2013;119:907–31.
4. Braddom RL. Physical medicine and rehabilitation. 4th ed. Philadelphia: Saunders; 2011.
5. Chung JW, Zeng Y, Wong TK. Drug therapy for the treatment of chronic nonspecific low back pain: systematic review and meta-analysis. Pain Physician. 2013;16:E685–704.
6. Cohen SP, Argoff CE, Carragee EJ. Management of low back pain. BMJ. 2008;337:a2718.
7. Cohen SP, Huang JH, Brummett C. Facet joint pain-advances in patient selection and management. Nature Rev Rheumatol. 2013;9:101–16.
8. Jacobs WC, Rubinstein SM, Koes B, Van Tulder MW, Peul WC. Evidence for surgery in degenerative lumbar spine disorders. Best Pract & Res Clin Rheum. 2013;27(5):673–84.

Joint Pain

18

Michael P. Schaefer and Meredith Konya

Key Concepts

- Ultrasound guidance is often very helpful for improving the accuracy of joint injections. Ultrasound is also useful for imaging tendons, ligaments, and soft tissues but is usually not indicated for diagnosing cartilage tears.
- X-rays in osteoarthritis typically show the hallmark signs of joint space narrowing, osteophytes, bony sclerosis, and subchondral cysts.
- Patients affected by rheumatoid arthritis typically exhibit symmetrical swelling of the metacarpal phalangeal and interphalangeal joints.
- Shoulder pain has many potential causes. Patients with large rotator cuff tears should be referred promptly to surgery. Early intervention with a corticosteroid injection and therapy is important for adhesive capsulitis (frozen shoulder).
- Most cases of elbow arthritis are caused by prior trauma or inflammatory arthropathies.
- Corticosteroid injections for epicondylitis may lead to further tendon degeneration and worse outcomes in long-term follow-up.
- Hip osteoarthritis may present with either groin or buttock pain. Pain from the joint may be easily misdiagnosed as radiculopathy as it often radiates to the leg or shin. Reduced range of motion is often the first sign of hip osteoarthritis.
- Knee effusion is indicative of intra-articular pathology such as arthritis or meniscus tear. Regular exercise should be the first-line treatment for knee osteoarthritis.
- Effusions in the ankle/foot joints are relatively uncommon and should raise suspicion for inflammatory joint diseases such as gout and pseudogout.

M.P. Schaefer, MD (✉)
Musculoskeletal Physical Medicine and Rehabilitation, Cleveland Clinic, Cleveland, OH, USA

Associate Professor of Medicine,
Cleveland Clinic Lerner College of Medicine,
Case Western Reserve University,
Cleveland, OH, USA
e-mail: schaefm5@ccf.org

M. Konya, MD
Musculoskeletal Physical Medicine and Rehabilitation, Cleveland Clinic,
Cleveland, OH, USA

Introduction

Musculoskeletal pain affects the muscles, ligaments, tendons, bones, and nerves. It can be acute (having a recent onset) or chronic (long-lasting), localized in one area or widespread. Pain from overuse is common and affects 33% of adults. Since many of conditions of the musculoskeletal pain such as facet joint of the spine are discussed in other chapters, we focus on pain of the joints of the extremities, which are typically results of

J. Cheng, R.W. Rosenquist (eds.), *Fundamentals of Pain Medicine*,
https://doi.org/10.1007/978-3-319-64922-1_18

overuse, osteoarthritis, rheumatoid arthritis, and trauma. Common symptoms include:

- *Joint pain*: Joint injuries and diseases usually produce a stiff, aching, "arthritic" pain. The pain may range from mild to severe and worsens when moving the joint. The joints may also swell. Joint inflammation (arthritis) is a common cause of pain. It may be very severe with inflammatory arthritis.
- *Tendon and ligament pain*: Pains in the tendons or ligaments are often caused by injuries, including sprains. This type of musculoskeletal pain often becomes worse when the affected area is stretched or moved.
- *Muscle pain*: The feeling of muscles around the joint being pulled or overworked. It may be accompanied by muscle spasms and cramps. Muscle pain can be caused by an injury, an autoimmune reaction, loss of blood flow to the muscle, infection, or a tumor.
- *Bone pain*: Joint pain may arise from bones around the joint. Bone pain is usually deep, penetrating, or dull. It most commonly results from injury. It is important to be sure that the pain is not related to a fracture or tumor.
- *Neuropathic pain:* Nerves innervating the joint may be sensitized due to chronic inflammation, repeated microtrauma, compromised blood supply, or surgical scars. Thus neuropathic pain may be part of joint pain. In addition, joint pain may be associated with *"tunnel" syndromes* due to nerve compression, such as carpal tunnel syndrome, cubital tunnel syndrome, and tarsal tunnel syndrome. These syndromes are described elsewhere.
- *Fatigue and/or sleep disturbances*

The diagnosis of joint pain is based on a thorough medical history, a hands-on examination looking for the source of the pain, and necessary tests that may include:

- Blood tests to confirm a diagnosis, such as rheumatoid arthritis
- X-rays to take images of the bones
- CT scans to get an even more detailed look at the bones
- Ultrasound to image tendons, ligaments, and soft tissues
- MRIs to further look at soft tissues such as muscles, cartilage, ligaments, and tendons

Joint pain is best treated by treating its cause. Other treatments include:

- Physical or occupational therapy
- Using a splint to immobilize the affected joint and allow healing
- Using heat or cold
- Reducing workload and increasing rest
- Reducing stress through relaxation and biofeedback techniques
- Acupuncture or acupressure
- Injections with anesthetic or anti-inflammatory medications in or around the painful sites
- Strengthening and conditioning exercises
- Stretching exercises
- Chiropractic care
- Therapeutic massage

Shoulder Joint Pain

The shoulder is a complicated joint consisting of the scapula and its articulation with the rib cage (scapulothoracic joint), clavicle through the acromioclavicular (AC) joint, glenohumeral joint, rotator cuff, subacromial bursa, biceps tendon, and overlying myofascial structures. Therefore, proper identification of the pain generator in the shoulder joint syndromes can be challenging. Fortunately, injections are quite helpful in both relieving symptoms and identifying the cause of patient's pain.

Acromioclavicular Joint Pain

This syndrome is common but often unrecognized. AC joint pain tends to localize to the superior aspect of the shoulder but can radiate to the scapula or anterior chest. It is exacerbated by overhead motions, lying on the affected side, or reaching (all similar to subacromial bursitis). However, painful AC joints are usually quite tender, and patients often have significant imaging findings around this joint or a history of shoulder separation. Also, patients that do excessive overhead lifting, particularly body builders and power lifters, cause damage to the distal clavicle and thus develop secondary AC joint pain.

Subacromial Bursitis

More properly known as the subacromial/subdeltoid bursa, this layer of bursal tissue and fluid provides cushioning and lubrication on the superior surface of the rotator cuff. Impingement of the humeral head on the under surface of the acromion or AC joint can cause bursal thickening and inflammation. As opposed to rotator cuff disorders, patients with subacromial bursitis usually have pain with passive end-range abduction and flexion (impingement signs), whereas rotator cuff patients have pain with active external rotation and abduction in the neutral position. However, there is often overlap between the two symptoms, and they commonly coexist.

Rotator Cuff Injury

The tendons of the rotator cuff may be subject to chronic, cumulative, and overuse conditions but also may be injured daily. The supraspinatus tendon is most commonly involved, followed by the infraspinatus tendon. Patients often present with pain and weakness on active abduction and/or external rotation. Large, full thickness rotator cuff tears may cause palpable atrophy in the subacromial space and over the scapula. These more severe, acute injuries should be addressed with surgical repair promptly to avoid tendon retraction which makes the repair challenging. Chronic, partial thickness, or small rotator cuff tears often can be managed conservatively.

Glenohumeral (GH) Joint Disorders

These consist of osteoarthritis, glenoid labrum tear, adhesive capsulitis, and glenohumeral instability.

Osteoarthritis

GH joint osteoarthritis often results from a history of trauma or dislocation but can be the result of a normal degenerative process as well. Patients may also develop this many years after rotator cuff injury, particularly if the rotator cuff injury is left untreated. Aside from imaging findings, patients usually have reduced range of motion; deep pain that may be anterior, lateral, or posterior; and pain that often is referred into the arm.

Glenoid Labral Tears

This injury is common in young, active patients with a history of shoulder subluxation or dislocation. The pain presentation is similar to that of rotator cuff injury, but specific provocation maneuvers can sometimes elicit a deep "clunk" or mechanical symptoms in the shoulder.

Glenohumeral Instability

Instability includes two subsets: multidirectional instability, which is more common in young female patients with a history of other joint laxity, and traumatic, unidirectional instability which is usually caused by injury with resultant capsule and labral defects. In general, multidirectional instability patients do poorly with surgical stabilization, whereas unidirectional patients respond well to surgery.

Adhesive Capsulitis (aka Frozen Shoulder)

Frozen shoulder usually presents with no apparent cause and can occur after a minor trauma. Diabetic patients, particularly with poor glucose control, are three to five times more likely to develop this condition. It usually presents with severe pain at onset, and followed by progressive stiffening over the ensuing 6 months. The natural history includes a "frozen" phase for 6–12 months and then a "thawing" phase that results in improvement over a period of 1–2 years. Early intervention with physical therapy, glenohumeral and subacromial corticosteroid injections may help to reduce the severity and duration of the condition.

Biceps Tendinitis

This condition usually involves the long head of the muscle, as its tendon passes through the bicipital groove of the humerus on the anterior shoulder. It may be exacerbated by impingement and is commonly mistaken as subacromial bursitis or glenohumeral arthritis. In trauma, the biceps tendon is commonly torn at the same time as the superior labrum. Patients usually present with tenderness over the bicipital groove and pain with active forward flexion of the shoulder.

Diagnosis of Shoulder Pain

History and physical examination are usually adequate to provide initial diagnostic information and to initiate treatment. Appropriate physical examination of the shoulder requires practice and demands careful interpretation by the examiner to identify the precise location of symptoms during provocative maneuvers. A careful examination of the cervical spine and myofascial structures should be included. When patients have significant strength deficits, atrophy, or history of trauma, a low threshold for initial X-rays and advanced imaging should be employed. Ultrasound can be used to make or confirm a diagnosis of rotator cuff tear; however, ultrasound is very user dependent, and diagnostic scanning should be done only by experienced providers. Ultrasound can simultaneously be used with diagnostic and therapeutic injections. MRI remains the goal standard for imaging of all the shoulder structures and is particularly better than ultrasound for the glenohumeral joint and labral tears. Labral tears are often unrecognized in standard MRI sequences, so injection of intra-articular contrast prior to imaging is commonly recommended for young patients with a history of trauma. In an older population, the rotator cuff is usually injured at the same time as the glenoid labrum, so standard MRI sequences may be enough to justify diagnostic arthroscopy at the time of rotator cuff repair.

Management of Shoulder Pain

The multiple conditions that cause shoulder pain often share similar management principles. Conservative measures such as ice, analgesics, and anti-inflammatories are adequate for patients with mild symptoms. Ice is particularly beneficial for the shoulder, whereas heat is more helpful for myofascial structures. Analgesics and NSAIDs are often needed for patients with moderate pain. For patients with severe pain, relief is best obtained with corticosteroid injection prior to the initiation of therapies. The accuracy of corticosteroid injections is greatly enhanced with ultrasound guidance.

For all conditions affecting the shoulder complex, appropriate scapular stabilization and positioning is the foundation for rehabilitation. This includes proper posture of the thoracic spine, as kyphosis often leads to scapular protraction and resultant impingement. Likewise, chronic pain in the shoulder predisposes to abnormal scapular positioning. Once the scapula is functioning appropriately, the rotator cuff may be strengthened to provide stability to the joint. Finally, patients may progress to more aggressive strengthening exercises, shoulder stabilization, and stimulation of functional activities.

Elbow Pain

There are three articulations within the elbow: humeroulnar, humeroradial, and proximal radioulnar joints which aid in flexion, extension, supination, and pronation. When the arm is fully extended, there is normally an anatomic valgus alignment, which is greater in women.

Lateral Epicondylitis

More commonly known as tennis elbow, lateral epicondylitis is actually a misnomer as the true pathophysiology is tendinosis. This tendinopathy is characterized by degenerative, not inflammatory, changes of the common extensor tendon as a result of repetitive wrist extension and forearm pronation/supination movements. This is the most common cause of elbow pain and results in microtearing of the extensor carpi radialis brevis (ECRB) tendon. Symptoms will present insidiously as tenderness at the tendon attachment to the lateral epicondyle and in the proximal tendon, with or without further radiation distally. Pain is worsened with resisted wrist extension. Weakness with grip strength may be noted. An entrapment neuropathy of the deep radial nerve may also occur in this region and should be considered in the differential diagnosis. Conservative treatments include avoidance of the aggravating activity, oral and topical NSAIDs, cryotherapy, and platelet-rich plasma (PRP) therapy. Therapy focuses on passive stretching and progressing to resistance training, counterforce bands, and other modalities (including electrical stimulation and iontophoresis). Corticosteroid injections can be considered if the patient continues to be symptomatic, however, despite short-term pain relief; these can lead to further tendon degeneration and worse outcomes in long-term follow-up. Surgical intervention may be indicated if other treatments fail and symptoms persist.

Medial Epicondylitis

Also known as golfer's elbow, medial epicondylitis has the same degenerative changes as in lateral epicondylitis; however, it affects the common flexor tendon. The changes are noted within the pronator teres (PT) and flexor carpi radialis (FCR) origins. Patients will present with tenderness over the medial epicondyle, and their symptoms can be reproduced with resisted wrist flexion and pronation. They will also note weakness with grip strength. A mild ulnar neuropathy may also develop. Conservative treatments include rest, ice, oral and topical NSAIDS, therapy/modalities, and immobilization. If modifications of poor ergonomics or throwing mechanics are indicated, these should be addressed as well. Corticosteroid injections are an option but should be used with caution so as to avoid further weakening of the tendon. Surgical intervention is rarely indicated.

Elbow Arthritis

Elbow involvement is common in rheumatoid and other inflammatory arthropathies, but the elbow is one of the joints least affected by osteoarthritis. Most patients with osteoarthritis have a history of trauma to the elbow (and therefore could be classified as post-traumatic arthritis). In the setting of a prior injury, ligamentous instability and abnormal wearing of the joint occur. Patients complain of pain, stiffness, and locking if a free fragment becomes trapped within the joint. In later stages, swelling may develop and put increased pressure on the ulnar nerve causing paresthesias. X-rays are usually diagnostic and commonly show osteophytes and a preserved joint space. Loss of full extension is most commonly noted early in the degenerative process. Treatment is conservative and includes oral NSAIDs, PT, activity modification, and potentially corticosteroid injections. Arthroscopy can provide symptom relief by removing loose bodies or degenerative tissues within the joint. Arthrodesis is an option for the elderly or those whom other treatment options have failed.

Wrist/Hand Pain

There are eight carpal bones within the wrist (proximal row, scaphoid, lunate, triquetrum, pisiform; distal row, trapezium, trapezoid, capitate, and hamate). The articulation between the rows is referred to as the midcarpal joint. There are five carpal metacarpal (CMC) joints, five metacarpal phalangeal (MCP) joints, four proximal interphalangeal (PIP) joints, four distal interphalangeal (DIP) joints, one interphalangeal joint

(IP) in the thumb, and a distal radial ulnar joint (DRUJ). The triangular fibrocartilage complex (TFCC) is located between the distal ulna and carpal bones and acts as the primary stabilizer of the DRUJ. Normally the wrist functions in flexion, extension, and radial and ulnar deviation.

Wrist/Hand Arthritis

The wrist and hand can be affected by both rheumatoid arthritis and osteoarthritis. In rheumatoid arthritis, articular cartilage is destroyed as a result of an autoimmune attack on the synovial tissue. Patients affected can exhibit swelling of the MCP and PIP joints only, ulnar deviation of the fingers, dorsal subluxation of the ulna, ulnar styloid erosion, and swan-neck and boutonniere deformities. X-rays will show periarticular osteopenia, erosions, and loss of the joint space. Osteoarthritis, on the other hand, is a noninflammatory process that results in articular cartilage deterioration and osteophytes at the bone margins. Patients can exhibit Heberden's nodes at the DIP and Bouchard's nodes at the PIP. There can be tenderness over the affected joint and crepitus with range of motion. Plain films aid in diagnosis and may show joint space narrowing, subchondral sclerosis, subchondral cysts, and osteophytes. Treatment includes lifestyle modification, NSAIDs, bracings, therapy, DMARDs/biologic agents (only for rheumatoid), or ultimately joint replacement.

Carpal Metacarpal Joint (CMC) Osteoarthritis

Osteoarthritis at the base of the thumb is the most common arthropathy of the wrist/hand. The first CMC joint allows for movement in multiple planes and is stabilized to the trapezium by multiple ligaments. Axial loading and ligamentous laxity contributes to the development of osteoarthritis at this joint. It can lead to significant pain, reduced range of motion, and notable deformities. Treatment is conservative and focuses on management of symptoms. Options include NSAIDs, built-up grips, intra-articular corticosteroid injections, and thumb spica splints. Viscosupplement (hyaluronic acid) injection may have a role. However, surgical referral for ligamentous reconstruction or fusion of the joint is appropriate for refractory cases.

Hip Pain

The hip consists of a deep acetabulum (socket) and spherical-shaped femoral head (ball). A hip joint is stabilized by the acetabular labrum, ligamentous capsule, and multiple muscles, including the gluteals, piriformis, obturator, gemelli, and quadratus. The other muscles of the hip including the adductors, rectus femoris, iliopsoas, and hamstrings also play a role in joint stability and contractures.

Hip Arthritis

Osteoarthritis of the hip joint is very common, and incidence increases with age. Other predisposing factors include congenital dysplasia (including femoral-acetabular impingement), prior injury, avascular necrosis of the femoral head, and joint infection. Hip arthritis may present with either buttock pain or groin pain and commonly refers pain down into the anterior thigh to the knee. Symptoms are worse with prolonged sitting or weight-bearing and can be severely disabling in advanced cases. The differential diagnosis should include referred pain from the spine, abdomen, and pelvis or from the multiple bursa/tendon attachments around the joint. Diagnosis is usually possible with physical examination. The most common finding is reduction and range of motion but also may include tenderness over the anterior joint. Examination is also remarkable for a characteristic antalgic gait pattern often called a Trendelenburg gait. This gait pattern is also commonly present with weakness in the hip abductors. In osteoarthritis, patients shift their center of mass directly over the joint to avoid pain from activation of the hip abductor muscles. The diagnosis of hip osteoarthritis is often confirmed with X-rays; however, an intra-articular injection with steroid often helps to differentiate this diagnosis from other pain generators. The use of a straight cane, physical therapy, and weight loss are all helpful to improve symptoms and function. Analgesic medications are often needed. Total hip arthroplasty is highly successful for cases that are refractory to conservative management and are commonly performed even in relatively young patients. Hip resurfacing procedures may also be attempted for young patients, because they have shorter recovery periods and sacrifice less bone tissue than a total hip arthroplasty.

Trochanteric Bursitis

Pain that localized to the lateral hip with tenderness over the greater trochanter is often called "bursitis," but it is probably more commonly caused by insertional tendinopathy of the gluteus medius and minimus. Regardless of the cause, this condition is usually treated with analgesics, corticosteroid injection, and/or physical therapy. Supervised therapy is often better than home exercise programs because of the intricacies with proper techniques and for improvement in patient compliance. In recent years, gluteal tendon rupture has been more readily diagnosed, and hip arthroscopy is useful to repair damaged tendons, particularly in cases that involve a traumatic onset.

Knee Pain

The knee consists of the articulation between the femur and tibia with both medial and lateral compartments and the articulation of the patella and femur, also known as the anterior compartment. The bony surfaces are lined with articular cartilage, whereas the medial and lateral menisci are made of meniscal cartilage. The knee is stabilized by medial and lateral collateral ligaments, anterior and posterior cruciate ligaments, and multiple smaller ligamentous and capsular structures that are beyond the scope of this review. The knee is also very dependent on the dynamic stability of the hip and ankle joints to maintain proper alignment. Therefore, a number of overuse and chronic pain syndromes in the knee are treated by therapy directed at the stability of the entire limb.

Knee Arthritis

By far the most common cause of knee pain is osteoarthritis. This is thought to be the leading cause of work-related disability in the USA and one of the leading public health problems nationwide. There is a significant relationship in the incidence of knee arthritis with obesity and with prior injury to the joint. Patients typically present with joint stiffness, swelling, and pain. The most important physical examination maneuver is detection of knee joint effusion. An effusion usually results in swelling above the patella on either side of the quadriceps tendon. Fluid wave and/or ballottement of the patella may or may not be present. X-rays typically show the hallmark signs of joint space narrowing, osteophytes, bony sclerosis, and subchondral cysts (Fig. 18.1). If there is significant warmth, large effusion, or history of infection, joint aspiration and synovial fluid analysis should be attempted to help confirm the diagnosis and provide pain relief. Treatment of knee arthritis, however, can usually be conservative, with an emphasis on home therapy exercises, continued aerobic physical activity, and weight loss. Second-line treatments include analgesics, corticosteroid or viscosupplement (sodium hyaluronate) injections, bracing, wedged insoles, and supervised physical therapy, including pool exercise. Alternative therapies, such as acupuncture, electrical stimulation, and vitamin supplementation such as glucosamine, chondroitin, and/or methylsulfonylmethane (MSM), have also shown some benefit but with conflicting evidence. Arthroscopy and joint replacement surgery should only be considered after a failure of conservative management.

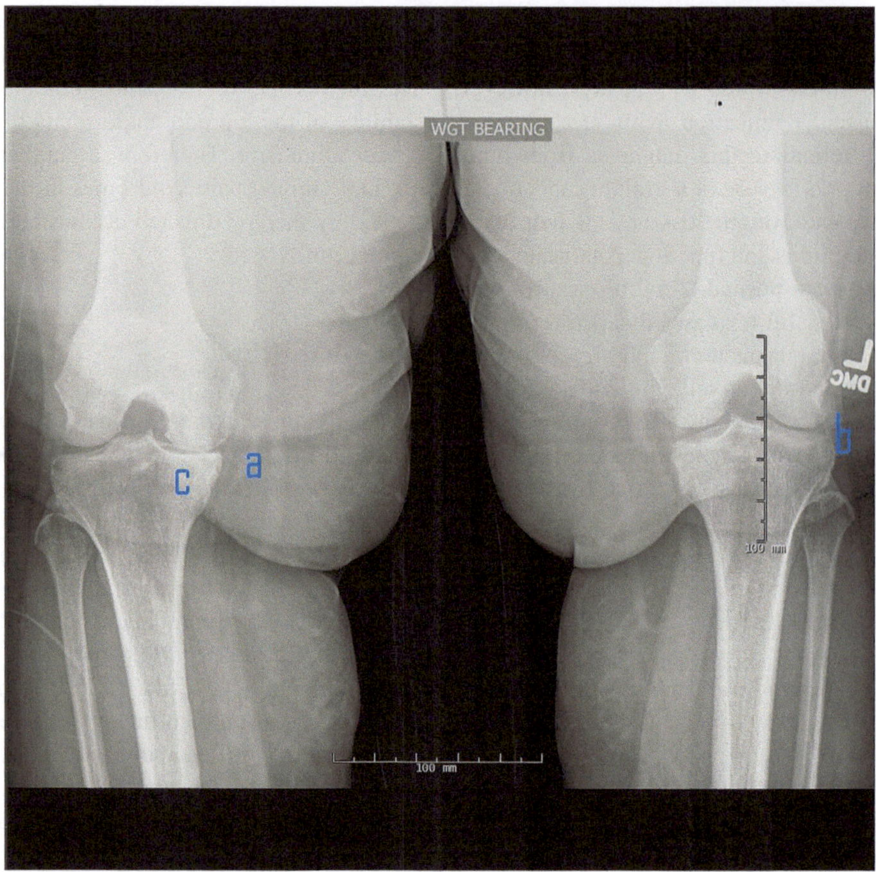

Fig. 18.1 Knee radiographs showing typical features of osteoarthritis: images are taken in posterior-anterior projection with the patient in 45° of knee flexion (also known as "notch" view). Note the severe joint space narrowing in the right medial compartment (*a*) and the associated subchondral sclerosis (*c*). The flexed knee positioning reveals joint space narrowing in the left lateral compartment (*b*) that was not visible on standard weight-bearing AP views without flexion. Also present are multiple small osteophytes at the joint lines, lateral deviation of the patella, mild varus alignment ("bowed legs"), and large amounts of adipose tissue of the thigh and legs due to the patient's obesity

Meniscus Injury

The typical mechanism of acute meniscus injury is a twisting motion during weight-bearing. Patients may complain of mechanical symptoms of locking, catching, or instability of the joint. The most sensitive and reliable physical examination maneuver is tenderness localized at the joint line. Other provocative tests such as the McMurray, Apley, and Thessaly tests may be helpful but should be done with caution to avoid aggravation of pain and extension of the meniscus tear. MRI is usually necessary to confirm this diagnosis. In many cases, there is concomitant osteoarthritis, and it may be very challenging to determine if the meniscus tear or the arthritis is more symptomatic. In the absence of mechanical symptoms or a traumatic mechanism, the meniscus injury is usually considered an incidental finding, and the patient should be treated for osteoarthritis with conservative measures instead of meniscectomy. Fortunately, conservative treatment of meniscus injury is similar to that of osteoarthritis. Even traumatic, isolated meniscus tears can be treated conservatively unless they are associated with mechanical symptoms or refractory to conservative care. The exception to this principle is a younger patient (less than 25 years old), as he/she has greater potential for primary meniscus healing if an arthroscopic repair is done promptly.

Ligament Rupture

Cruciate or collateral ligament ruptures in the knee are usually associated with twisting and varus/valgus sprains, typically in the weight-bearing knee. Female athletes are at least five times more likely to sustain anterior cruciate ligament injuries than males. Careful physical examination can often determine the extent of ligamentous laxity, but this takes considerable skill and experience, particularly in the setting of a painful knee. The examiner should keep in mind that meniscus ruptures commonly coexist with medial collateral and cruciate ligament injuries. The "terrible triad" knee injury includes rupture of the medial collateral ligament, medial meniscus, and anterior cruciate ligament combined. Any patient with ligamentous laxity after a knee injury should be immobilized and referred promptly to a sports medicine or orthopedic specialist. Multi-ligamentous knee injurys (knee dislocations) are at risk for neurovascular compromise.

Patellofemoral Pain

Patellofemoral pain syndrome, also known as "chondromalacia," is most common in young females and in endurance athletes. Patients typically complain of pain in the anterior knee that is exacerbated by sitting with the knee flexed for prolonged periods (aka "moviegoer's sign") and is relieved with knee extension. The most common etiology is maltracking of the patella that can be caused by a number of factors: quadriceps weakness, hip abductor weakness, tightness in the iliotibial band, femoral anteversion, high- or low-riding patella, thickening of the patellar retinaculum (plica syndrome), and pes planus (flat feet). Other times an abrupt change in physical activity, a patellar subluxation injury, or a blow to the anterior knee may initiate symptoms. Physical examination findings include swelling in the anterior knee and infrapatellar fat pad (usually without effusion), tenderness on the patellar margins, and visible maltracking with dynamic maneuvers. This condition is best treated with supervised physical therapy to address the multitude of predisposing factors. Prescription analgesics are occasionally necessary and knee joint injections are rarely needed. Patellar bracing, taping, or foot orthoses are often helpful.

Other Causes of Knee Pain

Less common causes of knee pain include quadriceps or patellar tendinitis, pes anserine bursitis, hamstring tendinopathy, Baker cyst, and distal iliotibial band syndrome. The pain medicine specialist should also keep in mind that hip pathology commonly results in referred pain to the knee. Other more rare etiologies include upper lumbar radiculopathy, avascular necrosis of the femur, tumor of the bone or synovium, and infection of the joint.

Foot and Ankle Pain

The ankle consists of the talocrural (ankle) joint and the subtalar joints. The most commonly injured structure in an ankle sprain is the anterior talofibular ligament. Therefore, any pain outside this region should be carefully evaluated in the setting of trauma. X-rays are indicated if a patient is unable to bear weight or if there is bony tenderness in the posterior malleoli, base of the fifth metatarsal, or anteromedial calcaneus. Chronic pain in the ankle or subtalar joints is usually related to osteoarthritis, but tendinopathies can also be long-standing and problematic. More acute injuries to the foot and ankle are outside the scope of this chapter but are summarized well elsewhere (Saleh 2013).

Ankle Joint Disorders

Effusions in the ankle/foot joints are relatively uncommon and should raise suspicion for inflammatory joint disease, especially gout and pseudogout. Joint aspiration (typically with ultrasound guidance) is helpful to make this diagnosis via synovial fluid analysis.

Heel Pain

Plantar heel pain is usually from plantar fasciitis, which involves swelling at the insertion of the plantar fascia on the calcaneus. The presence of a spur in this region is often incidental; therefore, the presence of a calcaneal spur does not indicate symptomatic fasciitis. Posterior heel pain is usually from Achilles tendonitis and is treated similarly.

Midfoot Pain

This pain most often comes from osteoarthritis in the multiple small articulations of the tarsal bones. X-rays are helpful to confirm this diagnosis and rule out stress fractures or other bony disorders such as osteomyelitis and avascular necrosis. Midfoot arthritis is best treated with supportive footwear, NSAIDs, and activity modification. Injections in this region can be challenging, even with guidance.

Forefoot Pain

This has many causes, the most common of which is an interdigital or "Morton's" neuroma. The differential diagnosis includes intrametatarsal bursitis and metatarsal stress fracture. Morton's neuromas commonly cause tenderness between the second and third or third and fourth metatarsals and are exacerbated by tight fitting shoes or high heels. Pain from these neuromas may radiate to the toes. Shoes with a wide toe box and/or metatarsal pad inserts help to off-load this area. Steroid injections are often helpful, and surgery with nerve resection may be curative.

Plantar Pain

Pain on the plantar aspect of the forefoot is most commonly called "metatarsalgia." This usually involves swelling and inflammation of the soft tissues under the metatarsal heads but may arise from the MTP joints, inflamed or fractured sesamoid bones, or from the distal insertions of the plantar fascia. Proper footwear is almost always curative, but foot orthoses may be necessary. Injections under the metatarsal head should be avoided due to the possibility of fat pad atrophy and tendon rupture.

Treatment of Foot Pain

Basic principles of foot and ankle treatment usually involve the application of supportive footwear, with or without braces or orthoses. The pain management physician should affiliate themselves with a good orthotic specialist or pedorthotist (foot-ankle bracing specialist). These clinicians are very well-versed in orthotic and footwear applications. Podiatry or Orthopaedic Consultation (foot-ankle subspecialist) should be sought for unusual or refractory cases. Physical therapy exercises to stretch the calf muscles and plantar fascia and stabilize the ankle are extremely important. Steroid injections are often helpful for acute flare-ups of many conditions, but oftentimes a brief period of immobilization in a walking boot (aka cam walker or pneumatic boot) will suffice and will help improve a patient's ambulation greatly.

Suggested Reading

1. Ahmad Z, Siddiqui N, Malik SS, Abdus-Samee M, Tytherleigh-Strong G, Rushton N. Lateral epicondylitis: a review of pathology and management. Bone Joint J. 2013;95-B(9):1158–64. https://doi.org/10.1302/0301-620X.95B9.29285. Review. PMID: 23997125 [PubMed – indexed for MEDLINE].

2. Cheng OT, Souzdalnitski D, Vrooman B, Cheng J. Evidence based knee injections for the management of arthritis. Pain Med. 2012;13:740–53.
3. Duckworth AD, Jenkins PJ, Roddam P, Watts AC, Ring D, McEachan JE. Pain and carpal tunnel syndrome. J Hand Surg Am. 2013;38(8):1540–6. https://doi.org/10.1016/j.jhsa.2013.05.027. PMID: 23890497 [PubMed – in process].
4. Gillis J, Calder K, Williams J. Review of thumb carpometacarpal arthritis classification, treatment and outcomes. Can J Plast Surg. 2011;19(4):134–8. PMID: 23204884 [PubMed].
5. Kozlow JH, Chung KC. Current concepts in the surgical management of rheumatoid and osteoarthritic hands and wrists. Hand Clin. 2011;27(1):31–41. https://doi.org/10.1016/j.hcl.2010.09.003. Epub 2010 Nov 20. Review. PMID: 21176798 [PubMed – indexed for MEDLINE].
6. Ntani G, Palmer KT, Linaker C, Harris EC, Van der Star R, Cooper C, Coggon D. Symptoms, signs and nerve conduction velocities in patients with suspected carpal tunnel syndrome. BMC Musculoskelet Disord. 2013;14(1):242. [Epub ahead of print] PMID: 23947775 [PubMed – as supplied by publisher].
7. Odum SM, Springer BD, Dennos AC, Fehring TK. National obesity trends in total knee arthroplasty. J Arthroplast. 2013;28(8 Suppl):148–51. https://doi.org/10.1016/j.arth.2013.02.036. Epub 2013 Aug 15.
8. Papatheodorou LK, Baratz ME, Sotereanos DG. Elbow arthritis: current concepts. J Hand Surg Am. 2013;38(3):605–13. https://doi.org/10.1016/j.jhsa.2012.12.037. Epub 2013 Feb 5. Review. PMID: 23391361 [PubMed – indexed for MEDLINE].
9. Rao S, Riskowski JL, Hannan MT. Musculoskeletal conditions of the foot and ankle: assessments and treatment options. [Review] Best Pract Res Clin Rheumatol. 2012;26(3):345–68. [Journal Article. Research Support, N.I.H., Extramural. Review] UI: 22867931.
10. Saleh A, Sadeghpour R, Munyak J. Foot and ankle update. [Review] Prim Care; Clinics in Office Practice. 2013;40(2):383–406. [Journal Article. Review] UI: 23668650.
11. Suarez JC, Ely EE, Mutnal AB, Figueroa NM, Klika AK, Patel PD, Barsoum WK. Comprehensive approach to the evaluation of groin pain. [Review] J Am Acad Orthop Surg. 2013;21(9):558–70. [Journal Article. Research Support, Non-U.S. Gov't. Review] UI: 23996987.
12. Taylor SA, Hannafin JA. Evaluation and management of elbow tendinopathy. Sports Health. 2012;4(5):384–93. PMID: 23016111 [PubMed].
13. Wluka AE, Lombard CB, Cicuttini FM. Tackling obesity in knee osteoarthritis. Nat Rev Rheumatol. 2013;9(4):225–35. https://doi.org/10.1038/nrrheum.2012.224. Epub 2012 Dec 18.

Myofascial Pain Syndrome

19

Jay P. Shah and Nikki Thaker

Key Concepts

- Myofascial pain syndrome (MPS) is a pain condition that may be acute, but it is most commonly chronic. MPS is often associated with myofascial trigger points (MTrPs) in muscle and connective tissue including fascia.
- MTrPs may be active, spontaneously painful nodules that when palpated recreate a patient's main pain complaint. Latent MTrPs, on the other hand, are only associated with local or referred pain when palpated. MTrPs can occur idiopathically or secondary to injury, overuse of muscle and/or surrounding fascia, and underlying medical conditions (e.g., musculoskeletal, visceral, and metabolic).
- Tissue damage is responsible for the release of inflammatory biochemicals intended to trigger the healing processes. However, these substances, including ATP, cytokines, catecholamines, and protons, can also serve to sensitize local nociceptors, lowering their activation thresholds and increasing their activity. This is called peripheral sensitization.
- Nociceptive bombardment of the central nervous system from the periphery can cause neuroplastic changes in the central nervous pain pathway including a reduction of activation thresholds and increased excitability. This can lead to abnormal functional and structural changes in the dorsal root ganglia, dorsal horn, and supraspinal cortical structures that result in central sensitization and chronic pain.
- Further, cortical structures like the limbic system and hypothalamus, influenced by hormonal fluctuations and stress, may play a role in top-down initiation or perpetuation of MPS.
- Management of MPS should take into account peripheral (e.g., MTrPs) and/or central (e.g., spinal segments) involvement and may include pharmacological and nonpharmacological techniques. Common treatment modalities include MTrP injections and dry needling, topical creams, relaxation, and narcotic medications.
- MPS can be perpetuated by nonmuscular and nonneurological dysfunction. Comorbidities, regardless of their origin, must be considered and addressed for pain to be successfully and comprehensively treated. Further, long-term treatment should include postural strategies and exercises to improve function and

J.P. Shah, MD (✉) • N. Thaker, BS
Rehabilitation Medicine Department, Clinical Center, Bethesda, MD, USA
e-mail: jshah@mail.cc.nih.gov

J. Cheng, R.W. Rosenquist (eds.), *Fundamentals of Pain Medicine*,
https://doi.org/10.1007/978-3-319-64922-1_19

biomechanics to prevent future tissue damage and pain reinitiation.

Epidemiology

Myofascial pain syndrome (MPS) is a pain condition that may be acute, but it is most commonly chronic. MPS is often associated with myofascial trigger points (MTrPs) in muscle and connective tissue including fascia. MPS is the most common type of muscle pain, estimated to account for 85% of visits to pain clinics.

Muscle Overuse or Trauma

- While the causes and effects of MTrPs are not well understood, the Cinderella hypothesis proposes a role for muscle in the development of MTrPs.
- During muscle contraction, small type I fibers are the first to be recruited and the last to be derecruited and therefore bear a higher metabolic burden than larger muscle fibers. During frequent submaximal exertions (e.g., typing and other fine motor tasks, cervical and postural muscle strain), these fibers can become susceptible to muscle damage.
- Sustained contractions may also impede blood flow, leading to regions of ischemia, hypoxia, and decreased ATP. These can then lead to acidity, increased Ca2+, and sarcomere contraction. Some research suggests that this damage and dysfunction can lead to the formation of MTrPs and their associated local and referred pain and muscle tenderness.

The Role of Sensitization in MPS

- The mimicking of patients' local pain complaint and referred pain associated with stimulation of active MTrPs suggests that peripheral and central sensitization play a role in MPS. Tissue damage is responsible for the release of inflammatory biochemicals intended to trigger the healing processes. However, these substances, including ATP, cytokines, catecholamines, and protons, can also serve to sensitize local nociceptors, lowering their activation thresholds and increasing their activity. This is called peripheral sensitization.
- Nociceptive bombardment of the central nervous system from the periphery can cause neuroplastic changes in the central nervous pain pathway including reduction of activation thresholds and increased neuronal excitability. This can lead to abnormal functional and structural changes in the dorsal root ganglia, dorsal horn, and supraspinal cortical structures, taken together as central sensitization. Hyperactivity in the dorsal horn at the corresponding segmental level of peripheral pain input is known as spinal segmental sensitization (SSS). When SSS affects connections to wide dynamic range (WDR) neurons, sensitization can cause an expansion of the pain perceptive field to include regions of the body that provide afferent input at the spinal level of the original pain source even though the original source of pain has not changed. For example, involvement of thoracic spinal levels (e.g., T1–T12) in SSS facilitates and perpetuates abdominal pain and somatovisceral symptoms via WDR neurons, commonly mimicking gastrointestinal conditions, such as peptic ulcer disease.
- Primary afferent nociceptive fibers trifurcate upon entering the dorsal horn. One branch enters the dorsal horn at that segmental level, one branch ascends, and one branch descends along the dorsal margin of the dorsal horn, and this can facilitate the expansion of the receptive field of pain.
- Together, peripheral and central sensitization can cause increased response to non-noxious stimuli (allodynia) and noxious stimuli (hyperalgesia), abnormal pain perception, and the transition from acute to chronic pain.
- Active MTrPs are associated with similar symptoms to sensitization, which suggests that the mechanisms of sensitization may play a role in the pain experience of active MTrPs and MPS. Persistent noxious stimulation, for example, from an active MTrP, causes the

release of substance P (SP) and glutamate at the synapse between the peripheral afferent and dorsal horn, opening postsynaptic calcium channels.
- The constant influx of calcium caused by persistent afferent input lowers excitation thresholds of dorsal horn neurons and can activate previously ineffective synapses. Calcium is a second messenger that can initiate gene transcription in the nucleus, leading to an increase in ion channels at postsynaptic bouton. This results in increased sensitivity of the neuron, creating a vicious cycle of stimulation, transcription, and sensitization that can be long term or permanent.
- The deluge of calcium can also induce apoptosis in cells like inhibitory interneurons that modulate pain sensation and balance out noxious input from the periphery. Loss of this inhibition allows nociceptive bombardment to go unchecked, leading to increased pain sensitivity and intensity.
- In addition to affecting neuronal sensitivity, SP and other vasoactive biochemicals can increase the permeability of the vasculature, allowing inflammatory mediators into tissue. When this causes inflammation, the process is known as neurogenic inflammation. When inflammation is already present, inflammatory mediators can aggravate the existing problem. Both of these processes increase tenderness, allodynia, and hyperalgesia in the area of inflammation. Because active MTrPs are often surrounded by inflammatory biochemicals, this mechanism may explain the clinical findings associated with active MTrPs.
- Active MTrPs and their surrounding muscle evince elevated local levels of endogenous biochemicals compared to latent MTrPs and normal muscle. Bradykinin (BK), serotonin/5-hydroxytryptamin (5-HT), norepinephrine (NE), SP, calcitonin gene-related peptide (CGRP), tumor necrosis factor-alpha (TNF-α), interleukin-1β (IL-1β), IL-6, IL-8, and protons (i.e., a more acidic pH) are significantly elevated at active MTrPs. These substances contribute to inflammation, sensitization, intercellular signaling, and persistent pain states, all of which are also associated with active MTrPs and MPS.

The Role of Emotions and Hormones in Pain Modulation

- The rostral ventral medulla (RVM) connects the periaqueductal gray in the midbrain and the dorsal horn and provides a key connection between the spinal and supraspinal pain pathways. The periaqueductal gray receives input from the limbic forebrain and hypothalamus, centers of emotion subject to hormonal fluctuations. Therefore, the RVM serves as a connection between emotional/hormonal brain regions and the spinal cord, perhaps modulating top-down pain perception and perpetuation. This would help explain the impact of negative emotions, stress, and hormonal fluctuations on the clinical findings of allodynia and hyperalgesia in MPS.
- The RVM has complimentary cell types: ON and OFF cells. ON cells increase pain perception and provide useful protective pain sensation during tissue damage and injury that would fade as tissue heals. OFF cells are likely inhibitory and provide antinociceptive sensation. Thus, a balance of ON and OFF cells modulates dorsal horn activity and controls pain perception.
- During chronic pain conditions, such as MPS, an imbalance in ON and OFF cell activity may lead to the perpetuation of pain sensation even after an initial injury or pain stimulus has resolved. Dysfunction at the RVM can lead to dysfunction at the dorsal horn, and a bombardment of ON cell activity can lead to maladaptive neuroplastic changes including neurogenic inflammation at the dorsal horn. This can cause individuals to feel local tissue tenderness in the absence of a pain stimulus, and this pain perceptive field can expand both ipsilaterally and contralaterally to the original pain focus.
- Neurons are not the only nervous system cells that can play a role in the development and maintenance of chronic pain. Like dorsal horn

neurons, microglia and astrocites are activated by persistent nociceptive bombardment from peripheral nociceptors. Microglia and astrocites can sensitize their surrounding neurons through the release of pro-inflammatory biochemicals. Thus, rather than directly participating in central sensitization as dorsal horn neurons do, dorsal horn glial cells can initiate and perpetuate sensitization from outside the pain pathway.

Clinical Features and Diagnosis

- MTrPs are commonly associated with MPS, though establishing a direct causal relationship has been elusive. MTrPs are palpable, tender nodules located in taut bands of skeletal muscle or fascia (Fig. 19.1). MTrPs are associated with local pain and tenderness and often referred pain to remote areas.
- MTrPs may be active, spontaneously painful nodules that when palpated recreate a patient's main pain complaint. Latent MTrPs, on the other hand, are only associated with local or referred pain when palpated. Generally, active MTrPs are especially sensitive to palpation and pressure because they are more closely related to the pain complaint.
- Recent studies have shown that ultrasound diagnostic imaging techniques can be used to visualize MTrPs and objectively measure their physical properties. On ultrasound, MTrPs appear as focal hypoechoic (darker) areas with a heterogeneous echotexture. They also show reduced vibration amplitude on elastography, indicating a localized area of stiffer tissue compared to the surrounding soft tissue. In

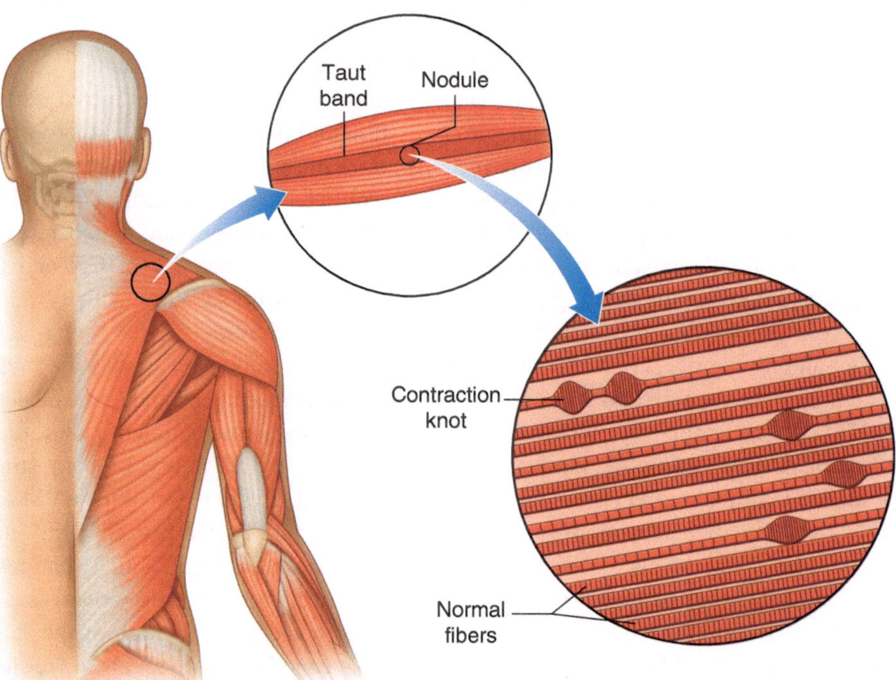

Fig. 19.1 Trigger points are nodules in taut bands of muscle and may be made up of one or more contraction knots (Adapted from Simons DG, Travell JG. Myofascial pain and dysfunction: the trigger point manual, vol. 1; 2nd ed., and Användare: Chrizz., In: Shah JP, Gilliams EA. Uncovering the biochemical milieu of myofascial trigger points using in vivo microdialysis: an application of muscle pain concepts to myofascial pain syndrome. J Bodyw Mov Ther. 2008;12(4):371–84)

addition, ultrasound reveals that MTrPs have a unique vascular environment, that active MTrPs have differences in local microcirculation compared to latent MTrPs and normal tissue, and that active MTrPs have a significantly larger surface area than latent MTrPs.

- MTrPs can occur idiopathically or secondary to injury, overuse of muscle and/or surrounding fascia, and underlying medical conditions (e.g., musculoskeletal, visceral, and metabolic).
- Proper palpation technique can allow a clinician to thoroughly evaluate MPS and monitor the efficacy of treatment strategies. Palpation provides clinicians with information about the presence and quality of MTrPs and the state of neurological sensitization.
- Active MTrPs provide a source of persistent peripheral noxious stimulation and may initiate the sensitization and pain perpetuation mechanisms described earlier in this chapter. Treatment for MPS that does not resolve active MTrPs may leave the dorsal horn vulnerable to resensitization, resulting in the reemergence of the original pain complaint.
- Though they do not produce spontaneous pain, latent MTrPs are also important treatment targets. Latent MTrPs may transition to active MTrPs, exacerbating and/or creating a new pain complaint.
- Even after MTrP treatment, pain may persist due to nervous system sensitization. SSS should be assessed by examining dermatomal, myotomal, and sclerotomal levels not only associated with the location of the pain but also adjacent and contralateral to the pain source.
- Sensitization at dermatomal levels is found by:
  - Assessing hyperalgesia. Exaggerated pain to a noxious stimulus indicates sensitization at a particular spinal level. To assess which spinal segments are sensitized, a paperclip or Wartenberg pinwheel may be pulled along the skin paraspinally. A patient report of increased sharpness or pain indicates presence of hyperalgesia at the given segment.
  - Assessing allodynia. Pain to a non-noxious stimulus is also indicative of sensitization. A pinch-and-roll test (Fig. 19.2), von Frey monofilament, or stiff paintbrush can be applied along the skin paraspinally. A report of pain at any of these non-noxious stimuli is indicative of allodynia.
- Sensitization affecting the myotome and sclerotome is assessed by palpating regions that are innervated at the same spinal segment as the pain focus. Identifying tenderness, taut bands, and MTrPs in and assessing the pain pressure threshold (PPT) of related

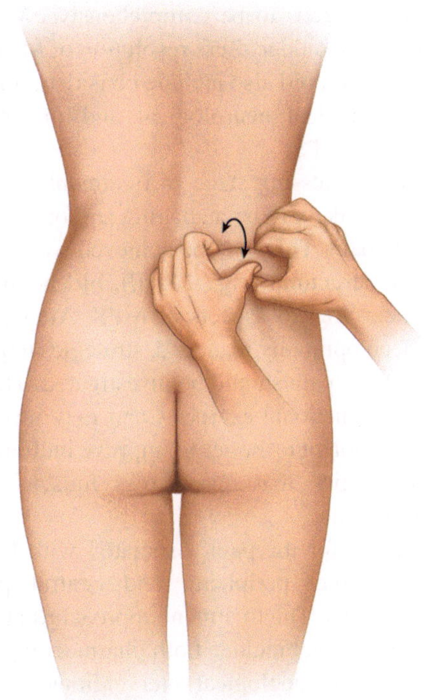

Fig. 19.2 In the pinch and roll test, tissue is firmly pinched between the thumb and forefinger. Rolling vertically across dermatomal boundaries will elicit allodynia in sensitized segments (Appeared in advanced techniques in musculoskeletal medicine and physiotherapy. Ed. Fermin Valera Garrido, Francisco Minaya Munoz. Publisher: Eslivier. 2016. "Acupuncture and needling techniques for segmental dysfunction in neuromusculoskeletal pain." Jay P. Shah, Nikki Thaker. Figure appears on page 249. Chapter is on pages 239–55)

musculature, tendons, entheses, bursae, and ligaments can reveal regions that are more sensitive to pain because of peripheral and central sensitization.
- Understanding the degree of sensitization is important in characterizing and effectively treating a patient's chronic pain state. Using these objective measures, clinicians elicit reproducible findings that allow for characterization of a patient's sensitization level.

Treatment

- Because MPS is a complex condition involving peripheral and central neurological and local and distant musculoskeletal systems, treatment needs to be comprehensive. While treatment should address resolution of MTrPs, treatment should also include consideration of the biochemical, neurological, and functional aspects of MPS.
- The most pressing stage of treatment for the patient is likely to be managing and/or resolving the pain. This may be achieved by targeting the structural (e.g., MTrP), biochemical, and neurological aspects of MPS. After pain has been optimally managed, strategies to prevent future pain should be investigated. These include functional exercises and may involve introduction of orthotics to improve inefficient biomechanics that may stress muscle and result in pain.
- Treatment for the pain associated with MPS should target peripheral and central pain mechanisms. The treatment approaches at the peripheral level include both pharmacological and nonpharmacological interventions.
- Pharmacological interventions are most commonly pain medications, including nonsteroidal anti-inflammatory drugs and narcotics. Topical creams like lidocaine and capsaicin are also used, and MTrP injections of lidocaine and botulinum toxin are increasingly studied and available.
- Nonpharmacological interventions are much more varied. Manual therapies, dry needling, and massage can provide important strengthening and stretching of affected tissue.
- Dry needling of MTrPs is an effective, nonpharmacological treatment strategy (Fig. 19.3). During dry needling, the patient and practitioner may notice a local twitch response (LTR), and this can be indicative of effective needling treatment. Though the mechanism of an LTR is unknown, elicitation can significantly decrease SP and CGRP to levels approaching those of normal muscle. These biochemical changes may contribute to the decrease in local pain commonly experienced after dry needling.
- When sensitization is present or local treatments are ineffective, segmental sensitization should be assessed and targeted for treatment. Treatments for SSS include manual therapies and dry needling at the segment, trans- and percutaneous electrical nerve stimulation (TENS and PENS, respectively), and paraspinous injections and needling.
- Relaxation techniques can also help patients address the psychosocial and emotional aspects of their pain. As discussed earlier in this chapter, stress and hormonal fluctuations can affect supraspinal pain pathways, creating top-down pain perpetuation. Optimizing mental health is therefore an important component of successful pain management.

Paraspinous Needling and Paraspinous Block Technique

- Paraspinous needling and blocks are indicated when pain is refractory to other treatment strategies. When sensitized dermatomal, myotomal, and sclerotomal segments do not overlap, targeting the individual segments that most closely match the pain source can address the SSS component of pain. Like other muscles, paraspinal muscles may also have MTrPs that provide nociceptive input to the central nervous system and may require treatment. If initial needling does not provide

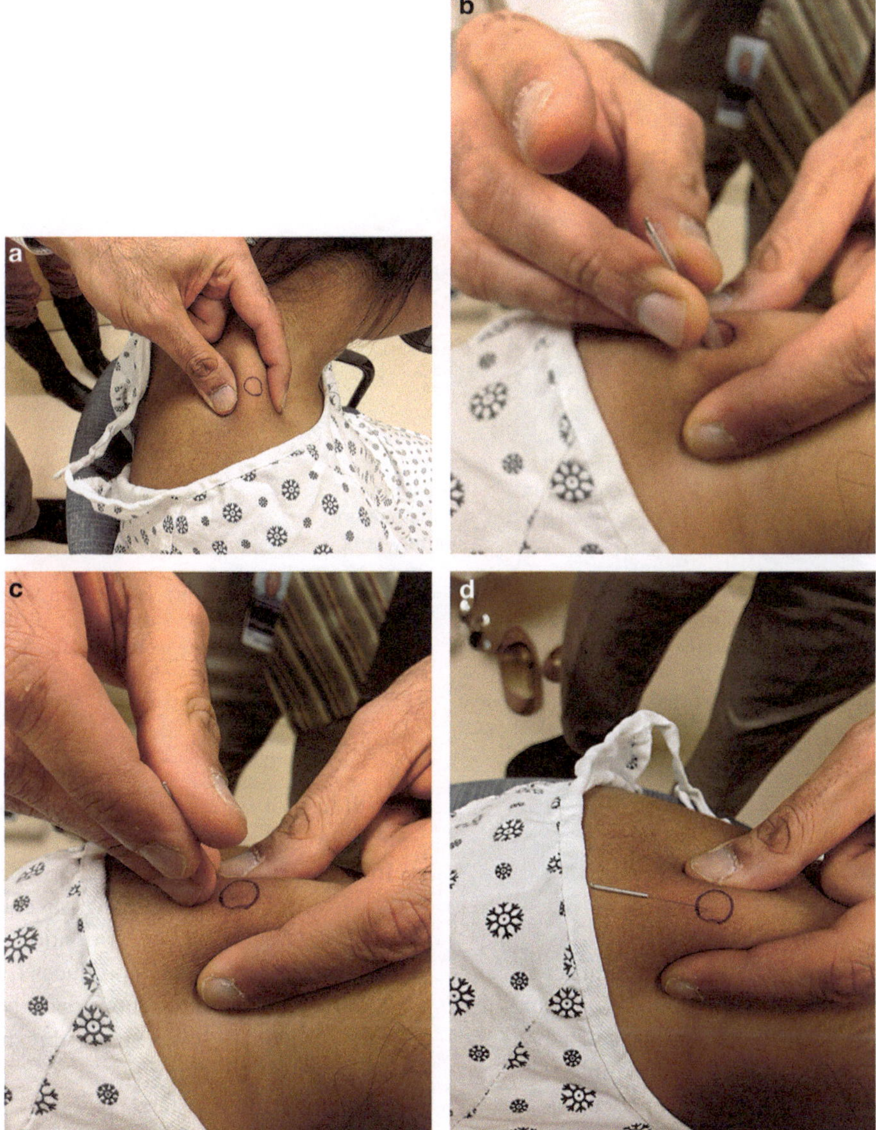

Fig. 19.3 When an MTrP is identified to be dry needled, it should be grasped firmly between the thumb and forefinger (**a**) An acupuncture needle should be inserted swiftly to minimize discomfort (**b**) Moving the needle up and down, the clinician is able to localize the MTrP with the needle and may elicit an LTR (**c**) Once the needle is in the MTrP, it is left in place for 1–2 min. (**d**) (Cite Shah JP, Thaker N, Heimur J, Aredo JV, Sikdar S, Gerber L. Myofascial trigger points then and now: a historical and scientific perspective. Phys Med Rehabil. 2015;7(7):746–61)

pain relief, targeting adjacent segmental levels can treat a larger area.

- In addition to needling, paraspinous blocks of lidocaine injections can provide relief similar to trigger point injections in other muscles. However, more research is necessary to validate paraspinous needling and block techniques (Fig. 19.4).

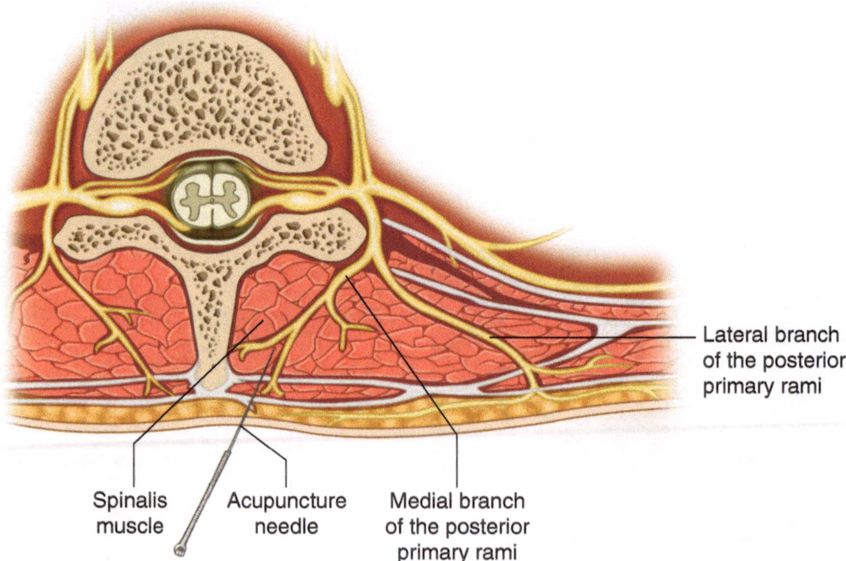

Fig. 19.4 During paraspinal needling, an acupuncture needle is inserted into the spinalis muscle. Much like with peripheral MTrP dry needling, the needle should be left in place for 1–2 min. Paraspinous blocks are achieved by inserting multiple acupuncture needles at a given segment (Appeared in advanced techniques in musculoskeletal medicine and physiotherapy. Ed. Fermin Valera Garrido, Francisco Minaya Munoz. Publisher: Eslivier. 2016. "Acupuncture and needling techniques for segmental dysfunction in neuromusculoskeltal pain." Jay P. Shah, Nikki Thaker. Figure appears on page 251. Chapter is on pages 239–255)

Prevention

Identify and Correct Perpetuating Factors

MPS can be perpetuated by nonmuscular and nonneurological dysfunction. Comorbidities, regardless of their origin, must be considered and addressed for pain to be successfully and comprehensively treated. Common conditions that can affect pain perception are summarized below:

- Vitamin D deficiency is a common comorbidity with musculoskeletal pain. It is associated with loss of type 2 muscle fibers and muscle atrophy.
- Iron is a critical element in energy production, and iron deficiency can lead to an energy crisis that may facilitate MTrP formation.
- Hypothyroidism, which produces a hypometabolic state, can cause hormonal dysfunction that results in lower pain thresholds and increased pain sensitivity.
- Functional and postural problems may also exacerbate pain and lead to musculoskeletal dysfunction that results in MPS. Compensating for these factors using orthotics or specific stretches or exercises can reduce their impact on pain.

Part V

Radicular Pain

20 Cervical Radicular Pain

Robert W. Hurley and Jennifer L. Chang

Abbreviations

CT Computed tomography
EMG Electromyography
MRI Magnetic resonance imaging
TNF Tumor necrosis factor

Key Concepts

- Radicular pain and radiculopathy are two discrete entities. Radicular pain is pain along a dermatomal pattern that is caused by the irritation of a nerve, whereas radiculopathy is a sensory or motor deficit resulting from a dysfunctional nerve pathway.
- Cervical radicular pain is mediated by the inflammatory response and the release of phospholipase A2, interleukins 1 and 6, TNF-α, and nitric oxide. Common causes of cervical radicular pain are neuroforaminal narrowing, disc herniations, or radiculitis.
- The diagnosis of cervical radicular pain can be accomplished by a thorough history and physical exam that includes provocative tests such as a Spurling test, a shoulder abduction test, and an axial manual traction test.
- Cervical radicular pain is commonly seen at C6 and C7. Imaging studies, electrodiagnostic studies, and diagnostic nerve blocks can help unravel the exact level of pathology.
- The American College of Radiology recommends a five-view radiographic examination for a patient with neck pain. A cervical magnetic resonance imaging (MRI) or computed tomography (CT) myelography with multiplanar reconstruction (if MRI is contraindicated) is recommended for patients with neurological symptoms.
- Electromyography (EMG) and diagnostic nerve blocks can further differentiate the exact nerve root level that is causing pain in patients with overlapping myofascial pain syndrome and multilevel findings on imaging studies.
- EMG findings in radiculopathy include fibrillation potentials, positive sharp waves, and prolongation of H reflex and F wave latencies.
- Conservative treatment for cervical radicular pain involves a multimodal approach that includes hot/cold compresses, physical therapy, topical medications, acetaminophen, nonsteroidal anti-inflammatory medications, and neuropathic medications.

R.W. Hurley, MD, PhD
Department of Anesthesiology and Public Health Sciences, Wake Forest School of Medicine, Winston-Salem, NC, USA
e-mail: rwhurley@ufl.edu; rhurley@mcw.edu

J.L. Chang, MD (✉)
Department of Anesthesiology and Pain Medicine, University of Florida Health,
1600 SW Archer Rd, MSB-500, Gainesville, FL 32608, USA
e-mail: jchang@anest.ufl.edu

J. Cheng, R.W. Rosenquist (eds.), *Fundamentals of Pain Medicine*,
https://doi.org/10.1007/978-3-319-64922-1_20

- Cervical interlaminar epidural steroid injections and pulsed radiofrequency of the dorsal root ganglion are successful interventions for cervical radicular pain. Cervical transforaminal epidural steroid injections are no longer recommended due to catastrophic complications noted in the literature.

Introduction

Cervical radiculopathy and radicular pain are often used interchangeably in the literature because they often coexist; nevertheless, there is an important distinction between the two. Cervical radiculopathy is defined by an objective neurologic change such as a sensory or motor deficit that results from dysfunction of one or more cervical spine nerves. Cervical radicular pain is a subjective, unpleasant sensation along the dermatomal distribution of a nerve that is caused by irritation and the resulting inflammatory response mediated by phospholipase A2, interleukins 1 and 6, TNF-α, and nitric oxide, among other mediators.

Epidemiology

The prevalence of cervical radiculopathy and cervical radicular pain has not been clearly defined. An epidemiological study conducted in Rochester, Minnesota, reported that the annual incidence of cervical radiculopathy in a population of 13–91-year-olds was 83 per 100,000. The prevalence was higher (203 per 100,000 individuals) among individuals between 50 and 54 years old. Males had a higher age-adjusted incidence (107 per 100,000 people) than females (64 per 100,000 people). It was also noted that the incidence of cervical radiculopathy was commonly seen in C7 and C6. Although this study aimed to determine the incidence of radiculopathy, it can be assumed that individuals with cervical radicular pain were also included in this study because sensory and motor deficits were only reported in 33% and 64% of this population, respectively.

Pathophysiology

According to the above epidemiological study, up to 75% of cervical radiculopathy is caused by the degeneration of the zygapophysial joints and uncovertebral joints (Fig. 20.1) and the reduction of disc height. These disease processes narrow the neuroforamen and cause nerve compression. Only 20–25% of cervical radiculopathy is due to disc herniation (Figs. 20.2 and 20.3).

Cervical radicular pain may also be caused by neuroforaminal narrowing, disc herniations, and radiculitis and therefore often occurs alongside cervical radiculopathy. However, the presence of neural compression does not always lead to cervical radicular pain and vice versa. This is evident as we encounter asymptomatic patients with large disc herniations and symptomatic patients without evidence of neural compression on imaging. Cervical radicular pain has been attributed to an inflammatory response that involves the release of inflammatory mediators such as phospholipase A2, interleukins 1 and 6, TNF-α, and nitric oxide secreted by a degenerated nucleus pulposus.

Clinical Features and Diagnosis

History

The diagnosis of cervical radicular pain is accomplished by a thorough history and physical exam. It is important to gather information about the location and quality (sharp, stabbing, dull, achy, and electrical) of the pain to help differentiate between cervical radicular pain, cervical facet pain, myofascial pain, and cervical discogenic pain.

Patients with cervical radicular pain typically report pain that begins in the neck and radiates along the upper extremity and often pasts the elbow. The pain is often described as a shooting or electrical pain. Depending on the affected cervical level, pain may radiate in a dermatomal pattern along the lateral forearm (C5), middle finger (C6 or C7), fourth and fifth finger (C8), or medial arm (C8) (Table 20.1).

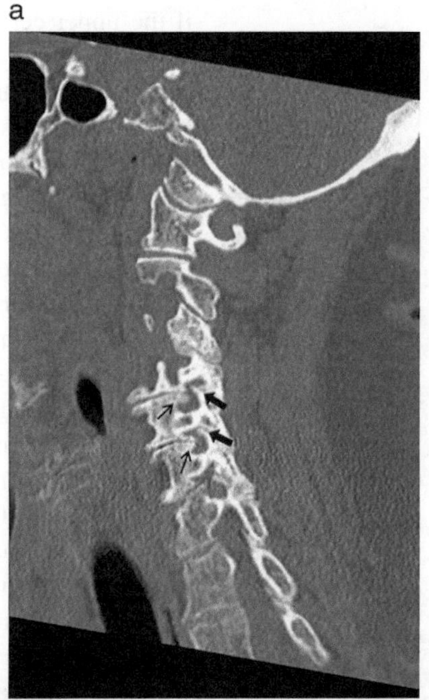

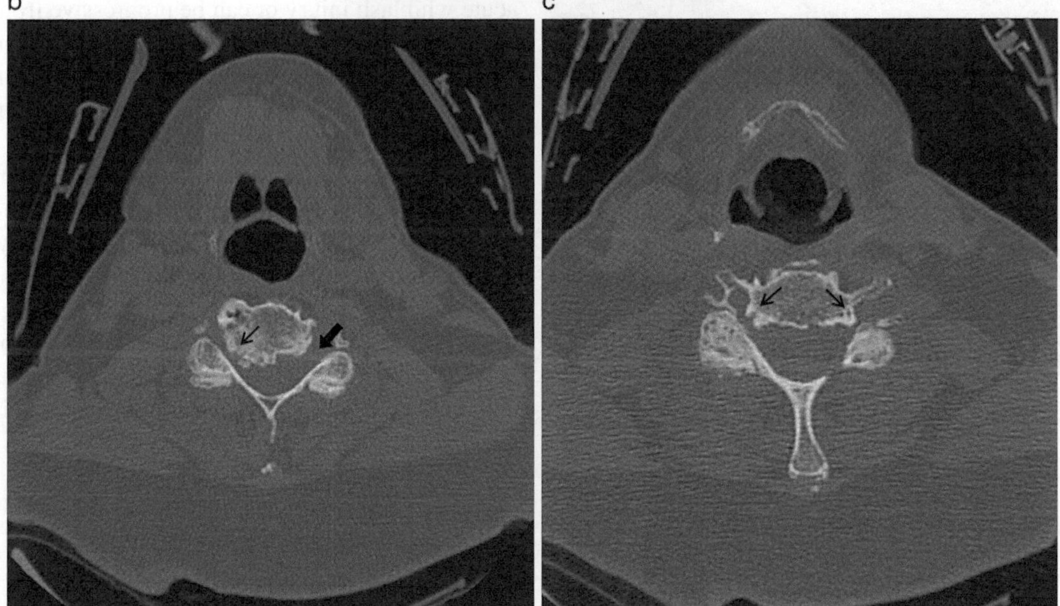

Fig. 20.1 Uncovertebral and facet osteophyte formation causing neuroforaminal narrowing. (**a**) Noncontrast computed tomography (CT) right of central parasagittal image of the cervical spine demonstrating uncovertebral osteophytes (thin black arrows) and facet osteophytes (*thick black arrows*) causing right neuroforaminal narrowing at C4-C5 and C5-C6. (**b**) Axial noncontrast CT image at C4-C5 demonstrating right uncovertebral and facet osteophyte formation causing severe right neuroforaminal narrowing (*thin black arrow*), compared with the normal diameter of the left neuroforamen (*thick black arrow*). (**c**). Axial noncontrast CT image at the level of C5-C6 demonstrating bilateral neuroforaminal narrowing from uncovertebral and facet osteophytes (*thin black arrows*) (Figure courtesy of Richard D. Beegle, MD, UF Health)

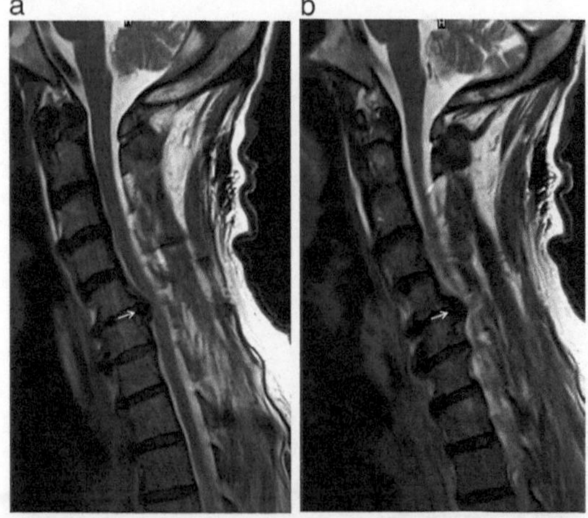

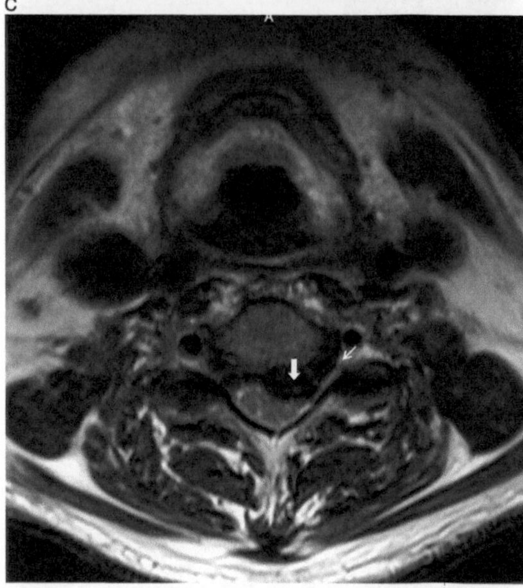

Fig. 20.2 Disc osteophyte complex with posterior disc extrusion causing central canal and neuroforaminal narrowing. (**a** and **b**) Two contiguous left central parasagittal T2-weighted magnetic resonance (MR) images of the cervical spine demonstrating a C5-C6 central disc osteophyte complex with posterior disc extrusion (*thin white arrows*) causing narrowing of the central canal. (**c**) Axial T2-weighted MR image at the level of C5-C6 demonstrating the left of a central disc osteophyte complex with posterior disc extrusion, narrowing of the central canal, and compression of the spinal cord (*thick white arrow*). There is severe left neuroforaminal narrowing (*thin white arrow*) (Figure courtesy of Richard D. Beegle, MD, UF Health)

Cervical facet pain often presents with an aching pain in the neck that frequently occurs with head rotation. The pain may cause headaches if the upper cervical facets are involved or may cause shoulder and upper arm pain if lower cervical facets are involved. Pain rarely extends below the elbows; if it does, it will occur in a nondermatomal pattern.

Cervical discogenic pain consists of vague and diffuse neck pain that is aggravated by head flexion, extension, and rotation. If the disc is affecting nerve roots, motor or sensory dysfunction may be notable.

The precipitating injury (trauma, whiplash, overuse, etc.), aggravating and alleviating factors (rotation, flexion, extension of the neck), environmental factors, and severity of the pain can further help differentiate between the common causes of neck pain. Patients with cervical radicular pain may note exacerbation of their pain with head extension toward the affected side, which further narrows the neuroforamen. Cervical facet arthropathy can occur after an acute whiplash injury or can be progressive from occupational overuse as seen in construction workers. Discogenic pain is worsened by flexion and extension and often wakes the patient up in their sleep.

In addition to the above characteristics of neck pain, it is extremely important to determine the presence of red flags in a patient's history. Fever, chills, night sweats, weight loss, or a history of cancer may be associated with malignancy. A history of intravenous drug abuse or HIV may point to an infectious cause such as osteomyelitis (Fig. 20.4) or an abscess that is causing neck pain.

Physical Examination

The physical examination should consist of a thorough neurological exam, including range of motion, strength, sensation, and deep tendon reflexes. Specific maneuvers to diagnose cervical radicular pain include the Spurling test, the shoulder abduction test, and the axial manual traction test.

The Spurling test is performed while the patient's neck is extended and rotated to the affected shoulder. If the examiner axially loads

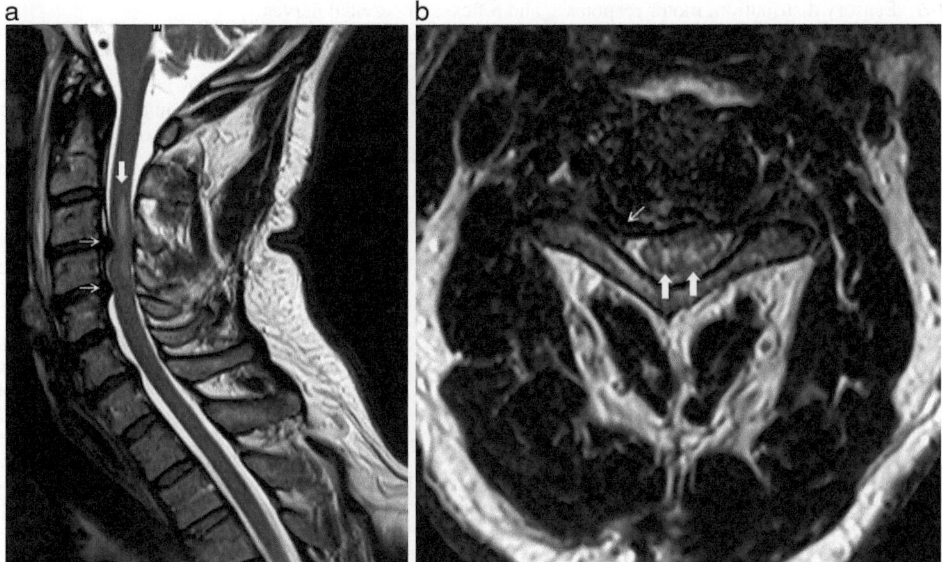

Fig. 20.3 Posterior disc osteophyte complexes causing central canal narrowing and cord ischemia. (**a**) Sagittal T2-weighted MR image of the cervical spine demonstrating disc osteophyte complexes at C3-C4 and C4-C5 causing central canal and neuroforaminal narrowing (*thin white arrows*). There is increased T2 signal in the spinal cord (*thick white arrow*) consistent with cord edema. (**b**) Axial T2-weighted MR image at the level of C3-C4 demonstrates a disc osteophyte complex worst in the right of central and right foraminal zones (*thin white arrow*) causing cord compression and severe right neuroforaminal narrowing. There is increased T2 signal in the gray matter of the spinal cord in a "snake eyes" configuration consistent with cord infarction (*thick white arrows*) (Figure courtesy of Richard D. Beegle, MD, UF Health)

the head in this position and the pain is reproduced, the test is positive for radicular pain. A Spurling test has high specificity (>90% specificity) but low sensitivity for a cervical nerve root compression. The shoulder abduction test is another highly specific test (90% specificity). This test is positive for cervical radicular pain if the radicular symptoms diminish when the patient lifts his/her affected hand above the head. The axial manual traction test is performed in the supine position. The examiner provides traction force of 10–15 kg axially. This test is positive if radicular symptoms diminish or disappear.

It is also important to investigate for the presence of red flags in a physical exam. The existence of weakness, bowel or bladder incontinence, or sensory deficits can be signs of spinal cord compression or myelopathy that may be a surgical emergency.

Imaging

In addition to the history and physical exam, imaging may provide further clues. The American College of Radiology recommends a five-view radiographic examination (anteroposterior, lateral, open mouth, and both obliques) as the initial evaluation of a patient with neck pain. Patients with normal radiographs, cervical spondylosis, or evidence of prior trauma need no further imaging as long as there are no neurological symptoms. If there are neurological signs or symptoms, the patient should undergo a cervical MRI. MRI is the preferred imaging modality over CT for identifying changes in the nerve roots, spinal cord, soft tissue, and intervertebral discs. However, if the patient has a pacemaker, extreme claustrophobia, or another contraindication to MRI, CT myelopathy with multiplanar reconstruction is recommended.

Table 20.1 Sensory distribution, motor responses, and reflexes of cervical nerves

–	C4	C5	C6	C7	C8	T1
Nerve	Dorsal scapular	Musculocutaneous (C5–C6)	Radial (C5–C6)	Radial (C6–C8)	Anterior interosseous (C7–C8)	Ulnar, deep branch (C8–T1)
Sensory	Shoulders	Lateral forearm, first and second finger	Middle finger	Middle finger	Fourth and fifth finger, medial forearm	Medial arm
Muscle(s) tested	Levator scapulae	Biceps	Extensor carpi radialis, longus, and brevis	Triceps	Flexor digitorum profundus	Dorsal interossei
Motor	Shoulder shrug	Elbow flexion	Wrist extension	Forearm extension	Middle finger flexion	Extension of fingers against resistance
Reflex	None	Biceps	Brachioradialis	Triceps	None	None

Adapted with permission from Chekka K, Moore JD, and Benzon HT. Physical examination of the patient with pain. In Benzon HT, Raja SN, Liu SS, Fishman SM, Cohen SP, editors. *Essentials of pain medicine*. Philadelphia: Elsevier Saunders; 2011. p. 25

It is important to remember that changes on imaging may not directly correlate with the pain syndrome. There are many "degenerative findings" that are asymptomatic. There is no relationship between the patient's clinical course and the size of the disc herniation. One limitation of imaging studies is that most are not obtained in an upright, weight-bearing posture.

Electrodiagnostic Studies

Electrodiagnostic studies, a collective term for EMG and nerve conduction studies, are additional diagnostic tools for determining the acuity of the injury and the anatomical site of pain. EMG involves needle insertion into the muscle and the evaluation of insertional activity, spontaneous activity, motor unit potentials, and recruitment. Nerve conduction velocities provide stimulus along sensory and motor nerves and measure the amplitude, latency, and conduction velocity of the response. Electrodiagnostic studies further narrow the anatomical site of pain to the nerve root, plexus, neuromuscular junction, and muscle and can help distinguish among peripheral neuropathy, plexopathy, radiculopathy, and nerve entrapment.

Radiculopathy is distinguished by the presence of fibrillation potentials, positive sharp waves, and prolongation of the H reflex and F wave latencies on EMG/nerve conduction velocity studies. Radiculopathy produces motor deficits but does not affect sensory nerve conduction because radiculopathy occurs within the spinal canal and is proximal to the dorsal root ganglion. EMG is less sensitive and more specific than MRI for radiculopathy and can identify which disc bulge causes nerve damage in a patient with multiple disc bulges on MRI.

Diagnostic Nerve Blocks

In patients with multilevel MRI pathology and overlapping myofascial pain syndrome, diagnostic nerve blocks can determine the exact nerve root that is causing pain. The C-arm is positioned 25–35° obliquely and 10° caudally so that the X-ray beams are parallel to the intervertebral foramen axis. By using a coaxial technique, the needle is placed directly above the caudal portion of the foramen. The C-arm is then changed to an anterior-posterior position where the needle tip is guided to the lateral part of the facetal column. Contrast dye is used to identify the nerve, and a local anesthetic is infiltrated. A reduction of 50% or more of the pain following this procedure confirms the nerve root as a source of the radicular pain.

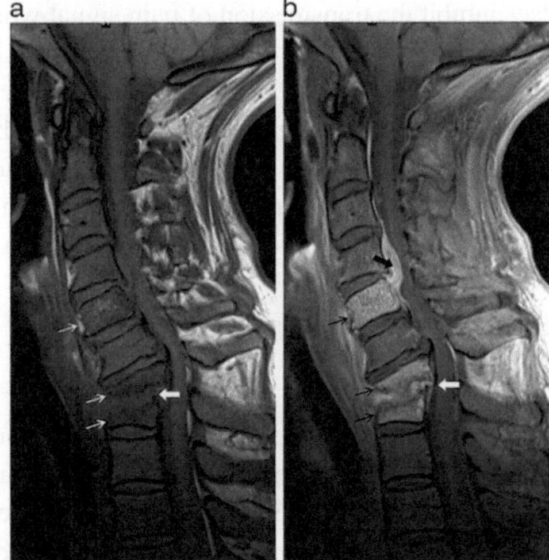

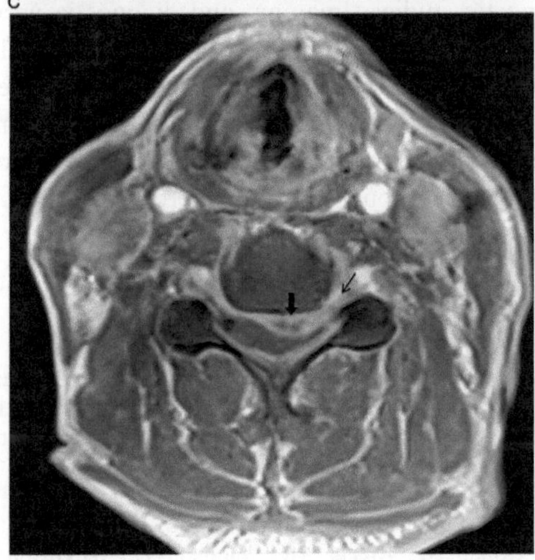

Fig. 20.4 Multilevel discitis/osteomyelitis causing cord compression and neuroforaminal narrowing. (**a**) Noncontrast T1-weighted sagittal MR image of the cervical spine demonstrates hypointensity of the C5, C7, and T1 vertebral bodies consistent with edema (*thin white arrows*). There is destruction of the inferior endplate of C7 and superior endplate of T1 with irregularity of the disc (*thick white arrow*). (**b**) T1-weighted sagittal MR image of the cervical spine after intravenous administration of gadolinium-based contrast demonstrates enhancement of the C5, C7, and T1 vertebral bodies (*thin black arrows*) and C7-T1 disc (*thick white arrow*). These findings are consistent with discitis/osteomyelitis. There is an enhancing epidural abscess posterior to C4-C5 causing narrowing of the central canal (*thick black arrow*). (**c**) Axial T1-weighted MR image at the level of C4-C5 after intravenous administration of gadolinium-based contrast demonstrates a peripherally enhancing epidural abscess narrowing the central canal and compressing the spinal cord (*thick black arrow*). There is extension of the epidural abscess into the left C4-C5 neuroforamen (*thin black arrow*) (Figure courtesy of Richard D. Beegle, MD, UF Health)

Treatment

Conservative treatment for cervical radicular pain stems involves a multimodal approach:

- Hot/cold compresses.
- Topical medications.
- Acetaminophen.
- Nonsteroidal anti-inflammatory medications.
- Medications for neuropathic pain such as gabapentin, pregabalin, carbamazepine, and oxycarbamazepine.
- Physical therapy with active exercise and stretching is superior to patient education about neck disorders.
- There is no evidence of efficacy with mechanical traction according to a Cochrane review.

Interventional Therapy

Cervical radicular symptoms are caused by inflammation of the spinal nerve root. Epidural administration of an anti-inflammatory medication such as a corticosteroid has been shown to decrease pain by tackling inflammatory mediators such as cytokines and prostaglandins.

Interlaminar cervical epidural injections are most often performed at the C7-T1 or T1-T2 levels. A cervical MRI is recommended to identify spinal stenosis or disc herniations that may be compressing the epidural space. A cervical interlaminar epidural injection is performed under fluoroscopic guidance in the anterior-posterior view. After sterile preparation and draping, the C-arm is positioned often with caudocephalad angulation to view the interlaminar space. Lidocaine is used for superficial infiltration, and a tuohy needle is advanced to the lamina of the inferior vertebrae. The needle is then walked off the bone in a superior and medial fashion. A loss-of-resistance syringe is placed, and the loss-of-resistance technique is performed under lateral fluoroscopic guidance. Once a loss of resistance is detected, contrast dye is injected to confirm epidural spread. The corticosteroid is then injected. This procedure should be aborted if paresthesia or cerebrospinal fluid is encountered.

Complications of cervical interlaminar epidural injections have been reported to be <1–16.8%. Due to the risk of epidural hematoma, patients must discontinue their anticoagulation therapy (duration is dependent on anticoagulant). Inaccurate needle placement can cause direct neural injury or accidental subdural and intrathecal injections. Infectious complications, although rare, include discitis, meningitis, and epidural abscess. Excess administration of corticosteroid is associated with elevated blood sugar, increased risk of infection, osteoporosis and osteopenia, and arachnoiditis.

Transforminal epidural steroid injections in the cervical spine are no longer recommended for cervical radicular pain due to catastrophic complications noted in the literature. Transient or permanent plegia and spinal cord infarction have been associated with inadvertent injection of local anesthetic or particular steroids into branches of the vertebral artery or anterior spinal artery.

In addition to epidural steroid injections in the cervical spine, pulsed radiofrequency treatment of the dorsal root ganglion has been reported. In a prospective study, this procedure provided 75% pain relief at 3 months and 50% at 6 months. On the other hand, systematic reviews have shown limited evidence of the superiority of radiofrequency treatment of the dorsal root ganglion over placebo and increased risk of harm. Pulsed radiofrequency treatment has been shown to be more effective than placebo in a single randomized control trial but remains a treatment reserved for very selected cases in which standard therapies have not been beneficial, as this technique carries some of the same catastrophic risks as the cervical transforaminal injections.

Side effects from radiofrequency ablation of the dorsal root ganglion include a temporary burning sensation at the affected area or a sensory change such as a hypoesthesia. Due to the close proximity of the dorsal root ganglion to the spinal cord, epidural space, and vertebral arteries, there has been accidental intrathecal, epidural, and intravascular injection of local anesthetic.

Spinal cord stimulation is the implantation of an electrode in the dorsal epidural space that delivers electrical pulses to the dorsal column of the spinal cord. According to the gate theory, these electrical pulses inhibit the transmission of pain signal while transmitting a vibratory sensation or paresthesia. Spinal cord stimulation also decreases the excitability of wide dynamic range neurons. This implantable system may be considered an option for managing cervical radicular pain, particularly in patients with a history of cervical spine surgery.

Summary

Neuroforaminal narrowing, disc herniations, and radiculitis can cause an irritation of the nerve and an inflammatory response that result in cervical radicular pain. History, physical exam, electrodiagnostic studies, imaging, and diagnostic nerve blocks can help diagnose cervical radicular pain. Treatment modalities include conservative therapy and interventional therapy such as epidural steroid injections, pulsed radiofrequency of dorsal root ganglions, and spinal cord stimulation.

Suggested Reading

1. Anderburg L, Annertz M, Rydholm BL, Saveland H. Selective diagnostic nerve root block for the evaluation of radicular pain in the multilevel degenerated cervical spine. Eur Spine J. 2005;15:794–801.
2. Carette S, Fehlings MG. Cervical radiculopathy. N Engl J Med. 2005;353:392–9.
3. Cohen SP, Bicket MC, Jamison D, Wilkinson I, Rathmell JP. Epidural steroids: a comprehensive, evidence-based review. Reg Anesth Pain Med. 2013;38:175–200.
4. Daffner RH, Weissman BN, Angevine PD, Arnold E, Bancroft L, Bennett DL, et al. Expert Panel on Musculoskeletal Imaging. ACR Appropriateness Criteria® chronic neck pain. [online publication]. National Guideline Clearinghouse Available at http://www.guideline.gov/content.aspx?id=23823.
5. Keyes RD. Nerve conduction studies and electromyography. Can Fam Physician. 1990;36:317–20.
6. Maus TP. Radiologic assessment of the patient with spine pain. In: Benzon H, Rathmell JP, Wu CL, Turk DC, Argoff CE, Hurley RW, editors. Practical management of pain. Philadelphia: Elsevier Mosby; 2014.
7. Radhakrishnan K, Litchy WJ, O'Fallon WM, Kurland LT. Epidemiology of cervical radiculopathy: a population-based study from Rochester, Minnesota, 1976 through 1990. Brain. 1994;117:325–35.
8. Van Zundert J, Huntoon M, Patijn J, Lataster A, Mekhail N, Van Kleef M. Cervical radicular pain. Pain Pract. 2009;10(1):1–17.

21 Thoracic Radicular Pain

Brian R. Monroe and Carlos A. Pino

Key Concepts

- While thoracic radicular pain is not as common as lumbar or cervical radicular pain, it accounts for up to 5% of referrals to outpatient pain clinics.
- Thoracotomies are very high risk with more than 80% of posterolateral thoracotomy patients having persistent pain after 1 year.
- Thoracic radicular pain is generally diagnosed based on history of trauma or surgery, however in the case of insidious or idiopathic onset, other causes should be considered including malignancy and central nervous system disease.
- Disc bulges are an uncommon cause of thoracic radicular pain. Unlike lumbar or cervical protrusions, thoracic disc bulges often lead to pyramidal tract symptoms rather than radicular pain.
- Steroids may be administered systemically or utilizing interventional techniques for symptomatic treatment of thoracic radicular pain. Caution should be observed with repeated doses.
- Neuromodulators such as the gabapentinoids and tricyclic antidepressants should be considered first-line therapy for patients with thoracic radicular pain.
- Opioids may be appropriate in selected patients for a limited time.
- Muscle relaxants have shown no benefit without concordant muscle spasm/spasticity. If used, a short duration is suggested.
- Physical therapy has not been shown to be effective in thoracic radicular pain but may help with other comorbidities in these patients.
- Interventional treatments have limited data supporting or refuting their use for thoracic radicular pain but are relatively low risk and should be considered.
- Without definitive pathology or signs of myelopathy, outcomes from surgical interventions are poor.

Epidemiology

Chest wall pain is a common clinical entity with some studies citing up to 5% of outpatient visits. While the differential for chest wall pain is large, a thorough history will generally delineate the cause. Thoracic radicular pain is defined as pain radiating in an area innervated by a nervus intercostalis. Usually, this pain is unilateral and rarely

B.R. Monroe, MD
Lewis Katz School of Medicine, Department of Anesthesiology and Pain Medicine Geisinger Health System, Danville, PA
e-mail: Bmonroe@geisinger.edu

C.A. Pino, MD (✉)
Department of Anesthesiology, University of Vermont College of Medicine, Burlington, VT, USA
e-mail: Carlos.Pino@UVMHealth.org

J. Cheng, R.W. Rosenquist (eds.), *Fundamentals of Pain Medicine*,
https://doi.org/10.1007/978-3-319-64922-1_21

covers more than one level. Thoracic radicular pain is particularly common after intra- and extrathoracic surgeries including CABG, mastectomies, and in particular thoracotomies. Persistent pain is seen in approximately 28% of patients after cardiac surgery. Women are particularly at high risk for post-thoracotomy pain. Postoperative pain control with epidural analgesia helps reduce the risk, but no surgical techniques have been shown to be preferable. A recent retrospective study found that more than 80% of posterolateral thoracotomy patients had persistent pain after 1 year, with 84% of patients reporting that the pain negatively affected their activities of daily living. Postherpetic neuralgia is a frequent cause of thoracic radicular pain (see Chap. 24).

Anatomy

The chest wall itself is made up of the 12 thoracic vertebrae, 12 ribs, the associated costal cartilages, and the sternum. Posteriorly, each rib articulates with the associated lateral vertebral body as well as with the associated transverse process at the first ten levels. Anteriorly the first 7 ribs articulate with the sternum; these are referred to as the "true ribs." Ribs 8–10 attach to each other and to the seventh rib at the inferior border of the sternum and are referred to as "false ribs." The joints that articulate with the sternum are true synovial joints and allow for chest wall movement with respiration. Ribs 11 and 12 do not articulate anteriorly and are referred to as "floating ribs." In about 0.5% of the population, an additional rib at C7 is present.

The intercostal nerves are formed from the anterior rami of the nerve roots from T1 to T11, and each has motor and sensory components. These nerves travel around the chest wall in the intercostal space. This space is formed by three muscle groups, the external, internal, and the innermost intercostals. The innermost intercostals are lined by the endothoracic fascia which contacts the parietal pleura. The intercostal nerve accompanies the artery and the vein within the intercostal grove on the inferior border of each rib. The vein is the most superior, the artery in the middle, and the nerve the most inferior. The T12 anterior ramus passes into the abdominal wall and forms the subcostal nerve. Additionally T1 has a branch into the brachial plexus and T2 to the medial cutaneous nerve of the arm, which can account for "referred" arm pain from the thorax.

Pathophysiology

The causes of thoracic radicular pain include neuropathic pain syndromes, musculoskeletal lesions, skin diseases, extrathoracic diseases, and psychogenic pain. The causes of neuropathic pain may include spinal cord pathology, actual injury to the nerve root causing a radiculopathy, or peripheral neuropathy. Postherpetic neuralgia is a common cause of neuropathic thoracic radicular pain. Musculoskeletal sources of pain can include bony lesions of the vertebrae such as a compression fracture leading to nerve root compression, rib pathology, and metastatic disease leading to nerve entrapment or direct invasion of the nerve. Muscular and bone injury after intrathoracic procedures are common. Diseases of the skin can also cause radicular pain, but this is usually associated with trauma or surgical manipulation that produces scarring near the path of the intercostal nerve. Extrathoracic causes of chest pain are common but they rarely cause radicular pain. Thoracic disc bulges causing pathology are rare accounting for less than 1% of all herniated nucleus pulposus. Unlike the lumbar spine where disc bulges may entrap an exiting or traversing nerve root, low cervical and thoracic bulges often result in pyramidal tract symptoms rather than thoracic radicular symptoms. Finally thoracic radicular pain can be a symptom of psychogenic pain.

Clinical Features

Patients with radicular thoracic pain generally present with radiating pain on one side of the chest along the path of one nervus intercostalis. The pain can begin acutely after a surgery or trauma or may be more insidious as in the case of neoplasm. Patients may use nearly any descriptors for the pain depending on the pathology. The pain may be described as constant, intermittent, dull, stabbing, sharp, electric, or burning, and these descriptors may give some insight as to the neuropathic versus nociceptive nature of the pain.

Diagnosis and Imaging

A clinical diagnosis of thoracic radicular pain is most often based on history of thoracic surgery or trauma with persisting pain. Even with a clear history supporting the diagnosis, other serious etiologies should be ruled out. A history of cough, hemoptysis, and weight loss can indicate a neoplastic process. Signs of myelopathy, lower extremity weakness, changes in bowel or bladder function, or pyramidal signs may indicate direct spinal cord injury or compression and depending on the time course of the symptoms may warrant immediate surgical evaluation.

Physical exam can be highly variable. Unfortunately, the thoracic dermatomes partially overlap making it difficult to isolate a single level on physical exam. Muscular dysfunction is also unlikely to be seen due to an overlap of the adjacent levels. The presence of local pain with sternal pressure may help differentiate sternal pain versus radicular pain, but in the event of rib pathology compressing a nerve root, this may elicit pain as well.

In the event of an unclear cause or the presence of any red flags, further steps should be taken to identify the cause of pain. X-rays are a simple and effective way to evaluate patients for bony abnormalities, including vertebral compression fracture and rib fractures. In the case of suspected radiculopathy, myelopathy, or neoplasm, an MRI of the thoracic spine may be indicated.

A diagnostic nerve root or intercostal nerve block can be performed in order to identify or confirm involvement of an individual nerve root or intercostal nerve. Diagnostic blocks are generally performed at the suspected level, the level above, and the level below in order to cover any overlap. These blocks are usually done on an outpatient basis under either fluoroscopic or ultrasound guidance to identify the anatomy and minimize the risk of complications, such as pneumothorax.

Treatment

Multiple treatments exist, but unfortunately thoracic radicular pain is particularly difficult to control. The largest studies have looked specifically at post-thoracotomy pain, and studies looking at treatments for other causes are extremely limited. It is generally agreed that for patients without myelopathy, conservative treatments should be started, including medication management (Table 21.1) and possibly minimally invasive procedures.

Medications

Steroids

Steroids may be administered orally or locally by means of interventional techniques as described below. There is little data on their use in thoracic radicular pain, but based on studies looking at lumbar radicular pain, they have been shown to be helpful in reducing pain. Orally, prednisone and methylprednisolone are the most frequently used steroids. Methylprednisolone is available as a dose pack, which is taken over 6 days with a declining daily dose starting at 24 mg and dropping by 4 mg daily. Prednisone dosing is highly variable ranging from several days to several weeks. A dose of steroid can substantially decrease pain due to inflammation, but the mechanism for treatment of noninflammatory pain is less clear. It is known that glucocorticoid receptors are present in lamina 1 and 2 of the dor-

Table 21.1 Medications frequently used for neuropathic pain

Medication	Dose
Gabapentin	300 mg TID–1200 mg TID
Amitriptyline	50–75 mg QHS
Duloxetine	60–120 mg QD
Venlafaxine	37.5–225 mg QD
Pregabalin	75–300 mg BID
Clonidine	0.1–0.3 mg BID

sal horn. While commonly prescribed, caution should always be used with steroid doses even for short bursts. Effects on the bone, skin, muscle, and fat, blood pressure, glucose levels, mental status, mood, and immune suppression can cause serious complications. Additionally exogenous glucocorticoids inhibit the hypothalamic-pituitary-adrenal axis. A single neuraxial injection can cause suppression for up to 3 weeks and a series of injections for up to 3 months.

Acetaminophen

Acetaminophen may be used alone or in combination with other medications. Although initially isolated in 1873 and used clinically for over a century, the mechanism of action for acetaminophen is not completely known. Acetaminophen is a weak inhibitor of prostaglandin synthesis in the brain leading to the antipyretic effects, but this is not thought to contribute to analgesia. Theories include modulation of the nitric oxide pathways, possible existence of a COX-3 enzyme, and potential suppression of central COX-1 and COX-2. Acetaminophen can be safely used in healthy individuals. In patients with malnourishment, renal disease, alcoholism, and hepatic disease, the potential risk should be compared to the benefit. Single doses of greater than 7.5 g and chronic doses of 3–4 g per day are associated with severe hepatic toxicity.

NSAIDs

These medications are some of the most commonly used drugs in the world. Their effects are derived from the inhibition of COX in the prostaglandin synthetic pathway. In the case of radicular pain with an inflammatory component, such as acute nerve compression, these drugs may provide adequate relief alone. Many formulations are available over the counter including ibuprofen and naproxen. Newer NSAIDs include the selective COX-2 inhibitors such as celecoxib, which is available by prescription only. NSAIDs must be used with caution in patients with history of gastrointestinal bleeding, renal disease, and heart disease. With acute injuries and inflammation, short-acting agents like ibuprofen are appropriate. For mild to moderate pain, 200–400 mg every 4–6 h as needed is appropriate, and individual doses of greater than 400 mg have not been shown to improve pain control, but higher doses may offer additional anti-inflammatory effect. A long-acting agent can be trialed when prolonged use is required. Naproxen can be bought over the counter and is effective with twice-a-day dosing. Dosing at 250–500 mg BID is appropriate but not to exceed 1500 mg per day. There is also a controlled release version of naproxen available that is once per day dosing. Meloxicam is a prescription only once-a-day option. Starting at 7.5 mg daily and titrating up as high as 15 mg daily are appropriate.

Gabapentinoids

The two most common medications in this category are gabapentin and pregabalin. Gabapentinoids act on alpha-2-delta-1 subunits of voltage-gated calcium channels in the central nervous system inhibiting the release of glutamate and substance P as well as downregulating N-type calcium channels in the spinal cord, to produce analgesia. Gabapentin works best when a constant blood level is maintained. Either three times daily dosing or a long-acting formulation should be used. Pregabalin can be employed in a BID dosing, but TID dosing is not unusual. Gabapentin and pregabalin can have harsh side effects most frequently causing sedation.

If a patient is intolerant to one drug, a lower dose or switching agents may minimize the side effects. These medications are most commonly used for neuropathic pain. While they have not been shown to specifically treat somatic pain, gabapentin has been demonstrated to decrease cutaneous pain sensations and central sensitization, which may play a significant role in chronic somatic pain.

Anticonvulsants

There are a large number of anticonvulsants that have been used for neuropathic and radicular pain, but their exact mechanisms of action on pain are poorly understood. The gabapentinoids as described above are the most frequently prescribed. Traditional anticonvulsants can be considered, but most require some form of chronic monitoring or have significant side effects. There are no studies at this time evaluating these medications for thoracic radicular pain. Anticonvulsants most commonly used include carbamazepine, phenytoin, lamotrigine, and topiramate.

Antidepressants

Antidepressants are frequently used for neuropathic and radicular pain. The exact mechanism is not well understood but it is thought to be related to their ability to inhibit presynaptic reuptake of serotonin and noradrenaline in the descending inhibitory pathways. Other theories include both central and peripheral changes in sodium channel signaling, NMDA receptor-blocking properties, and actions on H1, 5-HT, and muscarinic/nicotinic receptors. The doses for analgesia are often much lower than the doses required for antidepressant effects. The best-studied agent for neuropathic pain is amitriptyline, a tricyclic antidepressant. Tricyclics have significant anticholinergic side effects including sedation, and these medications should be avoided in patients with history of ventricular arrhythmia. When prescribed for pain, the side effect of sedation can be beneficial to patients whose sleep is altered by pain. Doses as low as 10–20 mg at night can be beneficial. Doses should be slowly titrated up to minimize side effects.

Another class of antidepressants with demonstrated benefit is the serotonin-norepinephrine reuptake inhibitors (SNRIs), which include venlafaxine and duloxetine. Studies have not shown any analgesic benefit for doses of duloxetine over 60 mg daily, but higher doses are commonly used when comorbid depression or anxiety is present. Other antidepressants, including agents like bupropion and the selective serotonin reuptake inhibitors (SSRIs), have not been shown to be effective for chronic pain.

Muscle Relaxants and Anxiolytics

There is no evidence that muscle relaxants, including the benzodiazepines, are beneficial for radicular pain. In the event of significant myofascial pain associated with muscle tightness and spasm with resulting radicular pain, they could be considered. Although there are no studies specifically on thoracic radicular pain, studies on low back pain have not shown them to be superior to NSAIDs and acetaminophen alone. If chosen, they should be used for a short duration (1–2 weeks) and limited to effective agents with minimal abuse potential or risks. Baclofen 10–80 mg and methocarbamol 1000–4500 mg total daily total dose are effective for muscle spasm.

Opioids

Opioids provide analgesia via direct effects on both the pre- and postsynaptic neurons within the spinal cord. The presynaptic cells have mu, delta, and kappa receptors that when activated lead to a decrease in calcium levels and a decrease in neurotransmitter release. The postsynaptic cell has mu receptors that, when activated, increase potassium conductance leading to hyperpolarization and inhibition of the postsynaptic potential. Opioids have long been considered the "gold standard" for pain control. However, in recent years the use of opioids in chronic pain has become controversial, with many experts cautioning against their use for longer than 3 months in non-cancer pain. The 2012 American Society of Interventional Pain Physicians (ASIPP) guidelines for opioid prescribing summarize the literature support for short-term use for pain and improvement of quality of life as "fair" but the use for greater than 3 months for both pain and quality of life as "limited." In the short term, opioids can provide benefits including analgesia, anxiolysis, cough suppression, euphoria, and sedation. Common side effects and risks include constipation, respiratory depression, nausea, vomiting, pruritus, tolerance, dependence, addiction, ileus, biliary spasm, mental clouding, and urinary retention. Long-term opioid use has been shown to increase hyperalgesia, central sleep apnea, and prolactin levels while decreasing cortisol, LH, FSH, testosterone, and estrogen. The risk of death increases in a dose-dependent manner. Opioid receptors are also found on immune cells and have been shown to suppress natural killer cellular activity and mitogen-induced lymphocyte proliferation and decrease inflammatory cytokine activation. Short-term opioids are appropriate when utilized during acute thoracic pain crisis, while the patient participates in conservative therapies or as a bridge to surgical intervention. Long-term opioids should only be used when conservative treatments have failed and full disclosure of the risks and benefits has been presented to the patient.

Sympatholytics

Clonidine is the most commonly used alpha-2 sympathomimetic agent. Within the dorsal horn, clonidine binds with alpha-2 receptors leading to decreased calcium levels and thereby directly inhibits transmission from both C- and A-delta fibers. It has been suggested that clonidine can increase acetylcholine in the CSF, which can also suppress transmission of pain signals. Because it is a potent antihypertensive, clonidine should be started slowly and titrated up as tolerated by the patient. Commonly starting at 0.1 mg BID and increasing by 0.1 mg per day weekly until the patient reaches 0.3 mg BID is well tolerated.

PT and Noninvasive Treatments

While increasing physical activity, strength, and endurance can benefit patients in multiple ways, physical therapy is poorly tolerated by patients with thoracic radicular pain and has not been shown to be beneficial. Massage and chiropractic manipulation has also not been shown to be beneficial. Studies on alternative therapies such as acupuncture are limited. Psychological treatments may be beneficial for those patients for comorbid depression and anxiety. There is a demonstrated relationship between psychological factors and development of post-thoracotomy pain.

Interventional

For patients with pain secondary to compression fractures, kyphoplasty and vertebroplasty may be beneficial. Two recent large studies did not find a long-term difference in patients who underwent these procedures versus placebo. These procedures have been widely criticized, but many specialists argue that, for a subset of patients with acute or subacute compression fracture, these treatments can provide substantial benefit.

Intercostal nerve blocks can be performed as a diagnostic tool or as a therapeutic intervention (Figs. 21.1, 21.2, and 21.3). These injections

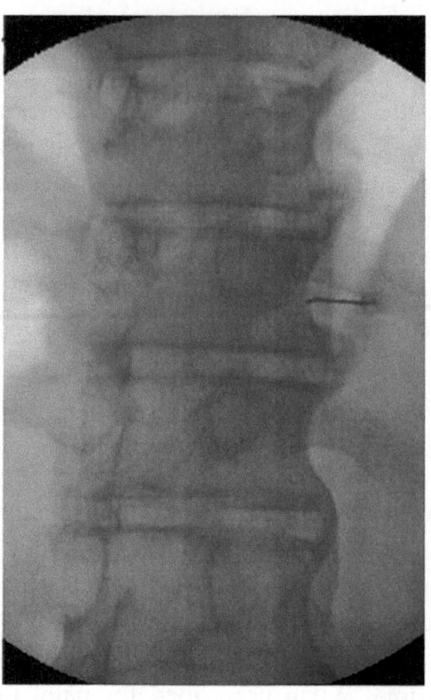

Fig. 21.1 Selective thoracic nerve root injection. This oblique view shows the approach to the nerve root below the rib head within the foramen

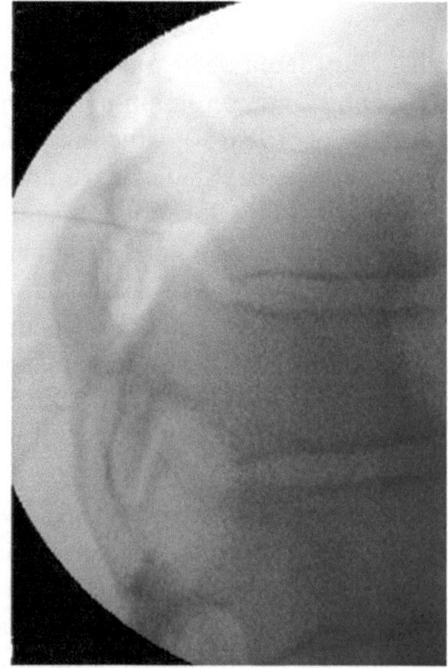

Fig. 21.2 Lateral view of a selective thoracic nerve root injection

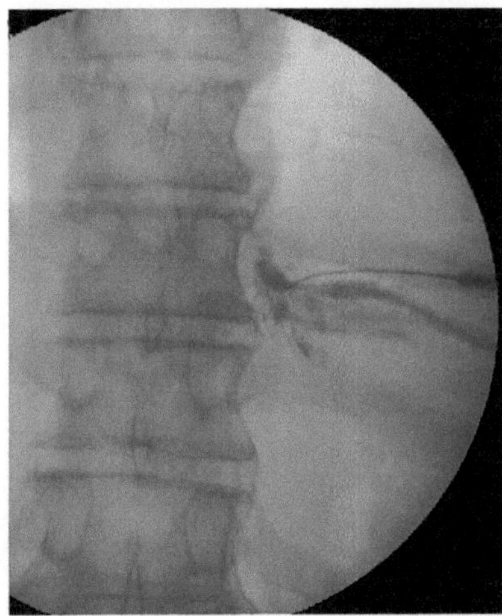

Fig. 21.3 Radiopaque dye is used to verify the position of the needle. Here the dye follows the path of the exiting intercostal nerve and tracks along the intercostal groove. Local anesthetic and steroid can now be placed to complete a therapeutic and diagnostic nerve block

may include a steroid in order to reduce inflammation, swelling, and irritation of the nerve. Unfortunately, there is no literature supporting or refuting the efficacy of these injections in the thoracic spine.

Epidural steroid injections can also be performed in the event of a central or foraminal origin of pain. The epidural space can be accessed through an interlaminar or a transforaminal technique. A recent review of the literature found that the data is "fair and limited" for the procedure.

Radiofrequency ablation (RFA) can be performed on the nervus intercostalis or the dorsal root ganglion (DRG) itself. This procedure is minimally invasive and performed on an outpatient basis. The procedure utilizes an electrode that is placed on the nerve or at the DRG and heated. The mechanism of action is unclear, but several small observational studies have reported clinical efficacy.

Pulsed radiofrequency (PRF) can also be performed. Similar to RFA, an electrode is placed near the DRG or intercostal nerve, and a series of pulse stimulations are applied rather than continuous heat. Small studies have shown this to be effective. No head-to-head studies of RFA vs. PRF have been performed.

Surgical

Surgical options for thoracic pain vary widely depending on the cause. It is generally agreed that when a definitive lesion or myelopathy is present, surgical intervention is appropriate. Depending on the cause, this may include laminectomy, fusion, discectomy, and rib resection. Unfortunately, many thoracic spine surgeries involve approaching through the chest, as the data for posterior laminectomies is poor. For radicular pain, it is less clear as patients often will improve with conservative treatment and time. For post-thoracotomy pain, scar revisions can be performed, but the outcomes are poor, and there is a chance of causing increased pain.

Suggested Reading

1. Benyamin RM, et al. A systematic evaluation of thoracic interlaminar epidural injections. Pain Physician. 2012;15(4):E497–514.
2. Haroutiunian S, et al. The neuropathic component in persistent postsurgical pain: a systematic literature review. Pain. 2013;154(1):95–102.
3. Mongardon N, et al. Assessment of chronic pain after thoracotomy: a 1-year prevalence study. Clin J Pain. 2011;27(8):677–81.
4. van Kleef M, et al. The effects of producing a radiofrequency lesion adjacent to the dorsal root ganglion in patients with thoracic segmental pain by radiofrequency percutaneous partial rhizotomy. Clin J Pain. 1995;11:325–32.
5. van Kleef M, et al. Thoracic pain. Pain Pract. 2010;10(4):327–38.

22 Lumbosacral Radicular Pain

Kent H. Nouri and Salahadin Abdi

Key Concepts

- Lumbosacral radicular pain is defined as pain caused by irritation of the exiting lumbosacral nerve roots, leading to a dysfunction of the sensory and/or motor fibers and causing radiating pain in a lumbar or sacral dermatomal pattern.
- The most common cause of lumbosacral radicular pain is intervertebral disc herniation, whereby the exiting nerve root is placed under tension by the displaced disc tissue. Another major cause of lumbosacral radicular pain is canal stenosis, either central or lateral in origin.
- Clinical signs of lumbar radiculopathy include worsening pain of a sharp, shooting, or burning quality, with or without paresthesias, in a dermatomal distribution characteristic of the nerve roots involved.
- The diagnosis of lumbosacral radicular pain is also one of exclusion. If imaging is warranted, an MRI is the diagnostic modality of choice.
- Selective nerve root blocks have been practiced as the "gold standard" of diagnosis, especially useful in patients with negative findings on radiography but with clinical signs of nerve root irritation.
- Conservative therapy including physical therapy and anti-inflammatory medications is recommended initially. If symptoms persist, interventional options such as selective nerve root blocks or transforaminal epidural injections of a mixture of steroid and local anesthetic under fluoroscopic guidance may provide therapeutic benefit.

Epidemiology

Lumbosacral radicular pain is defined as pain caused by irritation of the exiting lumbosacral nerve root(s), leading to a dysfunction of the sensory and/or motor fibers and causing radiating pain in a lumbar or sacral dermatomal pattern. While motor fiber irregularities including paresis, hyporeflexia, fatigue, and cramping may be present in varying degrees, sensory abnormalities predominate and include paresthesia, dysesthesia, and pain in the corresponding dermatomal distribution. The incidence of lumbosacral radicular pain varies between 9.9% and 25% of the population in numerous studies, with the most common risk factors being male gender, obesity, smoking, depression, and manual laborers with

K.H. Nouri, MD • S. Abdi, MD, PhD (✉)
Department of Pain Medicine, The University of Texas, MD Anderson Cancer Center, 1515 Holcombe Boulevard, Houston, TX 77030, USA
e-mail: sabdi@mdanderson.org

J. Cheng, R.W. Rosenquist (eds.), *Fundamentals of Pain Medicine*,
https://doi.org/10.1007/978-3-319-64922-1_22

flexion-based heavy lifting. The etiology of the nerve injury is most commonly due to disc herniation in those younger than 50 years old and secondary to lumbar stenosis and disc degeneration if older. Most complaints of lumbosacral pain do resolve without any treatment in 60% of the population within 3 months.

Pathophysiology

Anatomically the lumbar and sacral nerve roots follow a subarachnoid course through the cauda equina within the spinal canal, exiting through the intervertebral foramen. There are three anatomical elements which leave the lumbar and sacral nerve roots at a disadvantage to damage. The first is a lack of perineurium to provide tensile strength and thus a diffusion barrier, which their counterparts the peripheral nerve possess. The epineurium is also less plentiful and thus provides less of a compression defense for the nerve itself. And lastly there is poor lymphatic drainage to remove inflammatory mediators, leaving the nerve at a high risk for fibroblast invasion and intraneural fibrosis.

There are numerous anatomical abnormalities which may cause lumbosacral radicular pain. The most common cause is intervertebral disc herniation, whereby the exiting nerve root is placed under tension by the displaced disc tissue. This leads to an inflammatory response, which increases sensitivity and thus decreases the threshold of firing to a minor biomechanical insult. A stretch upon the nerve as small as 10–15% from its resting length is enough to cause neurophysiological dysfunction. Another major cause of lumbosacral radicular pain is canal stenosis, either central or lateral in origin. Spondylolysis or spondylolisthesis, whereby the vertebral body itself shifts away from the lumbosacral spine axis, pulls the nerve root taut and thus injures it. Less common anatomical causes of lumbosacral radicular pain include an arthritic facet joint with osteophyte formation and/or facet hypertrophy which can entrap the exiting nerve, facet joint cysts, ligamentum flavum damage/hypertrophy, vertebral body hyperostosis, and even tumor burden causing irritation.

Clinical Signs and Symptoms

Clinical signs of lumbar radiculopathy include worsening pain of a sharp, shooting, or burning quality, with or without paresthesias, in a dermatomal distribution characteristic of the nerve roots involved (Fig. 22.1). This pain is typically worse in the lower extremities than the lumbar spine itself. If due to a lumbar disc herniation, the pain will be of a quicker onset, worsened with flexion activities, prolonged sitting, and Valsalva maneuvers. If secondary to stenosis as a result of degenerative spine disease, the onset is more insidious, and pain will increase with extension-based activities including walking and prolonged standing, which can cause lower limb paresthesias, weakness, fatigue, and heaviness.

Diagnosis

The diagnosis of lumbosacral radicular pain is also one of exclusion, as many spine and lower extremity pain syndromes reside within the differential diagnosis. The physician should be prepared to rule out spinal pain secondary to facet arthropathy, sacroiliitis, intraspinal ligament damage, lumbosacral plexopathy, and cauda equina syndrome. Lower extremity pain may result from hip or knee arthropathy, piriformis syndrome, and meralgia paresthetica (lateral femoral cutaneous syndrome). Inflammatory issues confounding the diagnosis also include ankylosing spondylitis, Paget's disease, arachnoiditis, and spinal sarcoidosis, all discounted with a proper medical evaluation and workup.

Physical examination to diagnose the lumbosacral radicular pain, while not specific, can be sensitive. A detailed dermatomal mapping of complaints will provide evidence of nerve root involvement, as sensory deficits are a good indicator of the involved lumbosacral area. As Fig. 22.1 illustrates, L3 encompasses the medial thigh to knee, L4 medial to the tibial crest from the knee to sole of the foot, and L5 lateral to tibial crest from the leg to dorsum of the foot, and S1 covers the lateral malleolus to lateral side and plantar surface of the foot. The straight leg raise

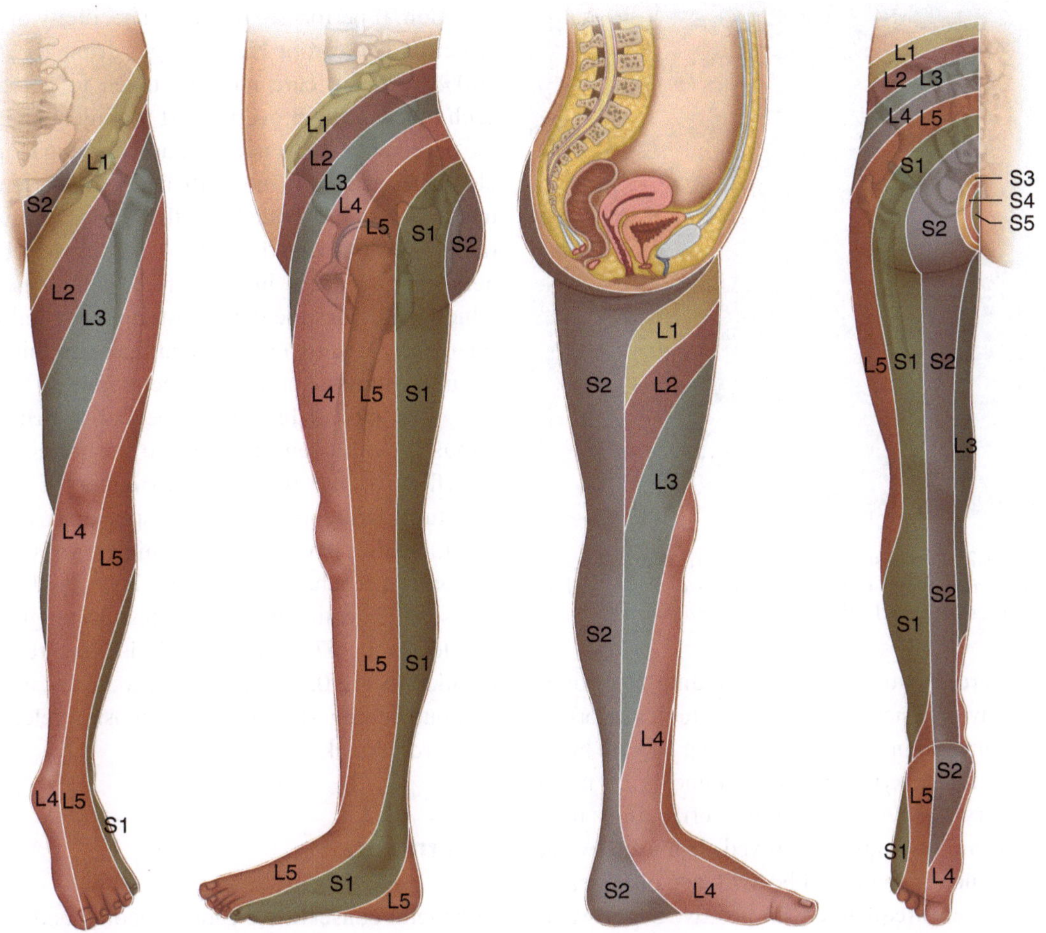

Fig. 22.1 Lower extremity dermatome map

test (a.k.a Lasegue test) may be performed, whereby the patient lies supine and the affected limb passively is raised from 20° to 60° with knee straightened. If pain is elicited with the Lasegue test, it is secondary to tension on the nerve, as there is no anatomical nerve root motion in this 20–60° arc. If pain is caused when raising the contralateral lower extremity in the same way (a.k.a the crossed straight leg raise test), it may be due to a space-occupying lesion within the intrathecal space, e.g., a disc herniation. The sensitivity and specificity of the straight leg raise test is 0.91 and 0.26, respectively, while for the crossed test has a sensitivity of 0.29 and a specificity of 0.88. A modified version of this test can be done while the patient is in sitting position and unable to lie supine.

If imaging is performed, MRI with contrast is the modality of choice, as it is highly sensitive for nerve injury albeit not specific (Figs. 22.2 and 22.3). In a study of asymptomatic patients by Boden et al., 28% were shown to have some form of MRI abnormality. Another study of asymptomatic patients by Jensen et al. showed 64% to have some form of intervertebral disc abnormality, 52% being a disc bulge, 27% disc protrusion, and 1% disc extrusion. CT may be used in patients for whom MRIs are unsuitable and can better delineate bony detail such as lumbar stenosis or bony pathology contributing to the radicular pain. Myelography is used as a last resort in patients unsuited for MRIs or CTs, as the accuracy is noted to be as low as 24%.

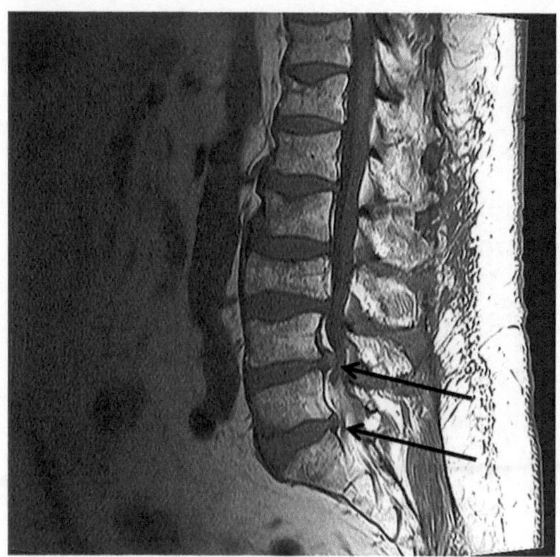

Fig. 22.2 Lumbosacral MRI of a 61 y/o male (*T1 weighted*). Sagittal view of herniations of the intervertebral discs between L4/5 and L5/S1 (*arrows*)

Neurophysiologic tests, including electromyography and nerve conduction studies, work as an adjunct to inconclusive imaging and are better suited for determining the prognosis of motor recovery. They are used to verify if a more peripheral etiology is involved. If muscle weakness is noted, there will be evidence of increased recruitment frequency with positive sharp waves and fibrillation potentials found in the deep paraspinal musculature. Wallerian degeneration secondary to axonotmesis will show a decrease in the evoked compound muscle activation potential amplitude compared to the contralateral muscles. Within the first month, early polyphasic motor unit potentials are present, indicating ephaptic activation of neighboring axons adjacent to the volitionally activated axons. The H-reflex, which is the nerve conduction study of the Achilles muscle stretch reflex arc, may also be used to differentiate between L5 and S1 radiculopathy. If the amplitude of evoked potentials is 50% larger than the contralateral non-affected muscle during neurophysiologic testing, motor function typically recovers well with conservative care alone.

Selective nerve root blocks have been practiced as the "gold standard" of diagnosis, especially useful in patients with negative findings on radiography but with clinical signs of nerve root irritation. If performed properly, specificity of the selective nerve root block ranges from 87% to 100%. Diligent care must be taken to perform each block without overflow of the injectate into the epidural space or adjacent neighboring neural elements, as runoff into either the sinuvertebral nerve or medial branch of the dorsal primary ramus may confound results. The sinuvertebral nerve is a sensory branch of the spinal nerve which innervates the dura, posterior longitudinal ligament, nerve root sleeve, and the outer third of annulus fibrosus of the adjacent intervertebral disc. The medial branch of the dorsal primary ramus provides sensory input to the facet joint. Overflow of the injectate into either of these structures will compromise the specificity of the block. Studies have shown that injection of 0.5 ml of contrast reached the adjacent level in 30% of cases, and injection of 1 ml reached the neighboring levels in 67% of cases. It is thus recommended to use 0.25–0.5 ml of a local anesthetic without adding steroid for diagnostic selective nerve root block.

Treatments

In general conservative care is recommended, as less than 15% of patients with lumbosacral radiculopathy require surgical intervention. As a first-line treatment, physical therapy is recommended, focusing on lumbosacral stabilization, activity modification, and core strengthening through "back school" rehabilitation. If the radicular pain is due to stenosis, Williams/flexion-based exercises are recommended. If due to disc herniation, McKenzie/extension-based maneuvers are preferred. Medications including NSAIDs and/or anticonvulsants are good first-line pharmacotherapeutic options as adjuvants to physical therapy in conservative care.

Interventional options include therapeutic selective nerve root blocks and transforaminal epidural injections of a mixture of steroid and local anesthetic under fluoroscopic guidance (Fig. 22.4). Patients with subacute radicular pain, primarily due to disc herniation, have a relatively good outcome with transforaminal injections.

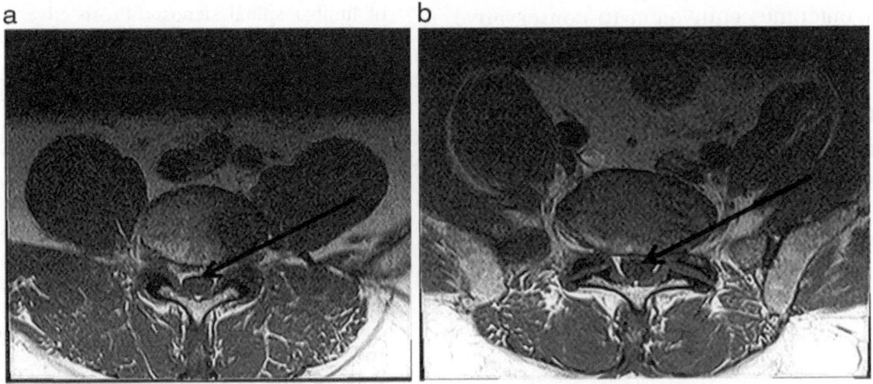

Fig. 22.3 Lumbosacral MRI of a 61 y/o male (T2 weighted). (**a**) and (**b**) Axial views of herniated intervertebral discs between L4/5 and L5/S1 (*arrows*) and foraminal stenosis

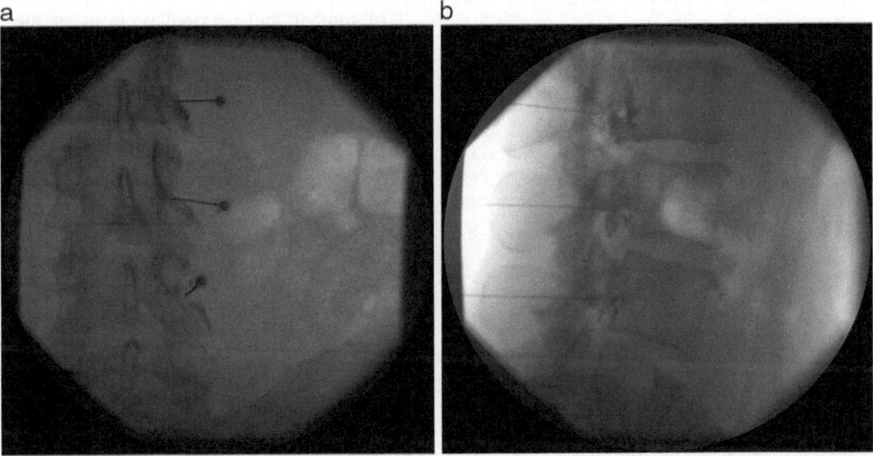

Fig. 22.4 (**a**) Anterioposterior fluoroscopic views of selective L2, L3 and L4 nerve root injections. (**b**) Lateral fluoroscopic views of L2, L3 and L4 selective nerve root injections

Interlaminar epidural injections were once the gold standard of interventional treatment for lumbosacral radiculopathy; however, studies have shown that by laterally targeting the affected nerve root in a transforaminal approach, outcomes improve due to medication spreading to the dorsal root ganglion and anterior epidural space. A detailed systematic review by Abdi et al. in 2007 showed that transforaminal epidural steroid injection is superior to the interlaminar approach for lumbar radiculopathy for a short term. However, the role of epidural steroid injection in treating spine disease including lumbar radiculopathy continues to be controversial. A recent publication in NEJM by Friedly et al. added more to this confusion.

Adhesiolysis has also been entertained as interventional treatment by releasing the entrapped nerve root, especially if this pathology develops post-surgery. Surgical options including discectomy, while once the mainstay of treatment, are now relegated to cases that have severe nerve root damage with resultant neurological deficits including motor abnormalities or have a more chronic duration with persistent pain which has failed to respond to conservative measures. Studies have shown that discectomy for lumbar disc herniation to improve lumbar radicular pain had 2-year outcomes equivalent to conservative care, and up to 70% of these surgically treated patients had residual neurological abnormalities postoperatively. It has been shown that spinal cord stimulation is superior over repeat surgery in patients with lumbosacral radiculopathy and failed back surgery syndrome who have failed first-line conservative therapy.

Summary

Lumbosacral radicular pain remains a challenge, as numerous anatomical abnormalities, including disc herniation and lumbar stenosis, may contribute to the problem. By focusing on the clinical symptoms and utilizing a proper diagnostic and therapeutic algorithm, the clinician can treat this patient population in an effective and safe manner to alleviate discomfort and prevent disability secondary to the pain.

Suggested Reading

1. Abdi S, Datta S, Trescot AM, et al. Epidural steroids in the management of chronic spinal pain: a systematic review. Pain Physician. 2007;10(1):185–212.
2. Boden SD, Davis DO, Dina TS, et al. Abnormal magnetic-resonance scans of the lumbar spine in asymptomatic subjects: a prospective investigation. J Bone Joint Surg. 1990;72A(3):403–8.
3. Bradley KE. Stress-strain phenomena in human spinal nerve roots. Brain. 1961;84:120.
4. Devillé WL, van der Windt DA, Dzaferagić A, Bezemer PD, Bouter LM. The test of Lasègue: systematic review of the accuracy in diagnosing herniated discs. Spine. 2000;25(9):1140–7.
5. Friedly JL, Comstock BA, Turner JA, et al. A randomized trial of epidural glucocorticoid injections for spinal stenosis. N Engl J Med. 2014;371:11–21.
6. Furman MB, Lee TS, et al. Contrast flow selectivity during transforaminal lumbosacral epidural steroid injections. Pain Physician. 2008;11:855–61.
7. Goodard MD, Reid JD. Movements induced by straight leg raising in the lumbosacral roots, nerves and plexus, and in the intrapelvic section of the sciatic nerve. J Neurol Neurosurg Psychiatry. 1965;28:12.
8. Guigui P, Cardinne L, Rillardon L, et al. Pre- and postoperative complications of surgical treatment of lumbar spinal stenosis. Prospective study of 306 patients. Rev Chir Orthop Reparatrice Appar Mot. 2002;88:669–77.
9. Haueisen C, Smith B, Myers SR, et al. The diagnostic accuracy of spinal nerve injection studies. Their role in the evaluation of recurrent sciatica. Clin Orthop. 198(198):179–83.
10. Herron LD. Selective nerve root blocks in patient selection for lumbar surgery – surgical results. J Spinal Disord. 1989;2:75–9.
11. Jensen MC, Brant-Zawadzki MD, Obuchowski N. Magnetic resonance imaging of the lumbar spine in people without back pain. N Engl J Med. 1994;331:69–73.
12. Johnson EW, Fletcher FR. Lumbosacral radiculopathy: review of 100 consecutive cases. Arch Phys Med Rehabil. 1981;62(7):321–3.
13. Johnson EW, Melvin JL. Value of electromyography in lumbar radiculopathy. Arch Phyl Med Rehabil. 1971;52(6):239–43.
14. Keegan JJ. Relations of nerve roots to abnormalities of lumbar and cervical portions of the spine. Arch Surg. 1947;55(3):246–70.
15. Murphy RW. Nerve roots and spinal nerves in degenerative disc disease. Clin Orthop Rel Res. 1977;129:46–60.
16. Ng L, Chaudhary N, Sell P. The efficacy of corticosteroids in periradicular infiltration for chronic radicular pain: a randomized, double-blind, controlled trial. Spine. 2005;30:857–62.
17. Schulz H, Lougheed WM, Wortzman G, et al. Intervertebral nerve-root in the investigation of chronic lumbar disc disease. Can J Surg. 1973;16:217–21.
18. Seimon LP. Low back pain: clinical diagnosis and management. Norwalk: Appleton-Century-Crofits; 1983. p. 3–114.
19. Tarulli AW, Raynor EM. Lumbosacral radiculopathy. Neurol Clin. 2007;25:287–405.
20. Taylor RS, Van Buyten JP, Buchser E. Spinal cord stimulation for chronic back and leg pain and failed back surgery syndrome: a systematic review and analysis of prognostic factors. Spine. 2005;30:152–60.
21. van Akkerveeken PF. The diagnostic value of nerve sheath infiltration. Acta Orthop Scand. 1993;64:61–3.
22. Weber H. The natural course of disc herniation. Acta Orthop Scan Suppl. 1993;251:19–20.
23. Weinstein JN, Tosteson TD, Lurie JD, et al. Surgical vs nonoperative treatment for lumbar disk herniation: the spine patient outcomes research trial (SPORT): a randomized trial. JAMA. 2006;296(20):2441–50.
24. Yildirim K, Kataray S. The effectiveness of gabapentin in patients with chronic radiculopathy. Pain Clin. 2003;15:213–8.
25. Younes M, Bejia I, Aguir Z, et al. Prevalence and risk factors of disc-related sciatica in an unrban population in Tunisia. Joint Bone Spine. 2006;73:538–42.

Part VI

Painful Disease States: Neuropathic Pain

Complex Regional Pain Syndrome

23

Michael Stanton-Hicks

Key Concepts

- Complex regional pain syndrome (CRPS) was formerly called reflex sympathetic dystrophy (RSD), "causalgia," or reflex neurovascular dystrophy (RND). As a result of a special consensus workshop in 1993, the term CRPS was adopted to describe a chronic systemic disease characterized by severe pain, swelling, and changes in the skin. This term does not imply any understanding of its mechanism.
- A large population-based study showed that the estimated overall incidence of CRPS was 26.2 per 100,000 person-years. Females were affected at least three times more often than males. The highest incidence occurred in females in the age group of 61–70 years. The upper extremity was affected more frequently than the lower extremity, and a fracture was the most common precipitating event even though it could occur after any type of injury, or even spontaneously.
- CRPS can be described as a painful inflammatory condition that occurs in most cases after trivial trauma to an extremity. The sympathetic nervous system is in some way involved with its pathophysiology. Neuropeptides, substance P, and CGRP, antidromically released from sensory terminals in the skin, evoke dilatation and protein extravasation in the tissue. The resulting signs – reddening, warming, and edema – are termed *neurogenic inflammation*.
- The diagnosis is essentially based on four different diagnostic categories – *sensory* (hyperesthesia, hyperalgesia, allodynia), *vasomotor* (temperature asymmetry and/or skin color changes and/or skin color asymmetry), *sudomotor/edema* (edema and/or sweating changes and/or sweating asymmetry), and *motor/trophic* (motor dysfunction and/or trophic changes). However, not all categories have to be met for each patient.
- The principals of therapy as currently recommended cover standard medical treatment used for neuropathic syndromes and other interventions directed at the current pathophysiology that may be necessary.

The original term to describe this syndrome reflex sympathetic dystrophy (RSD) was proposed by Evans in 1946. It was thought at the time that sympathetic hyperactivity underlies the signs and symptoms of the condition. However, many patients do not respond to sympathetic blocks; there is no evidence for a reflex mechanism, and dystrophy only occurs in a very small subgroup of patients. In 1993, as a result of a

M. Stanton-Hicks, MD (✉)
Department of Pain Management, Cleveland Clinic, 9500 Euclid Avenue, Cleveland, OH 44195, USA
e-mail: stantom@ccf.org

J. Cheng, R.W. Rosenquist (eds.), *Fundamentals of Pain Medicine*,
https://doi.org/10.1007/978-3-319-64922-1_23

special consensus workshop, the name of the syndrome was changed to complex regional pain syndrome (CRPS), a term that did not imply any understanding of its mechanism. Because some patients respond to block of the sympathetic nervous system to the affected extremity, the relief of pain that follows is termed sympathetically maintained pain (SMP). If no relief of pain occurs, the term sympathetically independent pain (SIP) is used. It is however understood that both SMP and SIP to a varying degree may coexist in the same patient. See Fig. 23.1.

Epidemiology

The largest study of 100,000 persons was undertaken in the Netherlands where a peak incidence of 61–70 years of age was found. The higher age range was most likely due to the occurrence of fractures at an older age which, together with sprain, is the most common cause of CRPS. The most recent study done in 2012 found that 7% of patients develop CRPS Type 1 after their injury and that none of these patients were free of symptoms 1 year later: 596 patients comprised this series. Two recent studies have found there to be no psychological factors or personality traits that predispose an individual to the development of CRPS Type 1.

Pathophysiology

CRPS can be described as a painful inflammatory condition that occurs in most cases after sprain or fracture and in a few cases after trivial trauma to an extremity. Our current understanding is that the sympathetic nervous system is in some way involved with its pathophysiology. The expression of α1-adrenoceptor mRNA was upregulated in DRG neurons after peripheral nerve injury or inflammation typical with that seen in CRPS Type 1. An increase in α1-adrenoceptors was seen in hyperalgesic skin of patients with CRPS Type 1. Inflammation is normally marked by a typical response of immune cells such as lymphocytes, phagocytes, and mast cells. These secrete proinflammatory cytokines. CRPS patients are associated with an increase in proinflammatory cytokines, TNF-α, IL-1β, IL-2, and IL-6, in local blister fluid, circulating plasma, and cerebral spinal fluid (CSF). Proinflammatory cytokines excite nociceptors and can induce long-term peripheral sensitization. Also found is an increase of calcitonin gene-related peptide (CGRP).

What is now known is that neuropeptides, substance P and CGRP, antidromically released from sensory terminals in the skin evoke dilatation and protein extravasation in the tissue. The resulting signs – reddening, warming, and

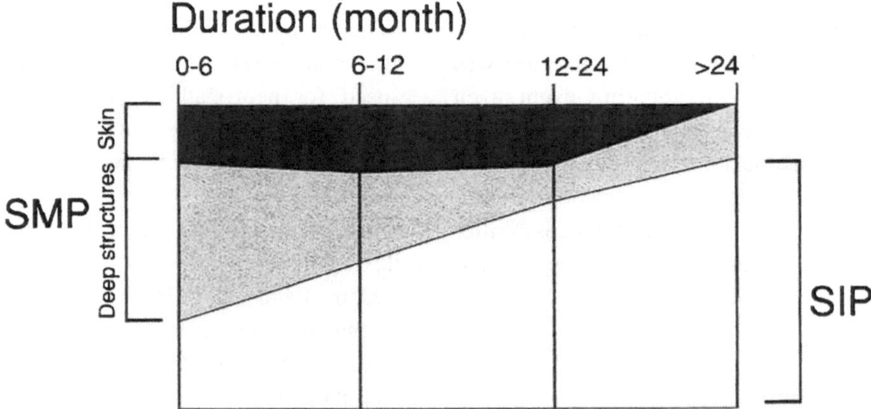

Fig. 23.1 The relationship between sympathetically maintained pain (SMP) and sympathetically independent pain (SIP) during the course of the CRPS. Also shown, the components of deep somatic sympathetic innervation (deep SMP) and superficial SMP (With permission: Wolters Kluwer Health, Inc., Jörn Schattschneider, Andreas Binder, Dieter Siebrecht, et al., Complex regional pain syndromes: the influence of cutaneous and deep somatic sympathetic innervation on pain. *Clin J Pain.* 2006;22(3):242, Fig. 1)

edema – are termed *neurogenic inflammation*. The importance of neuropeptides in CRPS pathophysiology is the recent association with the antihypertensive medication angiotensin converting enzyme (ACE) inhibitor therapy. ACE is responsible for metabolizing bradykinin and substance P to the inactive form and its inhibition leads to higher tissue levels of both neuropeptides and a possible increased risk for CRPS. The recent studies on lenalidomide and thalidomide emphasize the contribution of inflammation to the metabolic process of CRPS.

The production of free radicals in the affected limb is possibly responsible for the endothelial dysfunction observed in CRPS patients. The impaired endothelial function is a major factor in the pathogenesis of the trophic changes that are found in both superficial and deep tissues. Tissue acidosis is invariably followed by sensitization and activation of nociceptive afferents and therefore spontaneous pain sensation. Increased nociceptive activity will trigger central sensitization which in turn is responsible for allodynia and hyperalgesia. The increased CNS neuronal hyperactivity due to the nociceptive barrage particularly in the dorsal horn is one factor responsible for the pathogenesis of chronic pain in CRPS. Furthermore, temporal summation is significantly greater in CRPS patients because of repeated nociception from thermal and mechanical stimuli in the affected limb.

N-Methyl-D-aspartate (NMDA) receptors also contribute to central sensitization and are the reason why ketamine is used to reduce the associated pain. Another factor in central sensitization is glial activity particularly microglia and astrocytes. These are immunocompetent cells in the CNS which can help to drive and maintain allodynia and hyperalgesia. Glia are responsible for releasing a number of proinflammatory cytokines, nitric oxide (NO), excitatory amino acids, prostaglandins, and ATP. Elevated proinflammatory cytokines (IL-6, IL-β), glial fibrillary acidic protein (GFAP), MCPL, NO metabolites, glutamate, and calcium are found in increasing quantities in the CSF of patients with CRPS. The sensory, somatomotor, and autonomic changes observed in CRPS patients are likely the result of disordered CNS processing. Imaging studies of the somatosensory cortex (S1) have demonstrated reorganization that is related to the severity of pain, particularly the mechanical hyperalgesia found in CRPS. Other cortical changes associated with the motor system are also found in CRPS Type 1 and occur particularly in the primary motor and supplementary motor cortices which are related to the extent of motor dysfunction.

Interesting Clinical Aspects

The classical description of CRPS that included successive stages has been replaced by three clinical findings (see Table 23.1, Bruehl et al.). Pain however is always disproportional in intensity to what would be expected by the inciting event. Three distinct vascular dysregulation patterns are described:

- Patients with a *warm* type of regulation – generally the acute stage or less than 6 months. There is an associated increase in perfusion of the affected limb in comparison with the contralateral side.
- Patients with a *cold* type of regulation – chronic stage has lower skin temperatures and perfusion values than the unaffected side.
- Patients with an *intermediate* type in which the temperature and perfusion are either high or low depending on the degree of sympathetic dysfunction.

Edema is common in acute CRPS. It has been demonstrated that edema in CRPS Type 1 patients disappeared after spinal anesthesia, suggesting that sympathetic activity may maintain the edema

Table 23.1 Clinical findings

1.	Vasomotor and motor/trophic changes
2.	Pain and sensory abnormalities Particularly allodynia/hyperalgesia
3.	Florid or all aspects of syndrome Pain may be SMP or SIP Frequently both coexist in a variable manner

Adapted: Bruehl S, Harden RN, Galer BS, Saltz S, Backonja M, Stanton-Hicks M. Complex regional pain syndrome: are there distinct subtypes and sequential stages of the syndrome? *Pain* 2002; 95:119–124.

although the mechanism is unknown. Sympathetic afferent coupling is responsible for the release of peptides from peptidergic afferent neurons with unmyelinated fibers that cause vasodilatation and plasma extravasation.

Motor dysfunction is found in 97% of CRPS patients who were evaluated prospectively. Motor disorders include tremors, weakness, decreased range of motion, dystonia, and incoordination. Dystonia of the lower extremity typically is seen as an equinus foot deformity. In the upper limb it presents as finger flexion.

Patients with extensive hypoesthesia have increased thresholds for mechanical, cold, warm, and noxious heat stimuli. These phenomena are due to CNS changes. Half of CRPS patients can demonstrate these sensory changes in the ipsilateral quadrant or in a hemicorporeal distribution.

Maleki describes three patterns of spread in CRPS Type 1 – contiguous, independent, and noncontiguous such as mirror image spread. Van der Laan et al. described 7% out of 1006 patients developed severe complications of the lower extremity that included ulcers, edema, myoclonus, and dystonia.

Diagnosis

The standard IASP criteria which were published in 1994 have now been revised to include the following: four different diagnostic categories – *sensory* (hyperesthesia, hyperalgesia, allodynia), *vasomotor* (temperature asymmetry and/or skin color changes and /or skin color asymmetry), *sudomotor/edema* (edema and/or sweating changes and/or sweating asymmetry), and *motor/trophic* (motor dysfunction and/or trophic changes) (Table 23.2). If one sign is observed in two or more of these categories and at least one symptom is described in three of four categories, the resulting diagnosis of CRPS has a sensitivity of 0.85 and a specificity of 0.69. These modified diagnostic criteria (Budapest Criteria) have now been validated. The Committee for Classification of Chronic Pain Terms of the IASP has accepted these criteria for clinical and research diagnosis (Table 23.1). Additional diagnostic tests may be helpful to support the foregoing clinical diagnostic criteria. Because sweating abnormalities are relatively common (24%), they can be assessed by clinical examination. Table 23.3 lists some laboratory tests which may be useful to document the pathophysiological disturbances which occur in CRPS.

Management Approaches to CRPS

Without a definitive mechanism to address, treatment should follow an interdisciplinary approach that uses whichever modalities that are appropriate to treat the pathophysiology and achieve a restoration of function. Traditional measures that have been determined either by evidence or from experience should be applied in the management of CRPS. However, there is a paucity of evidence-based treatments. Many treatments are taken from experience gained from management of other neuropathic pain syndromes such as postherpetic neuralgia and diabetic neuropathy. The three greatest impediments to treatment that use physical modalities are allodynia, hyperalgesia, and the movement disorder.

Figure 23.2 illustrates the emphasis on rehabilitation, which is the core treatment for CRPS. Essentially the idea is that reactivation of the impacted tissue with desensitization and satisfactory pain management will begin the process of functional return. Because of induced pain resulting from pathological movement and mechanoreceptor dysfunction, it may be necessary to use isometric exercises before any attempt is made to move (range) the affected joint(s). Once early movement is achieved, this should be gradually increased against resistance (rROM). Passive movement is probably counterproductive to return of function. Sometimes it may be necessary to use mirror box treatment and mirror visual feedback (MV1). This has been found successful for both upper and lower extremity movement with laterality training and imaging of the movements by the patient. The premotor cortex may become active without involving other motor cortical areas. Sometimes

Table 23.2 *Budapest criteria*. At least one symptom in three of four categories and one sign in two or more categories (SENS. 0.99: SPEC 0.68)

Category	Symptom	Sign
Sensory	Hyperesthesia, allodynia	Hyperalgesia (PP) allodynia – Mech./thermal/deep
Vasomotor	Δ Skin/color Δ Temperature	>1 °C/Δ skin/color
Sudomotor Edema	Δ Sweating/edema	Δ Sweating/edema
Motor Trophic	Motor dysfunction ↓ROM Δ Trophic	Motor function ↓ROM (weak, dystonia, tremor)/trophic

Adapted: Harden et al. *Pain* (2010);150: 268–274

Table 23.3 Supplementary tests for CRPS

Tests	Sensitivity	Specificity	Helpful
1. Plain x-rays (late in disease) Gradl et al. (2003)	73	57	No
2. 3-phase bone scan (early disease) Wuppenhorst et al. (2010)	97	86	Possibly
3. Temperature side differences Wasner et al. (2002)	76	93	Yes, during sympathetic stimulation
4. Quantitative sensory testing Rommel et al. (2001)	High	Low	Impractical except research
5. Laser Doppler scintigraphy	High	High	Practical if equipment available
6. Quantitative sudomotor axon reflex test (QSART)	High	Fair	Requires special laboratory
7. Magnetic resonance imaging MRI Koch et al. (1991)	91	17	Impractical
8. FMRI cortical reorganization Maihofner et al. (2007)	Under investigation		
9. Magnetoencephalography Pahapill et al. (2013)	Under investigation		

it may be necessary to couple this with graded motor imagery (GMI). It may be necessary to use (GMI) over a period of 6 weeks. The theoretical basis for these programs is still evolving.

CRPS management should be in an interdisciplinary setting where psychological approaches are frequently required to assist patients with their treatment. The use of cognitive behavioral therapy (CBT) is often necessary in the early stages of treatment. The combination of behavioral therapy with CBT and GMI together accelerated the return of function in children. The three principles that should be followed are:

- Education regarding the nature of disease for patients and families.
- Patients whose condition has exceeded 2 months should be psychologically evaluated with or without CBT.
- Any psychiatric comorbidity or other live stressors should also be addressed.

Pharmacological Management

Any medications that are used for the treatment of patients with CRPS should be given on a symptomatic basis or for the treatment of known pathophysiology. These medications should be

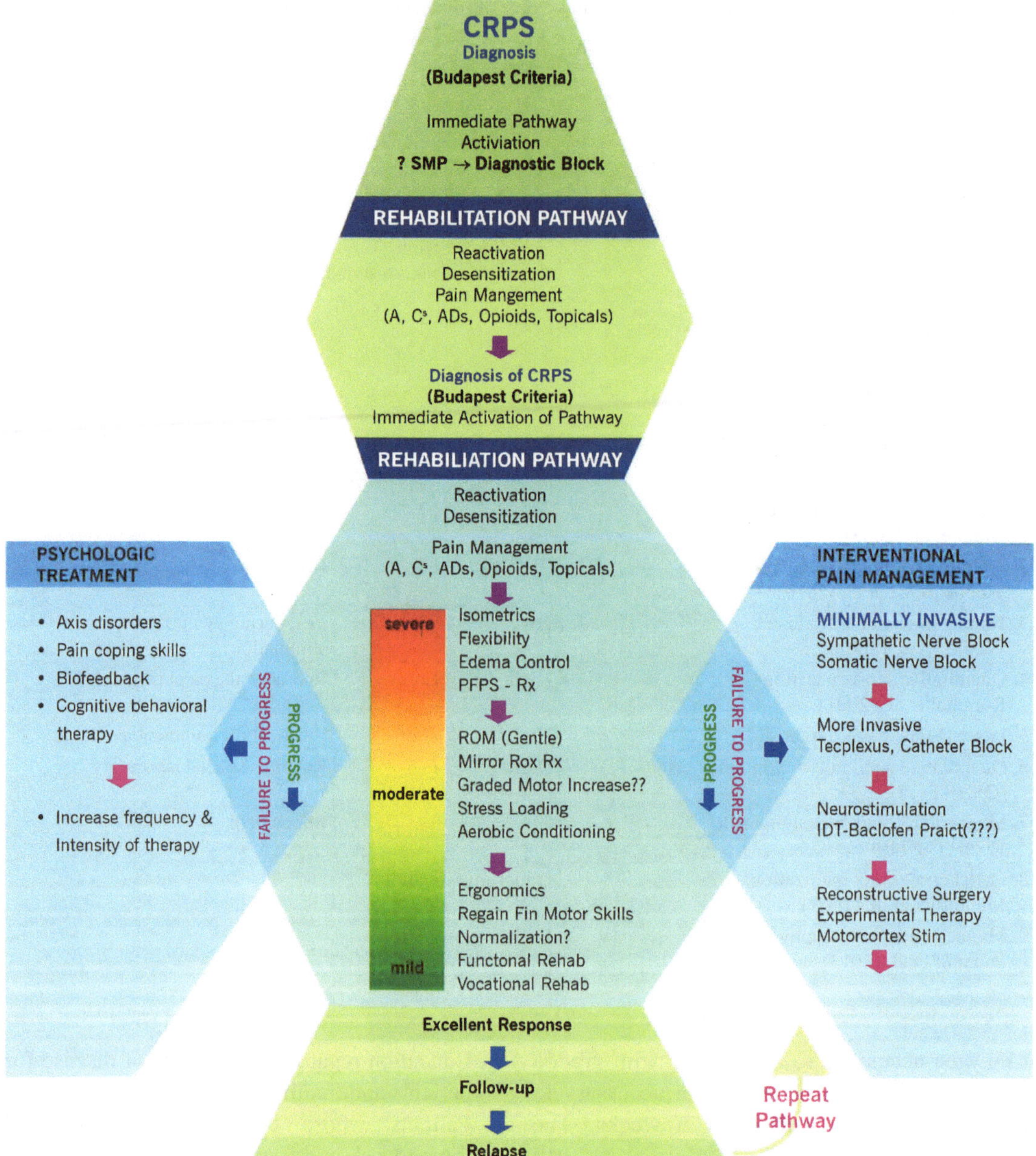

Fig. 23.2 Modified multidisciplinary care continuum for CRPS. The various treatment modalities are woven into the rehabilitation sequence; these are introduced in a time-contingent fashion. The severity gauge is a guide to the degree with which it may be necessary to introduce the different functional modalities throughout the course of functional restoration (With permission: John Wiley and Sons, Michael D. StantonHicks, Allen W. Burton, Stephen P. Bruehl, Daniel B. Carr, R. Norman Harden, Samuel J. Hassenbusch, Timothy R. Lubenow, John C. Oakley, Gabor B. Racz, P. Prithvi Raj, Richard L. Rauck, Ali R. Rezai. An updated interdisciplinary clinical pathway for CRPS: report of an expert panel. *Pain Practice*. 2002;1–16, Fig. 1)

considered facilitators whereby they assist the patient to undergo physical therapy. It should be understood that there are no FDA approved medications for CRPS. As already stated, many of the drugs used to treat CRPS are those already shown to be effective for other neuropathic pain. The following medications will be classified under their levels of evidence (Table 23.4).

- Corticosteroids should be tried early – a few weeks – following onset of CRPS. A 10-day tapering dose is frequently associated with immediate improvement of symptoms and well-being.
- Opioid use has not been studied in CRPS. These drugs are useful for treating acute pain and there have been a number of studies supporting their use in postherpetic neuralgia (PHN). Similarly, tramadol, morphine, oxycodone, and levorphanol have undergone blinded crossover studies in which they were found to be more effective than placebo in this indication (Level 2 evidence). There are however no long-term studies of opioid use in the treatment of neuropathic pain. If such drugs are used, they should only be a component of an interdisciplinary program.
- Calcitonin is normally used in the management of bone disorders associated with resorption or increased osteoclastic activity. It has been used to reduce pain in CRPS (Level 1 evidence in a systematic meta-analysis).
- Bisphosphonates have been found useful in providing some analgesia in early CRPS (Level 2 evidence). They are poorly tolerated due to side effects.
- Free radical scavengers (antioxidants) have been used for some 20 years. The basis for their use is damage caused by free radicals in both deep and superficial tissues. Dimethyl sulfoxide (DMSO) is compounded as a fatty cream and has been found effective in a small study of 32 patients.

Table 23.4 Level of evidence

Level	
1	Results of systemic review or meta-analysis
2	Reflects one or more well-powered randomized controlled clinical trials
3	Retrospective studies, open-label trials, pilot studies
4	Anecdotes, case reports, clinical experience

- Prophylactic vitamin C was shown to reduce the incidence of CRPS in patients with Colles fracture.
- A number of α1-adrenoceptor antagonists have been described in several studies. Phenoxybenzamine (Dibenzyline) was efficacious in 40 patients.
- Antiepileptics have found greatest utility in the treatment of CRPS. Gabapentin and pregabalin are among the most commonly used. Topiramate is a useful alternative to gabapentin and pregabalin because it frequently reduces the weight gain incurred by the former two agents.
- Antidepressants – mainly tricyclic antidepressants (TCAs) – have been studied extensively in the treatment of various neuropathic pains, e.g., diabetic neuropathy (Level 2 evidence). Desipramine, a selective norepinephrine blocker, can reduce pain in PDN and PHN (Levels 1 and 2 evidence). However, no studies of TCAs or serotonin reuptake inhibitors (SSRI) have been studied in CRPS. Antidepressants have some synergy as adjuvant medications with antiepileptics as well as their sedative and antidepressant properties.
- γ-Aminobutyric acid (GABA) receptor agonists may be useful in the treatment of the movement disorder, particularly tremor or dystonia in patients with CRPS. Both benzodiazepines and baclofen (GABA-A and GABA-B agonists) are useful for the treatment of the movement disorder of patients with CRPS. Baclofen may not be efficacious unless delivered by the intrathecal route.
- NMDA receptor blocking agents can be effective in moderating symptoms in either CRPS Type 2 or CRPS Type1. Ketamine, dextromethorphan, and memantine are such agents that have been found useful in the treatment of diabetic neuropathy. There are no prospective studies of dextromethorphan being used for CRPS. Ketamine has been studied in subanesthetic and anesthetic concentrations with promising results.
- Clonidine has been used either via transdermal, epidural, or intrathecal routes and oral

forms. Level 3 evidence is available for the use of transdermal clonidine in a small cohort.
- Topical lidocaine is supported by Level 2 evidence in the treatment of PHN and PDN. These compounds have also been studied in patients with CRPS (Level 3 evidence).

Interventional Measures

Sympathetic Blockade

Sympathetic block of the cervical thoracic or lumbar sympathetic chains may achieve complete pain relief in almost 80% of patients. As stated earlier in this chapter, this is mainly a diagnostic procedure to determine whether a patient has SMP or SIP. It is also important to emphasize that a technically successful sympathetic block can only be determined by temperature measurement (a temperature rise to 34 °C+ at a finger or toe pulp) or laser Doppler scintigraphy. There is no support for the continuing use of sympathetic blocks in the treatment of CRPS. If however on receiving a sympathetic block a patient obtains 1 or more weeks of pain relief, it may be useful to undertake another block in order to initiate physical therapy. A successful sympathetic block – meaning the patient has SMP – is supported by studies with Level 2 evidence.

Neurostimulation

Spinal cord stimulation can be effective in the treatment of neuropathic pain and has been used to treat pain of CRPS since 1987. SCS inhibits the release of dorsal horn excitatory amino acids, glutamate, and aspartate, via a local GABAergic mechanism. SCS also has a β fiber-mediated inhibition at the wide dynamic range (WDR) neurons. Also, antidromic activation of dorsal column fibers induces a presynaptic inhibition of WDR neurons. There are three RCTs and six long-term follow-up studies that support the use of SCS for CRPS.

- The most quoted study by Kemler et al. randomized 36 patients to receive SCS and physical therapy while the remaining 18 underwent physical therapy alone. The neurostimulator was implanted in those cases where the trial was successful. While no material change in function occurred, all patients had an improvement in the quality of life (QOL), and when the same patients were seen 2 years later, the SCS plus physical therapy group had a significant improvement in HQOL compared with the physical therapy group alone.
- In 2009, the health technology assessment under the auspices of the National Institute for Health and Care Excellence (NICE) in the UK published a report that determined the cost-effectiveness and clinical efficacy of SCS for use in treating neuropathic pain, CRPS Type I, and ischemic conditions. The results of SCS were superior to conservative medical management (CMM). A significant savings in cost were also reported.
- SCS has been used to facilitate exercise therapy in an interdisciplinary pediatric pain program. Because of severe allodynia that prevented the use of physical or occupational therapy, SCS as an extended trial for several weeks was used to help children to participate in the program.
- Peripheral nerve stimulation (PNS) has also been used as adjunct to the multidisciplinary treatment of patients with CRPS. In many cases, because SCS may not provide adequate regional analgesia, PNS should be a consideration for such applications.

Intrathecal Drug Delivery (IDD)

The intrathecal route for drug delivery may be necessary when both CMM and neurostimulation has failed to achieve either remission or symptomatic improvement. The opioids morphine, hydromorphone, fentanyl, and sufentanil have been used either alone or in conjunction with a local anesthetic such as bupivacaine or ropivacaine. Baclofen may be a consideration when dystonia or severe movement disorder of the upper extremity is associated with CRPS. One study found that baclofen was very successful in the treatment of dystonia in CRPS.

More recently, intrathecal ziconotide, an N-type calcium channel blocker, can be successful in treating neuropathic pain. While the side effect profile of ziconotide prevents many patients from using this drug, it can be successful in a small number of patients (about 35%) and lends support for a trial when other approaches have failed. Ziconotide can be trialed as either a bolus injection or through the use of a small intrathecal catheter over a period of 3 to 7 days.

Hyperbaric Oxygen

When indolent edema, skin breakdown, and open blisters remain refractory to all treatment measures in the affected extremity of patients with CRPS, hyperbaric oxygen should be considered. The one published RCT demonstrated significant improvement in joint movement and pain reduction in all patients that were studied. This author has experienced the complete resolution of similar clinical features in an adult and child.

Surgery

Surgery may be required in those patients who as a result of their disorder have developed tendon shortening, restricted ROM of joints, and dystrophic changes that prevent the therapist from achieving a full return of function. For example, the development of an equinus deformity of the foot may require tendon lengthening, and a similar approach may be necessary in the upper extremity. Amputation while not recommended in the treatment algorithm may be necessary for those cases in whom the pathological process is so florid that it is not possible to physically manage a patient or in those cases where osteomyelitis has supervened. These surgical procedures can be safely carried out under a regional anesthetic which from experience appears to prevent an exacerbation of the syndrome.

Summary

The treatment of CRPS requires an interdisciplinary and multimodal approach as early as possible after the onset of the syndrome. Physical functional maintenance or recovery of physical function should be the primary object of treatment. This approach has been defined by the IMMPACT recommendations that have been validated. Treatments are directed to regaining function, reduction of muscle spasm, and the use of whichever measures are most appropriate to address the associated severe pain. Pharmacological treatment is directed at a particular pathophysiology or current symptoms. Myofascial dysfunction, almost invariably present, together with allodynia and/or hyperalgesia, can adversely interfere with PT and OT, requiring the use of muscle relaxants, analgesics, and antidepressants. Severe allodynia may require a trial of anticonvulsants, desensitization, or some intervention such as SCS. When neurostimulation fails, it may be appropriate to use IDD in particular ziconotide.

Psychological management may be necessary either on an intermittent or continuing basis depending on the individual impact of this syndrome. Understanding the pathophysiology should help to select those medications and measures that will help to minimize the permanent impact of CRPS on affected tissues – severe ischemia, axonopathy, atrophy, skin breakdown, and central nervous system dysfunction.

CRPS in children requires a far greater use of behavioral treatments. In only a very few instances is there any need to use interventional measures (less than 6%). These however should not be withheld in the face of resistant allodynia/hyperalgesia and deteriorating function that prevent the continuing use of physical modalities. Within the foregoing framework, a high response to therapy can be achieved.

Suggested Reading

1. Beerthuizen A, Stronks DL, van't Spijker A, et al. Demografic and medical parameters in the development of complex regional pain syndrome type I: prospective study on 596 patients with a fracture. Pain. 2012;153:1187–92.
2. Bruehl S. An update on the pathophysiology of complex regional pain syndrome. Anethesiology. 2010;113:713–25.
3. Bruehl S, Harden RN, Galer BS, Saltz S, Backonja M, Stanton-Hicks M. Complex regional pain syndrome: are there distinct subtypes and sequential stages of the syndrome? Pain. 2002;95:119–24.
4. Cui JG, O'Connor WT, Ungerstedt U, Linderoth B, Meyerson BA. Spinal cord stimulation attenuates augmented dorsal horn release of excitatory amino acids in mononeuropathy via a GABAergic mechanism. Pain. 1997;73:87–95.
5. Daly AE, Bialocerkowski AE. Does evidence support physiotherapy management of adult complex regional pain syndrome type one? A systematic review. Eur J Pain. 2009;13:339–53.
6. de Mos M, de Bruijn AG, Huygen FJ, et al. The incidence of complex regional pain syndrome: a population-based study. Pain. 2007;129(1–2):12–20.
7. de Mos M, et al. The association between ACE inhibitors and the complex regional pain syndrome: suggestions for a neuro-inflammatory pathogenesis of CRPS. Pain. 2009;142:218–24.
8. Evans J. Reflex sympathetic dystrophy. Surg Clin N Am. 1946;26:780–90.
9. Flor H, Fydrich T, Turk DC. Efficacy of multidisciplinary pain treatment centers: a meta-analytic review. Pain. 1992;49(2):221–30.
10. Harden RN, Bruehl S, Perez RS, Birklein F, Marinus J, Maihofner C, Lubenow T, Buvanendran A, Mackey S, Graciosa J, Mogilevski M, Ramsden C, Chont M, Vatine JJ. Validation of proposed diagnostic criteria (the "Budapest criteria") for complex regional pain syndrome. Pain. 2010;150:268–74.
11. Hassenbusch SJ, Stanton-Hicks M, Schopa D, et al. Long-term results of peripheral nerve stimulation for reflex sympathetic dystrophy. J Neurosurg. 1996;84(3):415–23.
12. Kingery WS. A critical review of controlled clinical trials for peripheral neuropathic and pain complex regional pain syndromes. Pain. 1997;73:123–39.
13. Kiralp MZ, Yildiz S, Vural D, Keskin I, Ay H, Dursun H. Effectiveness of hyperbaric oxygen therapy in the treatment of complex regional pain syndrome. J Int Med Res. 2004;32:258–62.
14. Lohnberg JA, Altmaier EM. A review of psychosocial factors in complex regional pain syndrome. J Clin Psychol Med Settings. 2013;20:247–54.
15. Moseley GL. Graded motor imagery for pathologic pain: a randomized controlled trial. Neurology. 2006;67:2129–34.
16. North R, Shipley J, Prager J, et al., American Academy of Pain Medicine. Practice parameters for the use of spinal cord stimulation in the treatment of chronic neuropathic pain. Pain Med. 2007;(8 Suppl 4):S200–75.
17. Sanford M. Intrathecal ziconotide: a review of its use in patients with chronic pain refractory to other systemic or intrathecal analgesics. CNS Drugs. 2013;27:989–1002.
18. Schattschneider J, Hartung K, et al. Endothelial dysfunction in cold type complex regional pain syndrome. Neurology. 2006;67:673–5.
19. Schwartzman RJ, Alexander GM, Grothusen JR, et al. Outpatient intravenous ketamine for the treatment of complex regional pain syndrome: a double-blind placebo controlled study. Pain. 2009;147:107–15.
20. Stanton-Hicks M. Plasticity of complex regional pain syndrome (CRPS) in children. Pain Med. 2010;11:1216–23.
21. Stanton-Hicks M, Janig W, Hassenbusch S, et al. Reflex sympathetic dystrophy: changing concepts and taxonomy. Pain. 1995;63:127–33.
22. Turk DC, Dworkin RH, Allen RR, et al. Core outcome domains for chronic pain clinical trials: IMMPACT recommendations. Pain. 2003;106(3):337–45.
23. Uceyler N, et al. Differential expression patterns of cytokines in complex regional pain syndrome. Pain. 2007;132:195–205.
24. van Hilten R, van de Beek W, Hoff J, Voormolen J, Delhaas E. Intrathecal baclofen for the treatment of dystonia in patients with reflex sympathetic dystrophy. N Engl J Med. 2000;343:625–30.
25. Watkins LR, Milligan ED, Maier SF. Glial activation: a driving force for pathological pain. Trends Neurosci. 2001;24:450–5.
26. Xu J, Yang J, Lin P, Rosenquist E, Cheng J. Intravenous therapies for complex regional pain syndromes – a systematic review. Anesth Analg. 2015. (In press).
27. Zollinger PE, Tuinebreijer WE, Kreis RW, Breederveld RS. Effect of vitamin C on frequency of reflex sympathetic dystrophy in wrist fractures: a randomized trial. Lancet. 1999;354:2025–8.

24 Herpes Zoster and Postherpetic Neuralgia

Jianguo Cheng and Richard W. Rosenquist

Key Concepts

- Herpes zoster, also known as zoster and shingles, is caused by reactivation of the latent varicella zoster virus (VZV) that causes chicken pox. Once chicken pox resolves, VZV remains dormant in the dorsal root and cranial ganglia and can reactivate later in a person's life and cause herpes zoster. Approximately 95% of the US adult population have had varicella and thus can have herpes zoster. It appears predominantly in older adults, but may also occur in those that are immunocompromised. Most people typically have only one episode of herpes zoster in their lifetime. However, the second and even third episodes are possible.
- Postherpetic neuralgia (PHN) is defined as pain in the affected dermatome that is still present 1 month after the development of the vesicles. Between 10% and 40% of patients with herpes zoster develop PHN. The incidence increases with age.
- A herpes zoster vaccine consists of attenuated varicella virus at a concentration at least 14 times that found in chicken pox vaccine. It is effective to prevent herpes zoster and postherpetic neuralgia. A single shot of the vaccine can cut the risk of getting shingles by about 50%. Adults older than 60 should receive the herpes zoster vaccine as part of routine of medical care.
- The diagnosis of herpes zoster can be made based on characteristic skin lesions, pain, and itching in the involved dermatome. Differential diagnoses include contact dermatitis and herpes simplex virus infection.
- During the acute phase, an antiviral helps to reduce pain and complications and shorten the course of the disease. Antiviral medications should be started as early as possible, usually given orally within 72 h of the onset of lesions.
- The diagnosis of PHN is based on a history of herpes zoster, typical dermatomal distribution of the pain, and hyperalgesia and/or allodynia on physical examination.
- A large number of medications have been used to treat PHN, although only lidocaine patch, pregabalin, gabapentin, and 8% capsaicin patch are approved by the Food and Drug Administration (FDA) for this indication. Combination therapies are often necessary.
- Interventional options such as epidural injections, paravertebral blocks, selective nerve root blocks, sympathetic nerve blocks,

J. Cheng, MD, PhD (✉)
Departments of Pain Management and Neurosciences, Cleveland Clinic Anesthesiology Institute and Lerner Research Institute, Cleveland, OH, USA
e-mail: CHENGJ@ccf.org

R.W. Rosenquist, MD
Department Pain Management, Cleveland Clinic, Cleveland, OH, USA

J. Cheng, R.W. Rosenquist (eds.), *Fundamentals of Pain Medicine*,
https://doi.org/10.1007/978-3-319-64922-1_24

intercostal nerve blocks, trigeminal nerve blocks, spinal cord stimulation, and intrathecal therapy may be considered in refractory cases.

Herpes Zoster

Epidemiology

Herpes zoster (shingles) is a painful, blistering skin rash due to reactivation of the varicella zoster virus, the virus that causes chicken pox. About ~95% of the US adult population have had varicella and thus may develop herpes zoster. Herpes zoster occurs in ~1 million people in the USA annually. It is estimated that up to 1/3 of the population will have an episode of herpes zoster in their lifetime. Shingles may develop in any age group, but is more likely in people with (1) advanced age (age >60), (2) chicken pox before age 1, or (3) immunocompromise due to medications or disease. An adult or child who has not had chicken pox or the chicken pox vaccine may develop chicken pox, rather than shingles, after direct contact with the shingles rash.

Pathophysiology

Herpes zoster results from reactivation of varicella virus from its latent state in the dorsal root and cranial nerve ganglia and spread through the afferent nerve to the skin and in many cases the dorsal horn. The reason the virus suddenly becomes active again is not clear. Often, only one attack occurs, but the second and even third episodes are possible.

Clinical Features and Diagnosis

The first symptom of acute herpes zoster is usually one-sided pain, tingling, or burning. The pain and burning may be severe and is usually present before any rash appears. Red patches on the skin form in most people, followed by small blisters. The blisters break, forming small ulcers that begin to dry and form crusts. The crusts fall off in 2–3 weeks. Scarring is rare. The rash usually involves a narrow area from the spine around to the front of the abdomen or chest in one dermatome. Thoracic dermatomes are the most commonly affected sites, accounting for 50–70% of all cases. Other sites of herpes zoster include cranial, cervical, lumbar, and sacral dermatomes. The rash may involve the face, eyes (ophthalmic herpes), mouth, and ears. Other symptoms include paresthesia and motor deficits, usually within 2 weeks of zoster eruption and typically in the cervical and lumbosacral dermatomes (Fig. 24.1). In addition to acute HZ, there are a few clinical variations.

Subclinical Disease Asymptomatic viral replication is evidenced by the rise in varicella zoster virus antibody titers and detection of varicella zoster virus DNA in the cerebrospinal fluid by polymerase chain reaction (PCR).

Preherpetic Neuralgia Pain, pruritus, and paresthesia are usually reported by patients 7–21 days before rash eruption. This phase can be >100 days.

Zoster Sine Herpete (ZSH) Zoster sine herpete (ZSH) refers to a condition in which a dermatomal distribution of pain and/or motor deficits occurs in the absence of an antecedent rash. ZSH later became a distinct disease entity when PCR provided definitive virologic confirmation. Diagnosis is established by rising VZV titers, VZV DNA extraction from CSF, and viral isolation.

A diagnosis of herpes zoster can be made by looking at the skin and gathering a medical history. Complaints range from mild itching or tingling to severe pain in the involved dermatome. Fully developed herpes zoster is distinct and mimicked by few other diseases. When a clinical diagnosis of herpes zoster is not obvious, confirmatory laboratory tests may be needed. Blood tests may show an increase in white blood cells and antibodies to the chicken pox virus but cannot confirm that the rash is due to shingles. Differential diagnoses include contact dermatitis

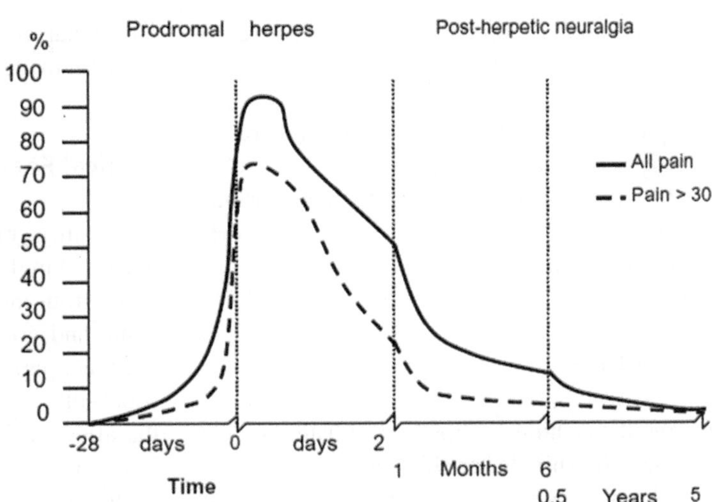

Fig. 24.1 Time course of pain in herpes zoster and postherpetic neuralgia (Data from van Wijck AJM et al. *Pain Practice.* 2011;11:88–97; with kind permission from Elsevier, Richard J. Whitley, Antonio Volpi, Mike McKendrick, Albert van Wijck, Anne Louise Oaklander, Management of herpes zoster and postherpetic neuralgia now and in the future, *J Clin Virol.* 2010;48)

and herpes simplex virus infection. Consultation with appropriate specialists may be necessary when the presentation of herpes zoster is atypical or complex. This is particularly true of active herpes zoster involving the V1 dermatome, which may result in corneal ulcers and loss of vision.

Treatment

An antiviral frequently helps to reduce pain and complications and shorten the course of the disease. Ideally, medications should be started within 24 h of feeling the pain or burning and preferably before the blisters appear. The drugs are usually given orally within 72 h of the onset of lesions. Prescribe acyclovir only if neither famciclovir nor valacyclovir is available, because acyclovir's complicated dosing schedule reduces the likelihood of compliance and its pharmacokinetic characteristics are inferior to those of famciclovir and valacyclovir.

- Famciclovir (500 mg orally 3 times a day for 7 days)
- Valacyclovir (1 g orally 3 times a day for 7 days)
- Acyclovir (800 mg orally 5 times a day for 7 days)

Intravenous acyclovir (10–15 mg/kg IV, every 8 h) should be administered in patients with herpes zoster that is complicated by central nervous system involvement, especially myelitis. For patients with severe herpes zoster ophthalmicus, intravenous acyclovir for initial therapy is also recommended.

Other medicines that are commonly used to treat herpes zoster include the following:

- Corticosteroids (such as prednisone), to reduce swelling and the risk of continued pain.
- Antihistamines to reduce itching (oral or topical).
- Analgesics to relieve pain.
- Zostrix, a cream containing capsaicin that may reduce the risk of PHN.
- Early initiation of tricyclic antidepressants may reduce the risk of PHN.

Non-pharmacological interventions to consider are as follows:

- Cool wet compresses can be used to reduce pain.
- Soothing baths and lotions may help to relieve itching and discomfort.
- Resting in bed until the fever goes down.
- The skin should be kept clean, and contaminated items should not be reused.
- Non-disposables should be washed in boiling water or otherwise disinfected before reuse.
- The patient may need to be isolated, while lesions are oozing to prevent infecting others who have never had chicken pox – especially pregnant women.

Interventional approaches to consider are as follows:

- Epidural injections or targeted nerve blocks may help to reduce pain.
- Repeated paravertebral blocks may not only reduce pain but also reduce the risk of PHN development.

Prevention

- Avoid touching the rash and blisters of persons with shingles or chicken pox.
- A herpes zoster vaccine is not the same as the chicken pox vaccine. It consists of attenuated varicella virus at a concentration at least 14 times that found in chicken pox vaccine.
- Adults older than 60 should receive the herpes zoster vaccine as part of routine medical care.
- A single shot of the vaccine can cut the risk of getting shingles by about 50%. It may also help prevent PHN and ophthalmic herpes.
- Because the vaccine contains a live virus, it cannot be given to people with a weak immune system.

Postherpetic Neuralgia

Epidemiology

Postherpetic neuralgia (PHN) is a zoster-related pain that is still present 1 month after the development of skin lesions. Between 10% and 40% of patients with acute herpes zoster develop PHN. The probability of PHN increases with age and is more likely to occur in people over age 60. The estimated number of PHN cases in the USA is between 500,000 and 1 million.

Pathophysiology

PHN occurs when nerve tissue has been damaged after an outbreak of herpes zoster. It is a common complication and is the result of damage that may involve the dorsal root and cranial nerve ganglia, the spinal cord, and the epidermis in discrete body segments.

Clinical Features and Diagnosis

The main symptom of PHN is pain in the area where shingles once occurred. The pain can range from mild to severe. It may be constant or come and go. The pain is often described as a deep aching, burning, stabbing, or an electric shock-like sensation. Skin discoloration along the affected dermatome is common (Fig. 24.2). The affected area is often very sensitive to touch or temperature changes (allodynia) and often displays an increased painful response to pin pricks (hyperalgesia). In some cases there is loss of peripheral sensation, and the patient may experience anesthesia dolorosa. The diagnosis is based on a history of herpes zoster, typical dermatomal distribution of the pain, and hyperalgesia and/or allodynia on physical examinations.

Treatment

Pharmacological treatment is the cornerstone of PHN therapy. A large number of medications have been studied and commonly used clinically,

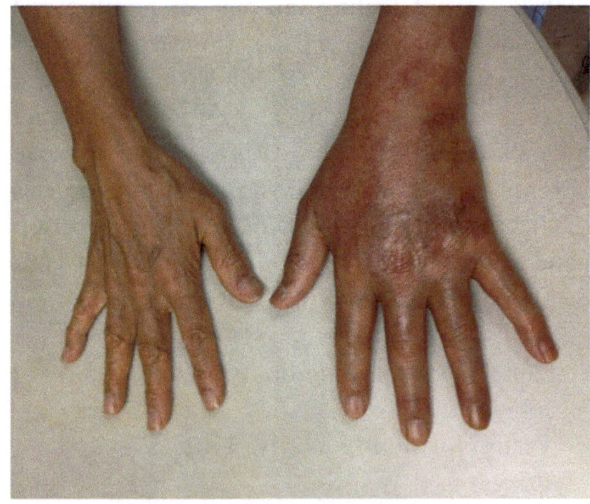

Fig. 24.2 Skin discolorations in postherpetic neuralgia. Dorsum of left hand affected by herpes zoster of the left C6 dermatome in a 69-year-old male patient (Photo courtesy of Kenneth D. Candido, M.D.)

although only lidocaine patch, pregabalin, gabapentin, and 8% capsaicin patch are approved by the Food and Drug Administration (FDA) for this indication:

- Anticonvulsant drugs may reduce the pain from damaged nerves. Gabapentin and pregabalin are the ones most often used.
- 5% lidocaine patches may relieve some of the pain for a period of time.
- 8% capsaicin patch has been demonstrated to be effective.
- Antidepressants such as amitriptyline may help reduce pain, as well as help with sleep.
- Analgesics, such as acetaminophen, nonsteroidal anti-inflammatory drugs (NSAIDs), tramadol, and opioids, are also commonly used.
- Combination therapies are often necessary.
- Interventional options such as epidural injections, paravertebral blocks, sympathetic nerve blocks, spinal cord stimulation, and intrathecal therapy may be considered in refractory cases.
- Psychological support is often helpful in persistent cases due to the chronicity of the pain.

Suggested Reading

1. Baron R, Wasner G. Prevention and treatment of postherpetic neuralgia. Lancet. 2006;367:186–8.
2. Center for Disease Control and Prevention [Internet]. 1600 Clifton Rd. Atlanta, GA 30333, USA. Shingles (herpes zoster): Available from http://www.cdc.gov/shingles/hcp/clinical-overview.html.
3. Cotton D, Taichman D, Williams S. Herpes zoster. Ann Intern Med. 2011;154:ITC31–15.
4. Dworkin RH, Schmader KE. Herpes zoster and postherpetic neuralgia. In: Benson HT, Raja SN, Molloy RE, Liu SS, Fishman SM, editors. Essentials of pain medicine and regional anesthesia: Elsevier; Philadelphia, Pennsylvian 19106. 2005. p. 386–93.
5. Ji G, Niu J, Shi Y, Hou L, Lu Y, Xiong L. The effectiveness of repetitive paravertebral injections with local anesthetics and steroids for the prevention of postherpetic neuralgia in patients with acute herpes zoster. Anesth Analg. 2009;109:1651–5.
6. van Wijck AJM, Wallace M, Mekhail N, van Kleef M. Evidence-based interventional pain medicine according to clinical diagnoses. 17. Herpes zoster and post-herpetic neuralgia. Pain Pract. 2011;11:88–97.

Peripheral Neuropathy

25

Daniel C. Callahan

Key Concepts

- Peripheral neuropathy is a dysfunction or disease of the peripheral nervous system. It may be inherited or acquired; progress insidiously or rapidly; involve sensory, motor, or autonomic nerves; and affect only specific nerves, multiple nerves, or all of them (polyneuropathy).
- Peripheral neuropathy is a broad classification that includes the symmetrical polyneuropathies (diabetic neuropathy), mononeuropathy (trigeminal neuralgia, radiculopathy, postherpetic neuralgia, etc.), and multiple mononeuropathies (mononeuritis multiplex).
- Peripheral nerves are classified by function (sensory, motor, mixed), nerve diameter (A-alpha, a-beta, A-delta, and C fiber), and whether they are myelinated or unmyelinated. Specific diseases have selective nerve fiber-type predominance, and it is essential to identify the nerve fiber types affected to form a limited differential diagnosis.
- Pathological processes that cause a peripheral neuropathy include trauma, metabolic, ischemic, infection, nutritional deficiency, paraneoplastic, radiation, genetic, toxic exposure, and idiopathic. Peripheral nerve dysfunction is a result of a limited number of pathological processes that include Wallerian degeneration, demyelination, and axonal degeneration.
- The generalized symmetrical polyneuropathy has a distal-to-proximal predominance of signs and symptoms and is the most common cause of a peripheral neuropathy seen in the pain clinic.
- Diabetes in the most common cause of generalized symmetrical polyneuropathy in the United States. Diabetic peripheral neuropathy is commonly used to describe a generalized symmetrical distal polyneuropathy. Diabetic polyneuropathy may affect large nerve fibers and/or small nerve fiber axons in a length-dependent fashion and exhibit a distal-to-proximal gradient of signs and symptoms.
- Onset, progression, anatomical topography, physical examination, and electrodiagnostic studies can determine which nerve fiber types have been affected.
- Diagnostic studies used to evaluate peripheral polyneuropathies include laboratory studies, electromyography (EMG), nerve conduction studies (NCS), peripheral nerve biopsy, skin biopsy, and QSART.

D.C. Callahan, MD (✉)
Department of Pain Management, Cleveland Clinic, Cleveland, OH 44195, USA
e-mail: dcallah@ccf.org

J. Cheng, R.W. Rosenquist (eds.), *Fundamentals of Pain Medicine*,
https://doi.org/10.1007/978-3-319-64922-1_25

- Identifying and treating correctable causes of polyneuropathy is imperative in preventing progression of the disease.
- Treatment of painful symmetrical polyneuropathy is primarily pharmacologic and includes tricyclic antidepressants (TCAs), selective serotonin-norepinephrine reuptake inhibitors (SNRI), antiepileptic drugs (AED), and topical medications.

Symmetrical Polyneuropathy

Overview

Peripheral neuropathy is a term used to describe any dysfunction or disease of the peripheral nervous system. Although it includes polyneuropathies, mononeuropathies, and multiple mononeuropathies, it is commonly used to refer to a symmetrical polyneuropathy.

Epidemiology

The heterogeneous etiology of this broad classification of nerve dysfunction makes epidemiological data difficult to obtain. The prevalence of peripheral neuropathy in the general population is 2.4% and as high as 8% in persons 55 years and older. The incidence is directly correlated with the duration of the disease, which explains the higher prevalence in the elderly population. The most common causes of painful symmetrical polyneuropathy are diabetes, alcohol, and HIV. Diabetic peripheral neuropathy is the single most common cause of peripheral neuropathy in the United States. It is found in up to 50% of patients with diabetes and has a prevalence of approximately 200 million cases worldwide. The cost in the United States is an estimated 11 billion dollars per year.

Pathophysiology

Pathological processes affecting the peripheral nerves include trauma, metabolic, ischemic, infection, nutritional deficiency, paraneoplastic, radiation, genetic, toxic exposure, and idiopathic. The actual site of nerve injury occurs at the nerve axon, Schwann cell, myelin sheath, or any combination of these. Nerve fibers are categorized by their function, size, and myelination. Motor nerve fibers are the largest in diameter and myelinated. Sensory fibers (Aβ-fiber) that serve proprioception, vibration, deep tendon reflexes, and light touch are large and myelinated. Sensory fibers serving pain, temperature, and itch sensation are smaller and can be myelinated (Aδ-fiber) or unmyelinated. Autonomic nerve fibers are small in diameter and unmyelinated. The nerve fiber types that are affected have important clinical implications since specific diseases tend to affect certain nerve fiber types.

Pain as a result of peripheral nerve injury is a multifactorial process of which there are several proposed mechanisms. In a small fiber neuropathy, injury to peripheral nerves can cause an increase in axonal sodium channel expression in the small fibers allowing for early depolarization and the occurrence of spontaneous pain. In large fiber peripheral neuropathies, injury to the A-beta fibers (vibration sensation, proprioception) decreases input to the interneurons of the spinal cord that inhibit nociceptive neurons, allowing pain impulses to travel unopposed. Peripheral nerves are composed of a multitude of nerve fibers. When a peripheral nerve is injured, the remaining uninjured nerve fibers increase expression of alpha-adrenoreceptors allowing C fibers subserving pain to respond to sympathetic nervous system activation.

Clinical Features and Diagnosis

Despite the numerous causes of a peripheral neuropathy, the differential diagnosis can be narrowed down by identifying important clinical features. A detailed history, physical examination, and a thorough understanding of which nerve fiber types and clinical modalities (sensory, motor, and autonomic) are being affected are essential to properly diagnose and treat peripheral neuropathies (Table 25.1). This point cannot

Table 25.1 Painful polyneuropathies: clinical features

Disease	Chronic onset	Acute onset	Large fiber	Small fiber	Modality	Axon affected	Myelin affected	Topography
Metabolic								
Diabetes	++++	++	++++	++	S > M > A	++++	+	Symmetric >> multifocal
Alcohol	++++	+	+	++++	S > M >> A	++++	+	Symmetric
Thyroid	++++	+	++++	+	M > S	++++	+	Symmetric
Nutritional[a]	++++	+	++++	+	S > M	++++	+	Symmetric
Infectious								
Leprosy[b]	++++	+++	+	++++	A > S >> M	++++	+	Symmetric > multifocal
HIV	++++	++	++++	++	S > A > M	++++	+	Symmetric > multifocal
Lyme	++	++++	++	++++	S > M > A	++++	++	Multifocal > symmetric
Autoimmune								
Lupus	++	++++	++++	++	S > M > A	++++	++	Symmetric > multifocal
Sjogren's	++	++++	+	++++	S > M > A	++++	+	Variable
AIDP[c]	–	++++	++++	–	M >> A > S	–	++++	Symmetric >> multifocal
Toxic								
Arsenic	+	++++	++++	+	M > S > A	+	++++	Symmetric >> Multifocal
Lead	++++	++	++++	+	M >>> S	+	++++	Symmetric > Multifocal
Hereditary								
Fabry's disease	++++	+	–	++++	S > A >> M	++	+++	Symmetric >> Multifocal
CMT[d]	++++	–	++++	+	M >> S >> A	–	++++	Symmetric

+, present; –, absent

[a]Vitamin B_1, B_6, B_{12}

[b]Leprosy is the most common cause of peripheral neuropathy outside the USA

[c]Acute inflammatory demyelinating polyneuropathy (Guillain-Barre syndrome)

[d]Charcot-Marie-Tooth

S sensory, *M* motor, *A* autonomic

be overemphasized because early identification and treatment is paramount to prevent progression of the disease. Peripheral neuropathies can be categorized by the onset, progression, topographical pattern of nerve involvement, and associated symptoms – e.g., autonomic signs and symptoms.

One of the most common types of peripheral neuropathies is the generalized symmetrical polyneuropathy, most commonly caused by diabetes. This may affect large nerve fibers and/or small nerve fibers. The nerve axons are predominately affected in a length-dependent fashion and exhibit a distal-to-proximal gradient of signs and symptoms.

- Symptoms begin insidiously in the feet and slowly progress to the mid-calf before involving the distal fingers. This is referred to as a "stocking-glove" distribution. The slow progression is a key clinical feature that distinguishes it from the acute onset and rapidly progressing polyneuropathies caused by a different set of diseases.
- Motor and sensory function is most often affected in the generalized polyneuropathies; however, one modality may predominate. In a patient with diabetic polyneuropathy, sensation is affected more than motor function.
- Sensory symptoms are described as burning, prickling, electrical, "pins and needles," and numbness. Proprioception (joint position sense) dysfunction in the setting of preserved motor function can cause a sensory ataxia.
- Motor symptoms are generally mild, and there may be some distal extremity muscle atrophy and/or weakness in more advanced stages of the disease.
- Autonomic dysfunction, as a result of small nerve fiber involvement, may result in resting tachycardia, changes in bowel/bladder function, transient swelling and/or changes in color of the distal extremities, hyperhidrosis, and anhidrosis just to name a few.

The physical examination is important in identifying the fiber types involved, modalities affected (motor, sensory, autonomic), and topographical pattern of nerve dysfunction.

- Vibration sensation is most often affected more than other modalities. Decreased vibration sensation and joint position sense identifies dysfunction of the large sensory nerve fibers and can be measured with a tuning fork. Decreased vibratory sensation in the toes or ankle malleoli compared to the patella objectifies a distal-to-proximal gradient.
- Despite the common complaint of numbness, pinprick and temperature sensation is often preserved on physical examination. Decreased pinprick and temperature sensation identifies small nerve fiber involvement.
- Ankle deep tendon reflexes are reduced compared to the patella.
- Motor weakness and atrophy in the distal extremities are seen in the more advanced stages. If motor symptoms are out of proportion to sensory symptoms, an alternate diagnosis should be sought.
- Color changes, distal extremity hair loss, hyperhidrosis, anhidrosis, resting tachycardia, and orthostatic hypotension without a compensatory tachycardia are objective signs of autonomic dysfunction and indicate small nerve fiber involvement as well.

Laboratory workup should be based on the suspected etiology of the peripheral neuropathy, which is guided by the results of the history, physical exam, and electrodiagnostic studies.

- Initial labs usually include hemoglobin A1-C (diabetes), TSH (hypothyroid), CBC, ESR, CRP (inflammatory causes), rheumatoid factor (collagen vascular diseases), vitamin B12, vitamin B6, folate (macrocytosis), serum protein electrophoresis, urine protein electrophoresis (monoclonal gammopathy, amyloidosis), and HIV-1 antibody (AIDs).
- If the initial labs are unrevealing, additional labs include urine heavy metals (lead, mercury, arsenic poisoning), hepatitis B and C antigen (polyarteritis), urine porphobilinogen (acute intermittent porphyria), antineutrophil

cytoplasmic inclusion bodies (Wegener's granulomatosis), *Borrelia burgdorferi* antibodies (Lyme disease), varicella zoster antigen, cytomegalovirus antibodies, angiotensin-converting enzyme (sarcoidosis), anti-Hu, and anti-GM_1 antibodies (paraneoplastic).

- In some cases cerebrospinal fluid (CSF) analysis may be necessary to identify the cause of a peripheral neuropathy. CSF studies should include CSF protein (Guillain-Barre, chronic inflammatory demyelinating polyneuropathy), CSF Lyme titers (Lyme disease), and white cell count.

Electrophysiologic studies consist of electromyography (EMG) and nerve conduction studies (NCS) and have considerable diagnostic value. These studies provide objective evidence of nerve dysfunction that may be too subtle to be found on neurological examination. In addition, they provide valuable information that limits the differential diagnosis and helps to direct further workup. Electrophysiologic studies can identify sensory and/or motor nerve involvement, differentiate axonal versus demyelinating processes, assess the degree of axonal loss and demyelination, identify chronic versus acute nerve dysfunction, as well as provide localizing information. Nerve conduction studies can also differentiate between an inherited and acquired cause of peripheral neuropathy. For example, electrophysiologic studies in a diabetic peripheral neuropathy would show sensory and motor nerve dysfunction, predominately an axonal pathophysiology, and a symmetrical, distal-to-proximal pattern of nerve dysfunction. Electrodiagnostic studies can only measure the large nerve fibers. It is therefore important to know that in a purely small fiber neuropathy, which can also be caused by diabetes, the EMG and NCS are normal.

Nerve biopsy is sometimes required to diagnose certain types of peripheral neuropathies. It involves removing and examining a sample of peripheral nerve tissue, most often from the sural nerve. This should be used only in specific situations where less invasive studies are not able to identify the etiology. Sural nerve biopsy has utility in providing histopathological appearances that help to identify diseases such as amyloid neuropathy, vasculitis, and sarcoidosis.

Skin biopsy is a safe, repeatable, and effective way to identify pathology in the small nerve fibers that is not evident on electrodiagnostic studies. Immunohistochemical staining can provide diagnostic information about intraepidermal small nerve fiber (IENF) density and morphological changes that occur early in the course of peripheral neuropathies. It is sometimes used to monitor progression of the disease.

Quantitative Sudomotor Axon Reflex Testing (QSART) is a noninvasive test that objectively evaluates the peripheral sympathetic cholinergic nervous system. The test is performed by iontophoresis of acetylcholine to stimulate small nerve fibers that innervate sweat glands and measure sweat output. This has been shown to increase the diagnostic yield of standard testing for small fiber neuropathy from 38% to 66%. QSART has limited availability and is most often used for research purposes.

Treatment

The most important factor affecting the treatment of a polyneuropathy is to identify and, if possible, correct the underlying etiology. In diabetic neuropathy, maintaining as close to normal blood glucose levels is the only treatment to prevent progression of the disease. Correcting thyroid levels and nutritional deficiencies, alcohol cessation, and reducing toxic exposure (lead, arsenic, mercury, chemotherapy) are among other important considerations.

Pharmacological treatment for pain is the primary treatment modality in most peripheral neuropathies. There are many classes of drugs used to successfully treat peripheral neuropathies, yet only duloxetine (Cymbalta), pregabalin (Lyrica), and tapentadol extended release have Federal and Drug Administration (FDA) approval. Many of these medications require laboratory monitoring at regular intervals.

- Antiepileptic drugs/membrane stabilizers such as gabapentin (Neurontin), pregabalin (Lyrica), topiramate (Topamax), and oxcarbazepine (Trileptal) are commonly used to treat neuropathic pain. Carbamazepine (Tegretol) and phenytoin (Dilantin) are less often used due to side effect profiles.
- Amitriptyline (Elavil), nortriptyline (Pamelor), imipramine (Tofranil), and desipramine (Norpramin) are among the tricyclic antidepressant (TCA) class of medications used to reduce neuropathic pain. TCAs are often limited by dose-dependent side effects. Of this class of medications, amitriptyline is the most commonly used, and desipramine has the least side effects.
- Serotonin-norepinephrine reuptake inhibitors (SNRI) such as duloxetine (Cymbalta) and venlafaxine (Effexor) are also commonly used. They target both serotonin and norepinephrine to alleviate painful symptoms of diabetic peripheral neuropathy. Cymbalta is considered first-line treatment for polyneuropathy.
- Tapentadol ER (Nucynta) is a centrally acting synthetic analgesic. It is presumed to act centrally at both μ-opioid receptor and as a norepinephrine reuptake inhibitor, although the exact mechanism is unknown. It is the only opioid medication that has FDA approval for diabetic peripheral neuropathy.
- Tramadol is a weak μ-opioid receptor agonist and has selective serotonin reuptake inhibitor properties. Tramadol at an average of doses of 210 mg per day in divided doses was found to be effective in treating diabetic peripheral neuropathy.
- Lidocaine is a local anesthetic that is available as a cream, patch, and an ointment. It has been shown to be effective in diabetic peripheral neuropathy in some small trials.
- Capsaicin cream is available as a topical cream and has been shown to have some benefit in painful diabetic peripheral neuropathy. Capsaicin is the active ingredient in hot chili peppers. It binds to the TRPV1 receptor on small nerve fibers, which is normally activated by heat. The sustained activation of the TRPV1 receptor over time causes a depletion of substance P, one of the primary neurotransmitters responsible for pain.

Transcutaneous electrical nerve stimulation (TENS) is a device that incorporates the use of electric current to stimulate the peripheral nerves to provide pain relief. It is a portable battery-operated device that is connected to the skin using two or more electrodes. The proposed mechanism of action by which TENS alleviates pain is by inhibition of nociceptive input at the presynaptic level through activation of low-threshold myelinated nerves in the skin. By activating afferent input from the large myelinated nerve fibers, nociception carried by small unmyelinated C fibers is inhibited from reaching the cortex (gate control theory). Some small-sample randomized controlled trials have demonstrated some benefit in pain reduction for diabetic peripheral neuropathy.

Spinal cord stimulation is an interventional treatment option that has been shown to be effective for diabetic peripheral neuropathy. It provides pain relief by electrically stimulating the dorsal columns of the spinal cord. Since it is an implantable device, it is reserved for neuropathic pain refractory to medical medication management.

Acute Painful Peripheral Neuropathy

Overview

The generalized symmetrical polyneuropathies discussed earlier in this chapter account for the vast majority of patients seen in the pain clinic suffering from neuropathic pain. The key clinical features are their symmetry, insidious onset, and slow progression. This is in contradistinction to an important, albeit less common, class of peripheral neuropathies that are acute in onset and can vary in both topography and progression. Acute onset describes symptoms that progress over days to weeks, whereas chronic onset generally refers to symptoms that progress over months to years. Trigeminal neuralgia and herpes zoster are examples of acute painful peripheral neuropathy. These topics are covered in detail in other chapters of this book.

Epidemiology

There are very few large population-based studies on the incidence and prevalence of peripheral neuropathy. Epidemiological data for acute painful peripheral neuropathy is lacking.

Pathophysiology

The majority of acute painful peripheral neuropathies are a result of ischemia (vasculitis, diabetes), infectious disease (herpes zoster, HIV, Lyme disease), and immune-mediated processes (Parsonage-Turner, Guillain-Barre syndrome).

Clinical Features and Diagnosis

Acute painful peripheral neuropathies tend to be more variable in topography than its chronic counterpart. They can affect the nerve roots, brachial plexus, and individual as well as multiple peripheral nerves and the cranial nerves. There are numerous acute peripheral neuropathies, and only a few are mentioned in this chapter for illustration.

HIV Neuropathy Peripheral neuropathy from HIV can present in several ways, of which the most common is a distal, symmetrical polyneuropathy. Acute onset of a burning sensation in the soles of the feet should raise suspicion for HIV. It is a common form of small fiber neuropathy and found in approximately 30% of people with AIDS. It is predominately a sensory neuropathy in which the physical examination and electrodiagnostic studies are often normal.

Neuralgic Amyotrophy (Parsonage-Turner Syndrome) Is a unique syndrome that presents with an acute onset of shoulder girdle pain. It is almost exclusively unilateral, associated with paresthesias, and occasionally will wake up the patient at night. The defining clinical feature is shoulder pain that resolves after several days that is subsequently followed by profound muscle weakness. It can be caused by infections, surgical procedures, and vaccinations. It is often mistaken as a result of arm positioning during surgery and regional anesthetic blocks. Physical examination usually reveals weakness in the deltoid, serratus anterior (wining of the scapula), biceps, and decreased reflexes. It is a self-limiting syndrome that tends to improve spontaneously after several weeks.

Mononeuritis Multiplex Is a painful, asymmetrical, acute or subacute onset, peripheral neuropathy that involves more than one distinct peripheral nerve. The peripheral nerves affected may occur simultaneously or sequentially. For example, a patient may present with a median mononeuropathy of the left upper extremity (carpal tunnel syndrome) and a peroneal neuropathy of the right lower extremity. Most often the axons of motor and sensory nerves are affected. It is found to occur with systemic diseases, infections, rheumatologic disorders, cancer, and diabetes. Patients will complain of pain and paresthesias in the distribution of the involved nerve, followed by sensory loss and motor weakness. The physical examination reveals motor weakness, sensory loss, and decreased or absent reflexes in the distribution of the involved nerve.

The differential diagnosis may be further limited by physical examination. Common findings in acute onset peripheral neuropathies are asymmetrical reflexes, sensory loss in a defined nerve distribution, proximal motor weakness, and cranial nerve involvement. Laboratory diagnostic studies are guided by the suspected etiology. Cerebral spinal fluid analysis and peripheral nerve biopsy play an important role in this class of diseases.

Treatment

As in the chronic symmetrical polyneuropathies, the treatment is predominately pharmacologic, and the same medications are used to ameliorate neuropathic pain. Acute onset peripheral neuropathies usually involve multiple specialties such as rheumatology, oncology, infectious disease, pain management, and neurology, to identify and treat the underlying disease.

Suggested Reading

1. de Vos CC, Rajan V, Steenbergen W, et al. Effect and safety of spinal cord stimulation for treatment of chronic pain caused by diabetic neuropathy. J Diabetes Complicat. 2009;23:40–5.
2. Dyck PJ, Kratz KM, Karnes JL, Litchy WJ, Klein R, Pach JM, et al. The prevalence by staged severity of various types of diabetic neuropathy, retinopathy, and nephropathy in a population-based cohort: the Rochester diabetic neuropathy study. Neurology. 1993;43(4):817–24.
3. Finnerup NB, Attal N, Haroutounian S, McNicol E, Baron R, Dworkin RH, Gilron I, Haanpää M, Hansson P, Jensen TS, Kamerman PR, Lund K, Moore A, Raja SN, Rice AS, Rowbotham M, Sena E, Siddall P, Smith BH, Wallace M. Pharmacotherapy for neuropathic pain in adults: a systematic review and meta-analysis. Lancet Neurol. 2015;14(2):162–73.
4. Harati Y, Gooch C, Swenson M, et al. Double-blind randomized trial of tramadol for the treatment of the pain of diabetic neuropathy. Neurology. 1998;50:1842–6.
5. Jin DM, Xu Y, Geng DF, Yan TB. Effect of transcutaneous electrical nerve stimulation on symptomatic diabetic peripheral neuropathy: a meta-analysis of randomized controlled trials. Diabetes Res Clin Pract. 2010;89(1):10–5.
6. Martyn C, Hughes R. Epidemiology of peripheral neuropathy. J Neurol Neurosurg Psychiatry. 1997;62:310–8.
7. National Institute for Health and Excellence (NICE). Neuropathic pain: the pharmacological management of neuropathic pain in adults in non-specialist settings. NICE Guidelines. 2010;96:1–155.
8. O'Connor AB, Dworkin RH. Treatment of neuropathic pain: an overview of recent guidelines. Am J Med. 2009;122(10 Suppl):S22–32.
9. Preston D, Shapiro B. Electromyography and neuromuscular disorders: Elsevier; Philadelphia, AP, 2005. p. 389–420.
10. Ropper A, Brown R. Adam's and Victor's principles of neurology: McGraw Hill; New York, NY, 2005. p. 1110–77.
11. Thaisetthawatkul P, Fernandes Filho JA, Herrmann DN. Contribution of QSART to the diagnosis of small fiber neuropathy. Muscle Nerve. 2013;48(6):883–8.
12. The Diabetes Control and Complications Trial Research Group. The effect of intensive treatment of diabetes on the development and progression of long-term complications in insulin-dependent diabetes mellitus. N Engl J Med. 1993;329(14):977–86.
13. Wulff EA, Wang AK, Simpson DM. HIV-associated peripheral neuropathy: epidemiology, pathophysiology and treatment. Drugs. 2000;59(6):1251–60.
14. Zhang WY, Po ALW. The effectiveness of topically applied capsaicin: a meta-analysis. Eur J Clin Pharmacol. 1994;46:517–22.

Peripheral Neuralgia and Entrapment Neuropathies

26

Justin T. Drummond, Sherif Zaky, and Salim M. Hayek

Key Concepts

- Peripheral neuralgias can develop from various etiologies. Identifying the provoking factor(s) is important for proper treatment planning. However, the diagnosis is often made clinically with inconclusive data results.
- Nerve damage can lead to chronic neuropathic pain due to hyperexcitability of the nervous system.
- Neuropathies often do not respond well to opioid management and are best treated using a multimodal approach. If mechanical entrapment of involved nerve is identified, surgical exploration and removal of offending factors may lead to improvement.

Introduction

Neuralgia is defined as an intense burning or stabbing pain caused by irritation of or damage to a nerve. Neuralgia usually follows an injury to the structure of the nerve that can result in atypical firing, neuroma formation, reorganization of nerve fiber interconnections, or central neuroplasticity that lead to chronic neuropathic pain. The medical concept of neuralgia was initially discussed by Francois Chaussier in 1801 as the term "névralgie" to indicate "an affection of one or more nerves causing pain which is usually of intermittent but frequently intense character." Peripheral neuralgias and entrapment neuropathies are often diagnosed on clinical grounds. Just as there are multifactorial etiologies, there are many treatment modalities directed to the pathophysiology. A discussion of common peripheral neuralgias and entrapment neuropathies ensues.

Meralgia Paresthetica

Anatomy

The lateral femoral cutaneous nerve, which is a purely sensory nerve, is a branch of the lumbar plexus (L2 and L3), emerges from the lateral border of the psoas muscle, and crosses the iliacus muscle obliquely toward the anterior superior

J.T. Drummond, MD (✉)
Comprehensive Pain Management Specialists, Cleveland Clinic Akron General, Akron, OH, USA
e-mail: jtdrummond@gmail.com

S. Zaky, MD, PhD
Pain Management & Anesthesiology, Firelands Physicians Group, Sandusky, OH, USA

S.M. Hayek, MD, PhD
Department of Anesthesiology, University Hospitals Case Medical Center, Cleveland, OH, USA

J. Cheng, R.W. Rosenquist (eds.), *Fundamentals of Pain Medicine*,
https://doi.org/10.1007/978-3-319-64922-1_26

iliac spine (ASIS). It passes beneath the inguinal ligament and then crosses over the sartorius muscle descending in a compartment between the sartorius muscle medially, tensor fascia lata laterally, and rectus femoris underneath (Fig. 26.1) dividing then into anterior and posterior branches with multiple possible variations.

Pathophysiology

Inflammation and irritation of the lateral femoral cutaneous nerve (LFCN) can lead to meralgia paresthetica (MP). The etiology may be either metabolic or mechanical (compression by the ASIS or inguinal ligament) in nature and can be related to the anatomical variations and subsequent development of neuromas.

Diagnosis

The name *meralgia* is derived from the Greek words *meros* for "thigh" and *algos* for "pain." It is typically noted by the patient as a burning, tingling sensation of the lateral or anterolateral thigh that can encompass the gluteal region, anterior thigh, and just inferior to the knee. Patients often complain that pain is worse with sitting or getting out of automobiles. On physical exam, patients often have touch sensitivity (allodynia) to the lateral thigh and may experience dysesthesia or even notice anesthesia of the same location to pinprick. Palpation along the inguinal ligament may also reproduce symptoms, and an injection of local anesthetic at the tender site/ in proximity to the lateral femoral cutaneous nerve with resolution of symptoms can provide a more definitive diagnosis.

Management

Conservative management is often successful with the removal of constricting items such as belts, casts, or braces at the waist. NSAIDs are also recommended for a short 7–10-day course with application of ice in an attempt to decrease the inflammation related to an acute entrapment of the nerve. Advocating weight loss and avoiding excessive hip extension until symptoms improve can also provide relief and long-term resolution of the pain. These conservative measures may relieve approximately 50% of symptoms. Blind injection at the site of tenderness or with the use of ultrasound guidance (Fig. 26.1) in proximity to the nerve using local anesthetic with

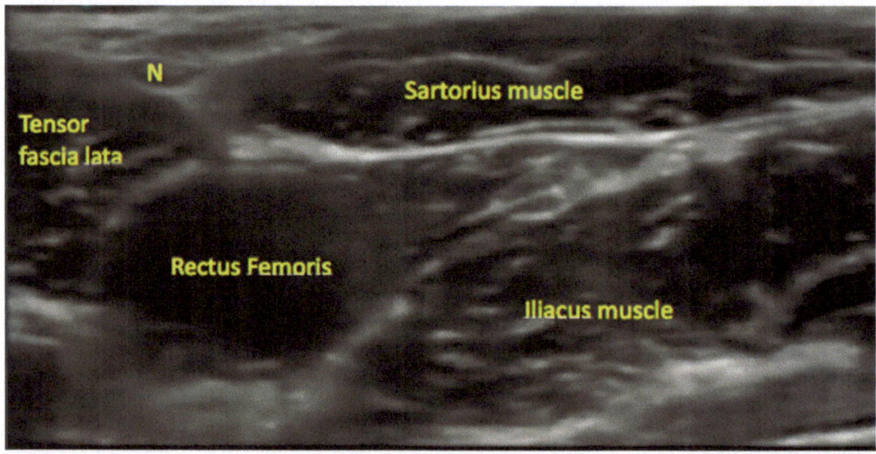

Fig. 26.1 Ultrasound image of the lateral femoral cutaneous nerve. The lateral femoral cutaneous resides in a compartment between the sartorius muscle medially and tensor fascia lata laterally. This compartment can be identified by placing the ultrasound probe below and parallel to the inguinal ligament, following the sartorius muscle laterally to its lateral border, and then scanned up and down to optimize the image. *N* lateral femoral cutaneous nerve

or without steroid can provide benefit as well, but repeat injections may be needed. If intractable pain occurs, surgery is an option with exploration and resection of the LFCN segment and burying the nerve into the fascia or periosteum, with minimal reoccurrence. However, locating the nerve can be challenging given the anatomical variations that frequently occur. Neurostimulation has been anecdotally effective in controlling meralgia pain. Cryoablation of the nerve is a treatment that has been used with successes.

Ilioinguinal Nerve Neuralgia

Anatomy

The ilioinguinal nerve is formed by the twelfth thoracic nerve root (T12) in conjunction with the first level of the lumbar plexus (L1 nerve root). This combination then splits into the ilioinguinal and iliohypogastric nerves. The course of the ilioinguinal nerve starts deep to the peritoneum and then surfaces lateral to the psoas major muscle before it penetrates the transverse abdominal muscle anterior to the iliac crest running in a fascial plane between the internal oblique and transverse abdominal muscles (Fig. 26.2). The nerve is frequently accompanied by the deep circumflex iliac artery and gives rise to motor fibers to the internal oblique muscle. The ilioinguinal nerve then joins the spermatic cord and exits via the external inguinal ring. The sensory distribution consists of the mons pubis and labium majus then cephalad to the anterior scrotum, base of the penis, and mostly superomedial thigh.

Pathophysiology

The most common location of injury occurs as the ilioinguinal nerve passes through the transverse abdominal muscle at approximately the anterior superior iliac spine. Injury is generally related to direct trauma to the nerve secondary to surgical interventions including open inguinal herniorrhaphy and during laparoscopic surgeries that leads to characteristic symptoms of nerve irritation.

Diagnosis

As with any chronic pain condition, an important diagnostic tool of ilioinguinal neuralgia consists of a detailed history and physical exam. Patients often complain of burning pain over the lower abdomen, which could travel within the sensory distribution to the superomedial thigh and scrotum. Provocation tests can help discern between genitofemoral and ilioinguinal neuralgias by tapping over the tender point to reproduce pain over the sensory innervation of the ilioinguinal nerve as well as asking the patient to extend at the hip. Because of the overlapping sensory distribution, local anesthetic injections targeting the specific nerve can be more definitive.

Management

If relief of symptoms occurs with nerve blockade (preferably on more than one occasion), exploration of the nerve could be considered. Most specifically, if related to previous surgical intervention such as mesh placement, alteration to the mesh or removal may be warranted. In some instances, a neurectomy may be appropriate and has been shown to provide relief with few side effects (loss of cremasteric reflex). If conservative medical management has failed, one may consider cryoablation after a successful nerve block, pulsed radiofrequency ablation, spinal cord stimulation, peripheral nerve stimulation, or even intrathecal therapy in refractory cases. There is limited or anecdotal evidence only in support of these interventions.

Genitofemoral Neuralgia

Anatomy

The genitofemoral nerve originates from the first and second lumbar nerve roots of the lumbar plexus to form sensory and motor fibers. The sensory distribution ultimately divides along the inguinal ligament into the femoral and genital branches, which have their own innervations. The femoral branch runs superfi-

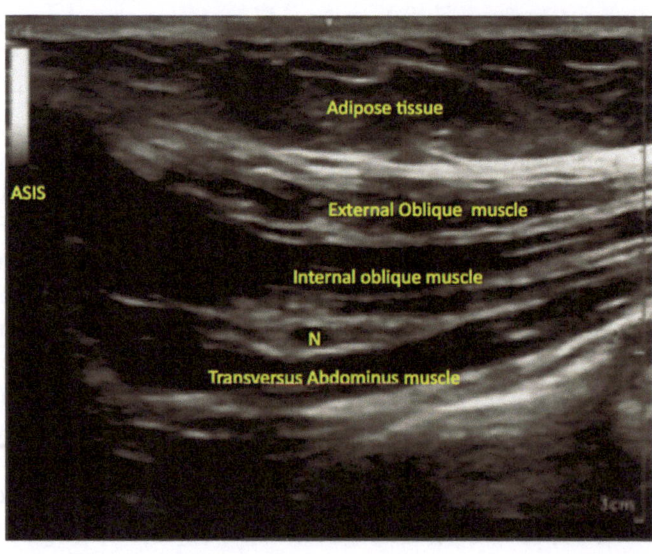

Fig. 26.2 Ultrasonography of a case of ilioinguinal entrapment neuropathy after abdominal surgery. *N* ilioinguinal nerve. *ASIS* anterior superior iliac spine

cial to the fascia iliaca and deep to fascia lata supplying the skin over the upper portion of the femoral triangle and inner thigh (Fig. 26.3). The genital branch enters the internal inguinal ring and supplies the cremaster muscle for the motor component and the sensory portion extending to the scrotum with the variation in women accompanying the round ligament of the uterus and supplying sensation to the skin of the mons pubis and labium majus.

Pathophysiology

Damage to the genitofemoral nerve can occur anywhere along the course of the nerve and has similar pathophysiology as the ilioinguinal nerve mentioned above.

Diagnosis

Patients with genitofemoral neuralgia often complain of burning pain in the groin with radiation to the upper medial thigh and genitalia. On exam, pain can be reproduced with the patient extending at the hip as well as asking the patient to bend forward at the waist. Patients may report improved discomfort laying down or flexing at the thigh. Because of the overlying distribution with the ilioinguinal nerve, nerve blocks may render better information as to the etiology of the pain.

Management

A diagnostic nerve block with local anesthetic can be performed initially to confirm the diagnosis of genitofemoral neuralgia. After a successful nerve block, further management of genitofemoral neuralgia is similar to that of the ilioinguinal neuralgia given the nature of the anatomy and similar characteristics of pathophysiology.

Carpal Tunnel Syndrome

Anatomy

The carpal tunnel is found on the palmar aspect of the wrist that is bounded by tendons from the flexor digitorum profundus and superficialis as well as the flexor pollicis longus alongside the median nerve, with the carpal canal ultimately surrounded by bone and muscle (Fig. 26.4).

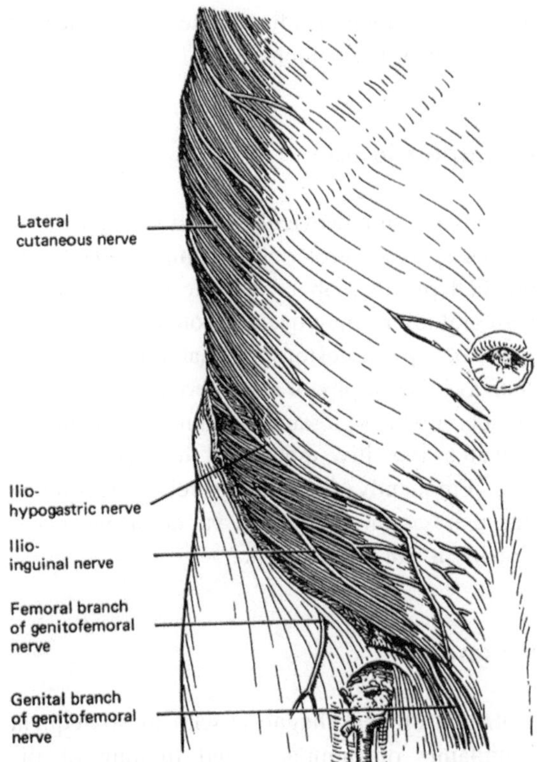

Fig. 26.3 The groin area is innervated principally by branches of the first lumbar nerve – the iliohypogastric and ilioinguinal nerves. These nerves innervate the skin area over the iliac crest (the lateral branch of the iliohypogastric nerve), the suprapubic region (the anterior branch of iliohypogastric nerve), and the front and side of the scrotum and upper medial thigh (the ilioinguinal nerve after it emerges from the inguinal canal) (With permission: Mahadevan V. Essential anatomy of the abdominal wall. In: Kingsnorth AN, LeBlanc KA, editors. *Management of abdominal hernias*. London: Springer; 2013. p. 25–53, Fig. 2.7)

Pathophysiology

The median nerve may become compressed by any of the tendons or surrounding tissue with consequent edema, which can result in clinical manifestations of carpal tunnel syndrome.

Diagnosis

Patients often complain of recurring pain with numbness and tingling in the distribution of the median nerve. Despite a reported prevalence of 3.8% of clinically diagnosed carpal tunnel syndrome and its socioeconomic impact as the most common entrapment neuropathy, there still is no definitive diagnostic modality. Physical exam findings are limited and have been shown to not correlate well with nerve conduction studies. Noting the muscle bulk of the thenar eminence is important in discerning a sign of myelopathy. Based on a systematic review, one of the most sensitive tests is the wrist flexion and carpal compression maneuver with 89% sensitivity. Tinel's percussion test has reported sensitivity as high as 75% as well as Phalen's test with ranging sensitivities of 43–83%, with variability based on the severity of nerve compression. Nerve conduction studies of the median nerve are often ordered as a measure for diagnosis and thought to be definitive; however, within the systematic review, there were variability and controversy in what was considered as abnormal sensory and motor latencies. Temperature may affect nerve conduction velocities and hence results.

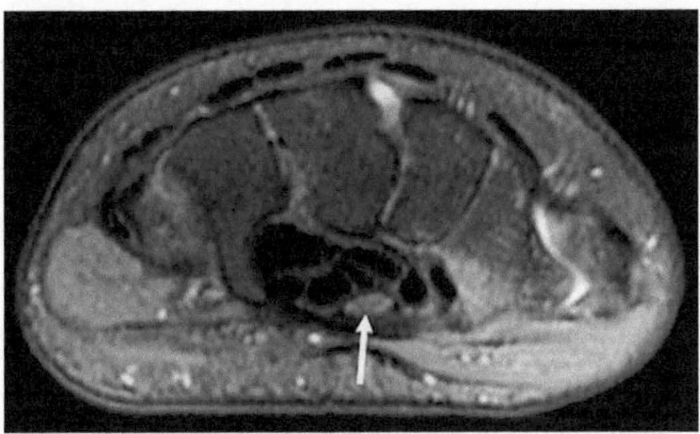

Fig. 26.4 MR axial image of the carpal tunnel displaying a single branch of the median nerve (*arrow*) inside the tunnel (From Pierre-Jerome C, Smitson RD, Shah RK, Moncayo V, Abdelnoor M, Terk MR. MRI of the median nerve and median artery in the carpal tunnel: prevalence of their anatomical variations and clinical significance. With permission: Springer, *Surgical and Radiologic Anatomy*, MRI of the median nerve and median artery in the carpal tunnel: prevalence of their anatomical variations and clinical significance, 2009, 32(3):315–22)

Management

With the questions that exist in diagnosis, the decision of medical management versus surgical intervention can become difficult. Often conservative management consists of recommending the use of wrist splints with 78% of patients perceiving "some" to a "great deal" of improvement in symptoms. Another option is the use of nonsteroidal anti-inflammatory drugs (NSAIDs) for a short duration with reported 74% improvement in symptoms. The combination of a splint and NSAIDs was able to elicit improvement in 85% of patients with carpal tunnel syndrome. Carpal tunnel injections with a combination of local anesthetic and steroid have been performed with short- or median-term symptom relief. In refractory cases, surgical decompression is certainly an option and is often discussed with patients prior to any electrodiagnostic studies. A prospective, randomized study demonstrated that both the open and endoscopic carpal tunnel release groups experience relief of pain and improvement of paresthesias in 98 and 99%, respectively, but with longer return to work time noted in the open group.

Thoracic Outlet Syndrome (TOS)

Anatomy

The neurovascular bundle consisting of the subclavian vessels and the brachial plexus courses through the interscalene triangle (bordered by the anterior/middle scalene and first rib), then enters the costoclavicular triangle (bordered by middle third of the clavicle, first rib, and upper scapula), and then finishes at the subcoracoid area inferior to the coracoid process and deep to the pectoralis minor tendon. The neural component of TOS, which is encountered in greater than 90% of the time, is related to the anatomy of the brachial plexus (C5–T1) as it courses out of the thoracic outlet with different divisions having correlating symptoms. The venous component is related to the relationship of the subclavian vein within the space formed by the anterior scalene muscle, costoclavicular ligament, and subclavius muscle that can lead to occlusion with hypertrophy or inflammation. Finally, the arterial form of TOS is related to an anomalous anterior scalene insertion or cervical/anomalous first rib leading to nearby subclavian artery compression.

Pathophysiology

Within the supraclavicular fossa and costoclavicular space, neurovascular compression of the brachial plexus, subclavian artery and vein, or vertebral artery may occur secondary to trauma, space-occupying lesions, or anatomic anomalies such as hypertrophy of the anterior scalene muscle, cervical rib pressure, or abnormal anatomy, as well as repetitive motions of the upper extremities. Frequently, the etiology relates to trauma that exposes an anatomical variation, but occasionally it can be idiopathic.

Diagnosis

TOS is a clinical diagnosis with most frequent complaints of numbness and tingling of the hands. The symptoms are often worsened with abduction of the arms, leading to occipital headaches, weak grip, vertigo, and cold hands. The traumatic etiology of TOS may be misdiagnosed as either cervical strain or cervical disc syndrome as complaints of neck pain and stiffness can be common as well. Symptoms can be reproduced by shoulder abduction via inward pressure on the brachial plexus. Examining the strength of the pulse in each upper extremity may be revealing especially during provocative tests (hyperextension test). Easy fatigability and paresthesias with the elevated arm test are also common findings. Imaging can be obtained such as cervical X-rays looking for degenerative disc disease, cervical ribs, and callous formation, to name a few. CT or MRI may reveal scalene muscle anomalies, brachial plexus compression, or space-occupying lesions such as a Pancoast tumor. Moreover, electrodiagnostic studies may assist with the diagnosis of neurogenic TOS. Diagnostic blocks of local anesthetic injected at the site of the anterior scalene muscle may relax the muscle and lead to reduction of pain.

Management

Management consists of muscle relaxants, NSAIDs, and physical therapy with moderate success rates. Physical therapy should focus on posture correction and neck stretching. The use of botulinum toxin can also provide symptomatic relief when injected into the scalene muscles to relax the tension causing the compression. Manipulative therapies and acupuncture are less effective. Some relief may be found temporarily with a transcutaneous electrical nerve stimulation unit (TENS). As noted in other neuralgias related to compression, once conservative treatment is no longer beneficial, supraclavicular cervicobrachial neurovascular surgical decompression may be warranted with moderate to high immediate symptom improvement; however, there is potential risk of complications such as brachial plexus neuritis as well as rare phrenic nerve injury.

Common Peroneal Entrapment

Anatomy

As the sciatic nerve descends in the posterior compartment of the thigh, it divides into common peroneal and tibial nerves. This division typically takes place in the popliteal fossa but can be as high as the subgluteal region. The common peroneal nerve (CPN) then descends in the popliteal fossa where it courses laterally to become superficial to the neck of the fibula within a tunnel formed by the soleus and peroneus longus muscles. It is within this tunnel that the CPN becomes vulnerable to compression injury. The CPN then divides into the deep and superficial branches distal to the fibular neck.

Pathophysiology

Peroneal nerve entrapment at the level of the fibula head is the most common entrapment syndrome in the lower limbs. It is due to the ease of external compression of the peroneal nerve, if not padded well in some positions under general anesthesia, while crossing legs, while sleeping in the elderly, and while following weight loss.

Diagnosis

A simple test is to observe if the patient is able to raise the forefoot off the ground while standing on heels. Not being able to do so is often accompanied by a sensory deficit in the lateral anterior tibial compartment. Tinel's sign may be positive and is elicited by tapping the peroneal nerve at the neck of the fibula, which produces pain and tingling in the distribution of the peroneal nerve supply. An important differential is a radiculopathy involving the L5 root. Features that define a L5 lesion include pain in the lower back with radiation along the lateral aspect of the lower extremity and additional loss of foot inversion and dorsiflexion. Another critical differential is spinal stenosis; patients often have pain in the buttocks radiating down the lower extremity and made worse when walking downhill and relieved by bending forward or sitting. MRI imaging of the spine can be very useful in delineating a diagnosis. Electrophysiological studies help distinguish these syndromes from peroneal entrapment. In entrapment cases, there is demyelination with conduction block in mild lesions and a marked loss of amplitude presumably secondary to axonal degeneration in more severe lesions.

Management

Because the majority of these lesions are caused by external pressure, a conservative approach of relieving the compression and a foot brace adjuvant can result in the resolution of the motor deficit within 3–6 months. Surgical decompression can be an alternative if conservative approaches are unsuccessful.

Morton's Neuroma

Anatomy

The third common digital nerve (TCDN), which is the most common nerve affected in Morton's neuroma, is formed by the medial and lateral plantar nerves and is found within the third web space becoming vulnerable to repeated movement of daily life (Fig. 26.5). The nerve sits inferior to the transverse intermetatarsal ligament and adjacent to the flexor digitorum longus and brevis. Because of the relatively fixed TCDN with the more mobile 4th metatarsal adjacent, a shearing stress can ensue. Wearing high-heel shoes further intensifies the stress on the susceptible nerve by placing the nerve closer to the transverse intermetatarsal ligament.

Pathophysiology

Theories about the pathophysiology of this neuralgia include ischemia, intermetatarsal bursitis, and entrapment. The compression and stretching may lead to focal ischemia and nerve damage consequent to sclerosis and narrowing of the arterial supply. The bursitis theory is based on the inflamed intermetatarsal bursa found dorsal to the 2nd and 3rd intermetatarsal space, leading to fibrosis and nerve irritation. Finally, the entrapment theory states that the digital nerve becomes compressed via the intermetatarsal ligament and the plantar aspect of the foot during the stance phase of walking. This theory is validated by the surgical technique of releasing the anterior edge of the intermetatarsal ligament without resection of the neuroma leading to prompt and consistent progression to relief.

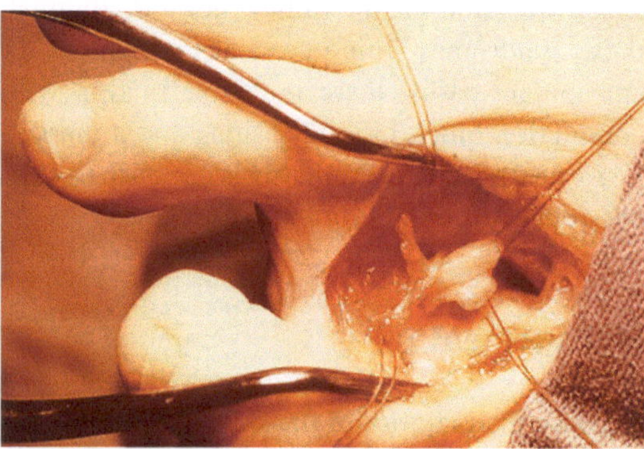

Fig. 26.5 A typical Morton's interdigital neuroma. Surgical dissection shows a thickened and inflamed common digital nerve (With permission: J. D. Heckman et al. (eds.), *Current Orthopedic diagnosis & treatment* © Current Medicine, Inc. 2000)

Diagnosis

Middle-aged women may complain of lancinating pain and numbness in the forefoot with radiation to the toes. The patients often describe pain with walking in high heels or pointed shoes with relief upon removing the footwear. The differential must include bursitis or synovitis with occasional diffuse pain that may encompass the ankles. Other differentials include lumbar radiculopathy, stress fracture, rheumatoid arthritis, and peripheral neuritis or neuropathy. Aside from history and physical exam, ultrasound may be used to find a hypoechoic mass within the intermetatarsal space. Local anesthetic injections at the site of point tenderness may be diagnostic without the need for further imaging such as MRI.

Management

Conservative treatments such as warm soaks, massage therapy, avoidance of high-heel and pointed shoes, and foot elevation may provide symptomatic relief. Placing cushions at the metatarsal and stiff-soled shoes has been successful. Anti-inflammatory medications have not proven to be successful, but an attempt at web space injections with steroid and local anesthetic can be attempted before surgical approaches to nerve resection, neurectomy, or intermetatarsal ligament release with or without neurolysis.

Suggested Reading

1. Alam C, Merskey H. What's in a name? The cycle of change in the meaning of neuralgia. Hist Psychiatry. 1994;5(20):429–74.
2. Atroshi I, Gummesson C, Johnsson R, Ornstein E, Ranstam J, Rosen I. Prevalence of carpal tunnel syndrome in a general population. JAMA. 1999;281(2):153–8.
3. Benzon, Raja, Fishman, Liu, Cohen. Essentials of pain medicine. 3rd ed. Elsevier. Philadelphia.
4. Benzon, Rathmell, Wu, Turk, Argoff, Hurley. Practical management of pain. 5th ed. Elsevier. Philadelphia.
5. Brown RA, et al. Carpal tunnel release. A prospective, randomized assessment of open and endoscopic methods. J Bone Joint Surg Am. 1993;75(9):1265–75.
6. Dellon AL. Somatosensory testing and rehabilitation. Bethesda: American Occupational Therapy Association; 1997. p. 84.
7. Dellon AL, Ebmer J, Swier P. Anatomic variations related to decompression of the common peroneal nerve at the fibular head. Ann Plast Surg. 2002;48(1):30–4.
8. Hassouna H, Singh D. Morton's metatarsalgia: pathogenesis, aetiology and current management. Acta Orthop Belg. 2005;71(6):646.
9. Homan MM, Franzblau A, Werner RA, Albers JW, Armstrong TJ, Bromberg MB. Agreement between symptom surveys, physical examination procedures and electrodiagnostic findings for the carpal tunnel syndrome. Scand J Work Environ Health. 1999;25(2):115–24.
10. Huang JH, Zager EL. Thoracic outlet syndrome. Neurosurgery. 2004;55(4):897–903.
11. Kimura J. Electrodiagnosis in diseases of nerve and muscle. Philadelphia: FA Davis; 1983. p. 83–4.
12. Massy-Westropp N, Grimmer K, Bain G. A systematic review of the clinical diagnostic tests for carpal tunnel syndrome. J Hand Surg. 2000;25(1):120–7.
13. Rab M, Ebmer J, Lee Dellon A. Anatomic variability of the ilioinguinal and genitofemoral nerve: implications for the treatment of groin pain. Plast Reconstr Surg. 2001;108(6):1618–23.
14. Ryan W, et al. Relationship of the common peroneal nerve and its branches to the head and neck of the fibula. Clin Anat. 2003;16(6):501–5.
15. Starling JR, Harms BA. Diagnosis and treatment of genitofemoral and ilioinguinal neuralgia. World J Surg. 1989;13:586–91.
16. Taylor-Gjevre RM, et al. Treatments for carpal tunnel syndrome who does what, when... and why? Can Fam Physician. 2007;53(7):1186–90.
17. Williams PH, Trzil KP. Management of meralgia paresthetica. J Neurosurg. 1991;74(1):76–80.
18. Woods WW. Thoracic outlet syndrome. West J Med. 1978;128(1):9.
19. Wu KK. Morton's interdigital neuroma: a clinical review of its etiology, treatment, and results. J Foot Ankle Surg. 1996;35(2):112–9.

Trigeminal Neuralgia

27

Samer Narouze

Key Concepts

- Classical trigeminal neuralgia is a unilateral disorder characterized by brief electric shock-like pains, abrupt in onset and termination, and limited to the distribution of one or more divisions of the trigeminal nerve. It is caused by neurovascular compression, most frequently by the superior cerebellar artery.
- Painful trigeminal neuralgia is previously termed symptomatic trigeminal neuralgia and secondary trigeminal neuralgia. It is secondary to a disease or lesion other than neurovascular compression such as trauma, herpes zoster, tumor, or multiple sclerosis.
- In addition to history and physical examination, MRI is essential in the investigation of trigeminal neuralgia.
- Classical trigeminal neuralgia is usually responsive, at least initially, to pharmacotherapy. The first medication of choice is carbamazepine or oxcarbazepine. Painful trigeminal neuropathy is less responsive to pharmacotherapy.
- When the pharmacological treatment is ineffective or intolerable, interventional options are considered, usually with high success rates. Options include radiofrequency ablation of the Gasserian ganglion, percutaneous balloon microcompression of the Gasserian ganglion, gamma knife (stereotactic radiation therapy) of the Gasserian ganglion, percutaneous glycerol rhizolysis, and surgical microvascular decompression.

S. Narouze, MD, PhD (✉)
Department of Anesthesiology, Ohio University, Athens, OH 45701, USA

Department of Neurological Surgery, Ohio State University, Columbus, OH 43210, USA
e-mail: narouzs@hotmail.com

Introduction

Trigeminal neuralgia is the most common form of facial neuropathic pain in elderly people with an annual incidence of four to five new patients per 100,000. Trigeminal neuralgia is more prevalent in women than men in a ratio of 1.5:1.

The International Classification of Headache Disorders 3rd edition (ICHD-3 beta version) describes trigeminal neuralgia as either "classical trigeminal neuralgia" or "painful trigeminal neuropathy" (Table 27.1).

Classical Trigeminal Neuralgia

This type was previously termed tic douloureux, *primary trigeminal neuralgia*, and *idiopathic trigeminal neuralgia*.

J. Cheng, R.W. Rosenquist (eds.), *Fundamentals of Pain Medicine*,
https://doi.org/10.1007/978-3-319-64922-1_27

Table 27.1 Classifications of Trigeminal Neuralgia

13.1 Trigeminal neuralgia
13.1.1 Classical trigeminal neuralgia
13.1.1.1 Classical trigeminal neuralgia, purely paroxysmal
13.1.1.2 Classical trigeminal neuralgia with concomitant persistent facial pain
13.1.2 Painful trigeminal neuropathy
13.1.2.1 Painful trigeminal neuropathy attributed to acute herpes zoster
13.1.2.2 Postherpetic trigeminal neuropathy
13.1.2.3 Painful post-traumatic trigeminal neuropathy
13.1.2.4 Painful trigeminal neuropathy attributed to multiple sclerosis (MS)
13.1.2.5 Painful trigeminal neuropathy attributed to space-occupying lesion
13.1.2.6 Painful trigeminal neuropathy

Pathophysiology

Classical trigeminal neuralgia is caused by neurovascular compression, most frequently by the superior cerebellar artery. Most patients have compression of the trigeminal root by tortuous or aberrant vessels as evident by posterior fossa exploration and magnetic resonance imaging (MRI). Imaging should be done to exclude secondary causes.

Description

Classical trigeminal neuralgia is a unilateral disorder characterized by brief electric shock-like pains, abrupt in onset and termination, limited to the distribution of one or more divisions of the trigeminal nerve. Pain is commonly evoked by trivial stimuli including washing, shaving, smoking, talking, and teeth brushing (trigger factors). Small areas in the nasolabial fold and/or chin may be particularly susceptible to the precipitation of pain (trigger areas). It also frequently occurs spontaneously. The pain usually remits for variable periods.

Diagnostic Criteria

A. At least three attacks of unilateral facial pain fulfilling criteria B and C.
B. Occurring in one or more divisions of the trigeminal nerve, with no radiation beyond the trigeminal distribution.
C. Pain has at least three of the following four characteristics:
   1. Recurring in paroxysmal attacks lasting from a fraction of a second to 2 min
   2. Severe intensity
   3. Electric shock-like, shooting, stabbing, or sharp in quality
   4. Precipitated by innocuous stimuli to the affected side of the face
D. No clinically evident neurological deficits.
E. Not better accounted for by another ICHD-3 diagnosis.

Clinical Presentation

- Classical trigeminal neuralgia usually starts in the second or third divisions (V2-V3), affecting the cheek or the chin. In <5% of patients, the first division (V1) is affected.
- The pain is strictly unilateral, right side more than the left with a ratio of 3:2. It may rarely occur bilaterally, in which case a central cause such as *multiple sclerosis* must be considered especially in young females.
- Following a painful paroxysm, there is usually a refractory period during which pain cannot be triggered. The pain often evokes spasm of the muscle of the face on the affected side (tic douloureux).
- Neurological examination is essentially normal in patients with classic trigeminal neuralgia. This is different from patients with secondary trigeminal neuralgia where there are some neurological deficits. In such cases trigeminal neuralgia is a symptom of another disease, e.g., multiple sclerosis or cerebellopontine angle neoplasm.

- Mild autonomic symptoms such as lacrimation and/or redness of the eye may be present.
- Between paroxysms, most patients are asymptomatic. However, in a subtype of the classical trigeminal neuralgia with concomitant persistent facial pain, there is prolonged background pain in the affected area. This has been referred to as "atypical trigeminal neuralgia" or "trigeminal neuralgia type 2." This type of TN responds poorly to conservative treatment and to neurosurgical interventions.

Investigations

MRI is essential to identify any neurovascular compression (idiopathic TN) and to rule out other pathology such as multiple sclerosis and posterior fossa tumors (secondary TN).

Painful Trigeminal Neuralgia

This type was previously termed *symptomatic trigeminal neuralgia* and *secondary trigeminal neuralgia*.

Prevalence

Herpes zoster affects the trigeminal ganglion in 10–15% of cases, with the ophthalmic division (V1) being affected in about 80% of patients. Herpes zoster is common in immunocompromised patients, occurring in about 10% of those with lymphoma and 25% of patients with Hodgkin's disease (see Chap. 24).

Description

It is head and/or facial pain in the distribution of one or more branches of the trigeminal nerve, often with neurological deficits. Pain is indistinguishable from classical trigeminal neuralgia but is caused by a demonstrable structural lesion other than vascular compression. A causative lesion is often demonstrated by special investigations and/or posterior fossa exploration. The pain is highly variable in quality and intensity according to the cause.

Painful Trigeminal Neuropathy Attributed to Acute Herpes Zoster

Description

Unilateral head and/or facial pain of less than 3 months' duration in the distribution of one or more branches of the trigeminal nerve is caused by and associated with other symptoms and/or clinical signs of acute herpes zoster.

Diagnostic Criteria

A. Unilateral head and/or facial pain lasting <3 months and fulfilling criterion C
B. Either or both of the following:
   1. Herpetic eruption has occurred in the territory of a trigeminal nerve branch or branches.
   2. Varicella zoster virus DNA has been detected in the CSF by polymerase chain reaction (PCR).
C. Evidence of causation demonstrated by both of the following:
   1. Pain preceded the herpetic eruption by <7 days.
   2. Pain is located in the distribution of the same trigeminal nerve branch or branches.
D. Not better accounted for by another ICHD-3 diagnosis

Clinical Presentation

The facial pain from acute herpes zoster is described as burning, stabbing, shooting, or tingling and is usually accompanied by cutaneous allodynia. Ophthalmic herpes may be associated with III, IV, and VI cranial nerve palsies. In rare situations, the pain is not followed by a rash (zoster sine herpete). The diagnosis may be confirmed by PCR detection of varicella zoster virus DNA in the cerebrospinal fluid.

Postherpetic Trigeminal Neuropathy

Description

Unilateral head or facial pain, caused by herpes zoster, persists or recurs for at least 3 months in the distribution of one or more branches of the trigeminal nerve with variable sensory changes.

Diagnostic Criteria

A. Unilateral head and/or facial pain persisting or recurring for >3 months and fulfilling criterion C
B. History of acute herpes zoster affecting a trigeminal nerve branch or branches
C. Evidence of causation demonstrated by both of the following:
   1. Pain is developed in temporal relation to the acute herpes zoster.
   2. Pain is located in the distribution of the same trigeminal nerve branch or branches.
D. Not better accounted for by another ICHD-3 diagnosis.

Clinical Presentation

Postherpetic neuralgia is more prevalent in the elderly. The first division of the trigeminal nerve (V1) is most commonly affected. The pain is usually burning and itching associated with variable sensory abnormalities and allodynia. Scars may be present as a result of healing from the previous herpetic eruption.

Painful Posttraumatic Trigeminal Neuropathy

It is previously termed *anesthesia dolorosa.*

Description

It is described as unilateral facial or oral pain following trauma to the trigeminal nerve. Other symptoms and signs of trigeminal nerve dysfunction may be present. The traumatic event may be mechanical, chemical (post-glycerol neurolysis), thermal (post-radiofrequency ablation), or radiation. Pain duration ranges widely from paroxysmal to constant and may be mixed.

Diagnostic Criteria

A. Unilateral facial and/or oral pain fulfilling criterion C
B. History of an identifiable traumatic event to the trigeminal nerve, with clinically evident positive (hyperalgesia, allodynia) and/or negative (hypoesthesia, hypoalgesia) signs of trigeminal nerve dysfunction
C. Evidence of causation demonstrated by both of the following:
   1. Pain is located in the distribution of the same trigeminal nerve.
   2. Pain has developed within 3–6 months of the traumatic event.
D. Not better accounted for by another ICHD-3 diagnosis

Painful Trigeminal Neuropathy Attributed to Multiple Sclerosis (MS) Plaque

Prevalence

About 7% of MS patients have a syndrome that is similar to classical trigeminal neuralgia. However, symptoms of trigeminal neuralgia are very rarely a presenting feature of MS.

Description

It is often described as unilateral head or facial pain in the distribution of a trigeminal nerve and with the characteristics of classical trigeminal neuralgia. It is caused by a multiple sclerosis plaque affecting the trigeminal nerve root and associated with other symptoms and/or clinical signs of multiple sclerosis.

Diagnostic Criteria

A. Head and/or facial pain with the characteristics of classical trigeminal neuralgia with or without concomitant persistent facial pain, but not necessarily unilateral.
B. Multiple sclerosis (MS) has been diagnosed.
C. An MS plaque affecting the trigeminal nerve root has been demonstrated by MRI or by routine electrophysiological studies (blink reflex or trigeminal evoked potentials) indicating impairment of the affected trigeminal nerve(s).
D. Not better accounted for by another ICHD-3 diagnosis.

Clinical Presentation

Symptoms of painful trigeminal neuropathy attributed to MS are more likely to be bilateral than those of classical trigeminal neuralgia. Other symptoms and signs of MS help to establish the diagnosis. Symptoms of trigeminal neuralgia are very rarely a presenting feature of MS.

Management of Trigeminal Neuralgia

Conservative Treatments

- Classical trigeminal neuralgia is usually responsive, at least initially, to pharmacotherapy (Table 27.2).
- The first medication of choice is carbamazepine or oxcarbazepine.
- The second medication of choice is baclofen.
- Other medications which can be tried, although there is no clinical evidence for their efficacy, are other anticonvulsants, e.g., gabapentin and pregabalin, among others.
- Patients with painful trigeminal neuropathy attributed to multiple sclerosis are less responsive to pharmacotherapy.

Interventional Treatments

When the pharmacological treatment is ineffective or intolerable, interventional options are considered (Fig. 27.1).

Surgical Approaches

Microvascular decompression (MVD): The vessels in contact with the trigeminal root entry zone are coagulated or separated from the nerve using an inert sponge.

Percutaneous Approaches

1. Gamma knife (stereotactic radiation therapy): This is a noninvasive treatment that allows high-dose irradiation of a small section of the trigeminal nerve. This leads to nonselective damage of the Gasserian ganglion.
2. Percutaneous balloon microcompression: The Gasserian ganglion is compressed by a small balloon, which is percutaneously introduced through a needle into Meckel's cavity. This leads to ischemic damage of the ganglion cells. The technique may be more suitable for treatment of V1 trigeminal neuralgia of the first branch as the corneal reflex tends to remain intact.
3. Percutaneous glycerol rhizolysis: Under fluoroscopy, in the sitting position with flexed head, the needle is introduced into the trigeminal cistern, visualized by X-ray. Contrast agent is then injected to determine the size of the cistern before an equal volume of glycerol is injected after aspiration of the contrast agent.
4. Percutaneous radiofrequency thermocoagulation of the Gasserian ganglion: This is usually considered for the elderly patient with high risk for surgical MVD (Figs. 27.2 and 27.3). The outcome may be less favorable than MVD, but it is less invasive with lower morbidity and mortality rates.

Table 27.2 Medical treatments for trigeminal neuralgia

Medication	Dosage	Comments
Carbamazepine	400–1200 mg/d	Monitor for multiple side effects and drug interactions Nausea, vomiting, leukopenia are common Available as extended-release (ER) and intravenous (IV)
Oxcarbazepine	300–1800 mg/d	Better tolerability than carbamazepine Need to monitor Na^+ level
Phenytoin	300–600 mg/d	Monitor for multiple side effects and drug interactions
Baclofen	40–80 mg/d	Short half-life Needs frequent dosing Helpful in MS patients
Clonazepam	1–4 mg/d	Anxiolytic, anticonvulsant, muscle relaxant, and sedative effects Monitor for multiple side effects and drug interactions Cognitive and motor impairments are common
Valproate	500–1500 mg/d	Time to pain relief: weeks Monitor for multiple side effects and drug interactions Available as intravenous (IV)
Lamotrigine	100–500 mg	Monitor for serious allergic reactions Need to adjust the dose with carbamazepine, phenytoin, clonazepam, valproate
Gabapentin	900–4800 mg/d	Time to pain relief: weeks Helpful in MS patients Limiting side effects are cognitive impairments and weight gain
Pregabalin	100–600 mg/d	Better tolerability than gabapentin
Topiramate	100–400 mg/d	Limiting side effects are cognitive impairments May cause weight loss

5. Pulsed radiofrequency ablation of the Gasserian ganglion: Although it would seem a safer alternative than the commonly used thermal RFA, its efficacy is questioned in a randomized controlled study.

Gasserian Ganglion Neuromodulation

Gasserian ganglion electric stimulation was reported either via a subtemporal craniotomy or a percutaneous approach. Technical difficulties and lead migration are the main factors that this approach is not widely used.

Choice of Treatment

- There are few systematic reviews comparing various treatment approaches.
- The first choice of treatment should be always conservative management.
- For those who failed pharmacological treatment, interventional management can be considered (Fig. 27.1).
- In general, younger patients with MRI evidence of vascular compression should be considered for MVD. The other minimally invasive procedures are generally considered to be less effective with higher relapse rate.

Fig. 27.1 Algorithm for the management of trigeminal neuralgia (With permission: Springer, *Algorithms for the Diagnosis and Management of Head and Face Pain*, Samer N. Narouze MD, PhD, Jan 1, 2014, pp. 9–14, Fig. 2.5)

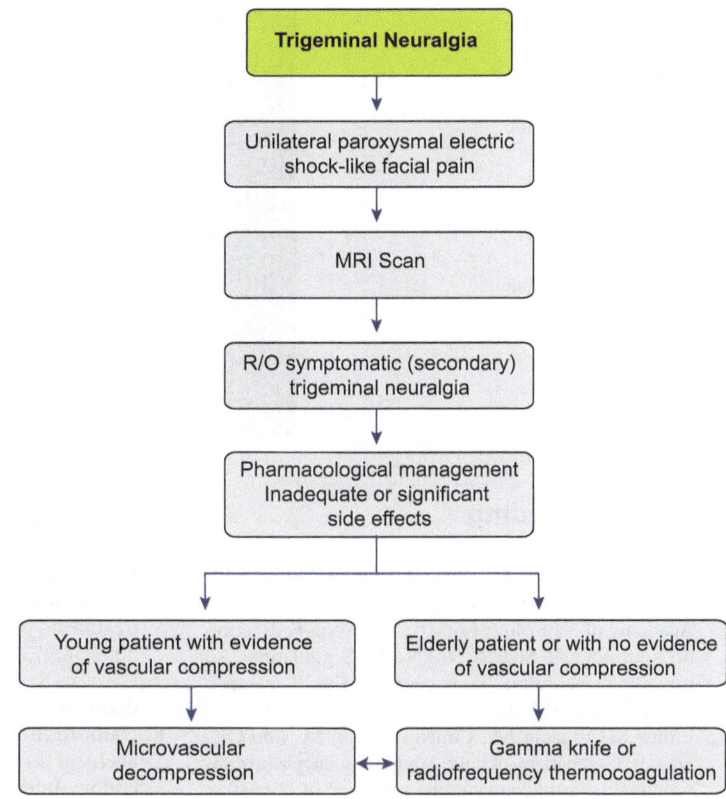

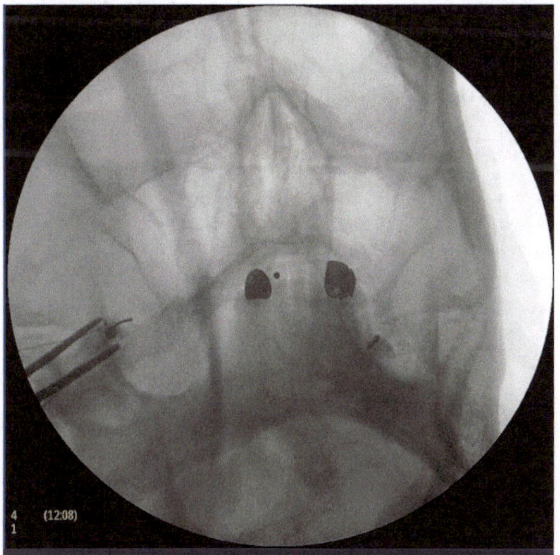

Fig. 27.2 Trigeminal ganglion thermal radiofrequency ablation: Oblique submental view showing the needle tip inside the foramen ovale (Reprinted with permission, Samer Narouze, MD, PhD, Ohio Pain and Headache Institute)

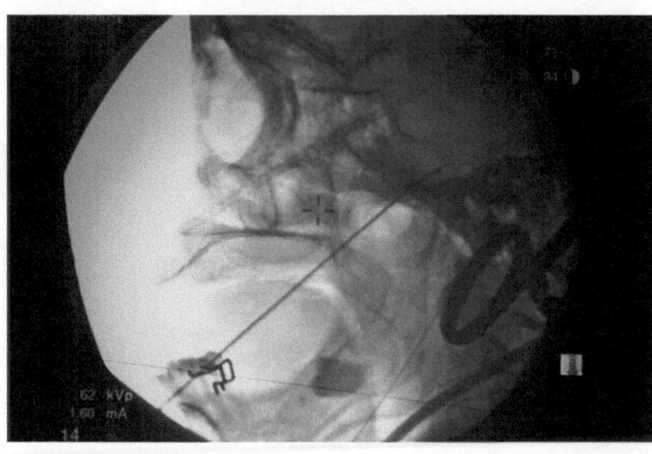

Fig. 27.3 Trigeminal ganglion thermal radiofrequency ablation; lateral view showing the needle going through the foramen ovale with the needle tip overlying the petrous bone (Reprinted with permission, Samer Narouze, MD, PhD, Ohio Pain and Headache Institute)

Suggested Reading

1. Cruccu G, Gronseth G, Alksne J, Argoff C, Brainin M, Burchiel K, Nurmikko T, Zakrzewska JM, American Academy of Neurology Society; European Federation of Neurological Society. AAN-EFNS guidelines on trigeminal neuralgia management. Eur J Neurol. 2008;15(10):1013–28.
2. Erdine S, Ozyalcin NS, Cimen A, Celik M, Talu GK, Disci R. Comparison of pulsed radiofrequency with conventional radiofrequency in the treatment of idiopathic trigeminal neuralgia. Eur J Pain. 2007;11:309–13.
3. Headache Classification Committee of the International Headache Society (IHS). The international classification of headache disorders. 3rd edition (beta version). Cephalalgia. 2013;33(9):629–808.
4. Jannetta PJ, McLaughlin MR, Casey KF. Technique of microvascular decompression. Technical note. Neurosurg Focus. 2005;18:E5.
5. Jorns TP, Zakrzewska JM. Evidence-based approach to the medical management of trigeminal neuralgia. Br J Neurosurg. 2007;21(3):253–61.
6. Lopez BC, Hamlyn PJ, Zakrzewska JM. Systematic review of ablative neurosurgical techniques for the treatment of trigeminal neuralgia. Neurosurgery. 2004;54:973–82. Discussion 982–973
7. Narouze S. Complications of head and neck procedures. Tech Reg Anesth Pain Manag. 2007;11:171–7.
8. Narouze S. Algorithms for the diagnosis and management of head and face pain. In: Narouze S, editor. Interventional management of head and face pain. New York: Springer Science + Business Media; 2014.
9. Rozen TD. Trigeminal neuralgia and glossopharyngeal neuralgia. Neurol Clin. 2004;22:185–206.
10. van Kleef M, van Genderen WE, Narouze S, Nurmikko TJ, van Zundert J, Geurts JW, Mekhail N. Trigeminal neuralgia. Pain Pract. 2009;9(4):252–9.

Central Pain Syndromes 28

Alexander Bautista and Jianguo Cheng

Key Concepts

- Central pain syndrome (CPS) is a neurological condition caused by damage to or dysfunction of the central nervous system (CNS). This syndrome can be caused by stroke, multiple sclerosis, tumors, epilepsy, brain or spinal cord trauma, or Parkinson's disease.
- The character of the pain associated with this syndrome differs widely among individuals partly because of the large variety of potential causes. It may affect a large portion of the body or may be more restricted to specific parts. A constant burning pain sensation may be the predominant symptom but not pathognomonic of CPS.
- The pathophysiology is variable and is generally poorly understood. Alterations of sensory pathway and impaired inhibitory mechanism may be involved in CPS. The syndrome often begins shortly after the causative injury or damage, but may be delayed by months or even years, especially if it is related to post-stroke pain.
- Thorough history and physical examination is the key to specific and accurate diagnosis of CPS. No single ancillary test is highly sensitive and specific to diagnose CPS.
- Improvement of function and rehabilitation is the main goal for treatment. Having a multidisciplinary approach in managing CPS increases success rate and satisfaction.
- The use of polypharmacy which includes membrane stabilizers, antidepressants, NMDA antagonist, and low doses of opioids can be useful in treating CPS. Drug therapy is directed to find the most effective drug or combination with minimal side effects. Amitriptyline, gabapentin, and pregabalin are recommended as first-line treatment, and lamotrigine and opioids are considered second- and third-line treatment.
- Neuromodulation, neuroablation, and intrathecal analgesic therapy may be considered in cases where traditional and conservative therapies have not been effective.

Introduction

Central pain syndrome (CPS) refers to the perception of pain resulting from a pathologic entity or lesion(s) or malfunction within the central nervous system. Common causes include stroke,

A. Bautista, MD (✉)
Anesthesiology and Pain Medicine, University of Oklahoma Health Sciences Center, Oklahoma City, OK, USA
e-mail: alexander-bautista@ouhsc.edu

J. Cheng, MD, PhD
Departments of Pain Management and Neurosciences, Cleveland Clinic Anesthesiology Institute and Lerner Research Institute, Cleveland, OH, USA

J. Cheng, R.W. Rosenquist (eds.), *Fundamentals of Pain Medicine*,
https://doi.org/10.1007/978-3-319-64922-1_28

phantom limb pain, multiple sclerosis, tumors, epilepsy, brain or spinal cord trauma, and Parkinson's disease. The extent of pain and the areas affected are related to the cause of injury in the presence or absence of a painful stimulus.

Epidemiology

CPS may originate from the brain and the spinal cord (see Table 28.1). Central pain of brain origin is predominantly manifested in stroke patients. Approximately 795,000 people suffer a stroke annually in the USA, and almost 10% of stroke patients may eventually have central pain. The incidence of phantom limb pain (PLP) after amputation due to trauma or peripheral vascular diseases is 60–80%. The leading cause of CPS of spine origin is trauma. It is present in 30–50% of patients with SCI. However, pain can also result from tumors and iatrogenic, inflammatory, and demyelinating lesions in the spinal cord. The incidence of CPS in such conditions varies and is estimated to range from 5% to 95% of patients.

Central pain is also prevalent in patients with multiple sclerosis (MS) and chronic degenerative CNS disease such as Parkinson's disease (PD) and epilepsy. Pain in MS is very common, with prevalence in patients ranging from 43% to 86%. In addition to central pain, these patients have different types of pain, including dysesthesias in the extremities, complex regional pain, trigeminal neuralgia, and pain secondary to tonic spasms. The elderly population is more commonly affected in stroke and Parkinson-related CPS, while MS, epilepsy, and SCI have a predilection to affect younger patients. CPS has a male predominance with the exception of MS which affects a vast majority of female patients.

Table 28.1 Common diseases associated with chronic central pain syndrome

Poststroke chronic pain
Spinal cord injury
Multiple sclerosis
Parkinson's disease
Epilepsy
Syringomyelia
Phantom limb pain

Pathophysiology

The mechanisms of central pain can be as diverse as its causes. Often times the mechanisms are not well understood. However, depending on the causation, a common pathway for these disease entities would be the perturbation of the somatosensory system in the CNS. The imbalance in the sensory input and alteration of synaptic connections will lead to pain perception by patients. Following injury, the neuroplastic and hypersensitivity changes may result in activation of *N*-methyl-D-aspartate (NMDA) receptors. Other physiologic hypotheses may include loss of spinal inhibitory mechanism and the presence of pattern generators along the spinothalamoparietal tract and its projections. For example, CNP in MS is thought to be secondary to damage to myelinated nerves in the central nervous system and propagated by two main mechanisms: the generation of ectopic impulses at demyelinated lesions and the disinhibition of afferent A-δ and C-fiber pain pathways by interruption of descending inhibitory pathways from the brain. Central sensitization of the dorsal horn neuron may also play a role in the development of mechanical and thermal allodynia which are commonly seen in SCI. Alterations of primary nociceptive fibers which display continuous firing and hyperexcitability may contribute to the central sensitization and development of chronic pain.

Patients with Parkinson's disease may experience central pain as stabbing, burning, scalding, or lancinating pain, which is unprovoked in unusual locations such as the face, mouth, genitalia, pelvis, anus, or abdomen. While conduction along the peripheral and central pain pathways may be normal, with or without primary central pain, the patients may exhibit a lack of habituation of sympathetic sudomotor responses to repetitive pain stimuli, suggesting an abnormal control of pain on the autonomic centers. The observation that such abnormalities were diminished by treatment with levodopa (L-dopa) suggests that the dysfunction may occur in dopaminergic centers regulating the autonomic functions and inhibitory modulation of pain inputs.

The mechanisms of central pain in SCI may have contributions from segmental pathologies such as nerve root entrapment and/or syringomyelia (a hollow fluid-filled cavity or syrinx) in the spinal cord. At a cellular level, dendritic spine remodeling occurs in second-order wide dynamic range (WDR) neurons and accompanies neuropathic pain after SCI, suggesting a synaptic model of long-term memory storage and persistent neuropathic pain. In addition, chronic central pain appears to be associated with hyperexcitable nociceptive primary afferent neurons, which may contribute to central sensitization. The release of glutamate, proinflammatory cytokines, adenosine triphosphate (ATP), reactive oxygen species, and neurotrophic factors triggers activation of postsynaptic neuron and glial cells. Interactions between neurons, glial cells, and immune cells further contribute to the underlying cellular mechanisms of central pain after SCI.

The pathophysiology of phantom limb pain is associated with the elimination or interruption of sensory nerve impulses by destroying or injuring the sensory nerve fibers after amputation or deafferentation. Stump pain is strictly a peripheral pain phenomenon and is seen in more than half of the patients with PLP. PLP does not only occur post-limb amputation but also post-mastectomy (phantom breast syndrome) as well as post-enucleation of the eye. After amputation, there is no input from the amputated part of the body. The brain may remap the part of the body's sensory circuitry to another part of the body. For example, sensory input from another part of the body such as the nose may be reconnected to the cortical representation of a missing limb. When the nose is touched, it may feel to the patient as if the missing limb is also being touched. Other abnormal sensations such as pain can also result within the complex neural networks of the brain.

Clinical Features and Diagnosis

Clinical Features

The character of central pain syndrome differs widely among individuals partly because of the variety of potential causes. It may affect a large portion of the body or may be more restricted to specific areas, such as hands or feet. Pain is typically constant, is moderate to severe in intensity, and is often made worse by touch, movement, emotions, and temperature changes. The patients may experience one or more types of pain sensations, the most prominent being burning. Other complaints such as "pins and needles," pressing, lacerating, and aching pain are also common. Numbness in the affected areas may coexist with the pain, usually most severe on the distant parts of the body, such as the feet or hands. Central pain syndrome often begins shortly after the causative injury or damage, but may be delayed by months or even years, especially if it is related to poststroke pain or SCI. The pain is less frequently on a dermatomal distribution but corresponds to the site of the lesion. It may be perceived as superficial, deep, or both in different degrees.

Diagnosis

The diagnosis of CPS is based on comprehensive history and accurate physical examinations and necessary lab tests and imaging studies. Information from these sources will help localize the central lesion or dysfunction as the first step of the diagnosis. Characterization of the lesion or dysfunction will help determine the respective neurological disorders. In addition to this diagnostic framework, one needs to obtain a comprehensive pain history and characteristics. This should be accompanied by pain-specific sensory examination (touch, temperature, and pinprick sensation), musculoskeletal evaluation, and psychological assessment.

Specialized sensory testing may also be needed. Occasionally, a differential block can be used to assess afferent function in relation to the pain complaints.

Studies using magnetic resonance imaging (MRI) and positron emission tomography (PET) scans may demonstrate anatomical lesions and provided associated information. Functional magnetic resonance imaging, diffusion tensor imaging, or single-photon emission computed tomography may be used to reveal activity patterns and connectivity of the brain in relation to central pain syndromes. For example, a study using PET scan technology revealed a striking loss of opioid receptor availability in the hemisphere contralateral to the pain (especially in the thalamus, anterior and posterior cingulate cortex, insula, S2, and lateral prefrontal cortex) in patients with poststroke pain. The loss of opioid receptor availability may result in a reduction of effectiveness of endogenous, opioid-mediated, analgesic mechanisms, leading to central pain syndrome.

Treatment

Treatment of central pain is difficult and challenging. The first priority is to effectively manage the inciting neurological disorder such as stroke, SCI, MS, or Parkinson's disease. The goal of pain management is to reduce pain (not necessarily eliminate it) and facilitate improvement in function and rehabilitation. To achieve this goal, a multimodal and multidisciplinary approach should be instituted which includes, but not limited to, physical therapy, behavioral/psychological therapy, pharmacotherapy, and interventional therapy.

Physical Therapy and Rehabilitation

This will help improve functionality in patients with CPS. It may help the patient psychologically as the patient gains more independence with life. The use of alternative treatments like ultrasound, massage, and acupuncture has been used, but data regarding its long-term benefit is still lacking. Anecdotal reports with the use of transcutaneous electrical nerve stimulation (TENS) have been promising as an adjunct to pharmacotherapy especially in patients with SCI. TENS may relieve SCI patients with muscular or segmental pain.

Behavioral/Psychological Therapy

Lowering stress levels and learning coping mechanisms appear to reduce pain in patients with CPS. The use of biofeedback, hypnosis, and cognitive behavioral interventions may play a role in managing patients with central pain state.

Pharmacotherapy

Drug therapy is directed to find the most effective drug or drug combination with minimal side effects. Amitriptyline, gabapentin, and pregabalin are recommended as first-line treatment, and lamotrigine and opioids are considered second- and third-line treatment.

- Anticonvulsant drugs: In recent years, anticonvulsant medications have been widely utilized in the management of neuropathic pain. Most of these drugs act on sodium channel receptors with the exception of gabapentin which presumably relieves pain via calcium channel blockade. Side effect profiles include CNS, renal, cardiac, GI toxicity, and, rarely, suicidal ideation.
  - Gabapentin 300 mg in increments to TID dosing up to a maximum of 3600 mg: Maintain at effective dose for at least 2 weeks and then reevaluate.
  - Pregabalin: Start at 25 mg and increase by 25 mg every 2–3 days in divided doses up to 600 mg. This has a faster onset than gabapentin.
  - Lamotrigine slows titration up to effective dose 600–800 mg or side effects.
- Antidepressant drugs: These agents are thought to enhance descending inhibitory pathways. At higher doses, patients may benefit from its mood-altering effects as well.

They are contraindicated in patients with acute porphyria, cardiac, and severe liver disease. These agents should not be stopped abruptly.

  - Amitriptyline: Start with 10–25 mg daily at bedtime, and increase slowly up to 150 mg daily if necessary.
  - New agents and other congeners (nortriptyline, clomipramine), aminergics (duloxetine, desipramine), SSRIs (fluoxetine), SNRI (venlafaxine, milnacipran), and selective norepinephrine blockers (reboxetine) have been used with no or trivial effects in patient with CPS.

- Opioids: Patient usually exhibits refractoriness to these medications, requiring very high doses. Long-term use may be associated with hyperalgesia and dependence which may be difficult to treat.
- Antiarrhythmic drugs: These drugs are considered as third- or fourth-line agents since they are not usually well tolerated and can be proarrhythmic in certain populations. However, its antihyperalgesic and antiallodynic effect may be helpful in certain situations.
  - Intravenous lidocaine 1 mg/kg (10 min) to 5 mg/kg (over 30 min–5 h) diluted in saline. Continuous blood pressure and ECG monitoring are mandatory.
  - Mexiletine slows titration up to effective dose 1000 mg or side effects.
- NMDA blockers: Blockade of these receptors has shown to reverse hypersensitivity states in animal studies. Ketamine is best reserved for parenteral in-hospital administration for refractory cases.

Interventional Therapies

- Neuromodulation: This is often considered as a last resort. The effectiveness remains to be established by well-designed clinical studies. The high cost and inherent risk of this approach should also be considered.
  - Stimulation of the primary motor cortex for intractable deafferentation pain, as well as central stroke pain, has been used successfully. Although the mechanism of pain relief is uncertain, motor cortex stimulation is felt to be the treatment of choice in post-stroke pain, thalamic pain, or anesthesia dolorosa of the face.
  - Repetitive transcranial magnetic stimulation of the primary motor cortex (M1) has also been used successfully. It is a good but transient relief.
- Intrathecal therapy: Continuous intrathecal infusion of medications has been used in a wide array of chronic pain states. Drug delivery by this route may be more effective than systemic/oral route. However, this may pose risk of infection, hemorrhagic complication, and reactive arachnoiditis. Intensive monitoring and regular follow-up are mandatory.
  - IT lidocaine/bupivacaine may reduce pain in SCI patients, but the effect is temporary.
  - IT midazolam.
  - IT baclofen: Reduces allodynic response and has utility in spastic patients. Its use is limited by inherent drug complication and development of tolerance in long-term use.
  - IT clonidine: May be beneficial due to its alpha-2 agonist effect that modulates central pain; however, long-term pain relief more than 3 months limits its use.
  - IT morphine/hydromorphone/fentanyl: Generally effective in acute pain states; however, long-term efficacy is still lacking.
  - IT ziconotide: Is a non-opioid intrathecal drug, is a synthetic form of cone snail toxin, and provides little or no relief with a very narrow therapeutic index.
- Ablative neurosurgery: This should only be considered when all other forms of treatment have been exhausted. Dorsal root entry zone lesion (DREZ) may be considered for patients with SCI. However, the evidence is weak, and the reported outcomes are unimpressive.

Suggested Reading

1. Attal N, Cruccu G, Baron R, Haanpää M, Hansson P, Jensen TS, Nurmikko T. European Federation of Neurological Societies. EFNS guidelines on the pharmacological treatment of neuropathic pain: 2010 revision. Eur J Neurol. 2010;17:1113–e88.
2. Bermejo PE, Oreja-Guevara C, Diez-Tejedor E. Pain in multiple sclerosis: prevalence, mechanisms, types and treatment. Rev Neurol. 2010;50:101–8.
3. Bowsher D. Central pain: clinical and physiological characteristics. J Neurol Neurosurg Psychiatry. 1996;61:62–9.
4. Brewer RP. Raj's practical management of pain. In: Benzon HT, Rathmell JP, Wu CL, Turk DC, Argoff CE, editors. Pain in selected neurologic disorders. 4th ed. Philadelphia: Elsevier; 2008. p. 585–93.
5. Nicholson BD. Evaluation and treatment of central pain syndromes. Neurology. 2004;62(5 Suppl 2):S30–6.
6. Brummett CM, Raja SN. Essentials of pain medicine. In: Benzon HT, Raja SN, Liu SS, Fishman SM, Cohen SP, Hurley RW, Narouze S, Malik KM, Candido KD, editors. Central pain states: Elsevier; 2011. p. 370–7.
7. Canavero S, Bonicalzi V. Central pain syndrome pathophysiology, diagnosis and management. 2nd ed. Cambridge: Cambridge University Press; 2011.
8. Cioni B, Meglio M. Motor cortex stimulation for chronic non-malignant pain: current state and future prospects. Acta Neurochir Suppl. 2007;97(pt 2):45–9.
9. Dworkin RH, O'Connor AB, Kent J, Mackey SC, Raja SN, Stacey BR, Levy RM, Backonja M, Baron R, Harke H, Loeser JD, Treede RD, Turk DC, Wells CD. International association for the study of pain neuropathic pain special interest group. Interventional management of neuropathic pain: NeuPSIG recommendations. Pain. 2013;154(11):2249–61.
10. Hirayama A, Saitoh Y, Kishima H, et al. Reduction of intractable deafferentation pain by navigation-guided repetitive transcranial magnetic stimulation of the primary motor cortex. Pain. 2006;122:22–7.
11. Lammertse D, Falci S. Surgical management of central pain in persons with spinal cord injury: the dorsal root entry zone (DREZ) procedure. Top Spinal Cord Inj Rehabil. 2001;7(2):41–50.
12. Lazorthes Y, Sol JC, Fowo S, Roux FE, Verdié JC. Motor cortex stimulation for neuropathic pain. Acta Neurochir Suppl. 2007;97(pt 2):37–44.
13. Lefaucheur JP, Drouot X, Menard-Lefaucheur I, et al. Neurogenic pain relief by repetitive transcranial magnetic cortical stimulation depends on the origin and the site of pain. J Neurol Neurosurg Psychiatry. 2004;75:612–6.
14. Rasche D, Ruppolt M, Stippich C, Unterberg A, Tronnier VM. Motor cortex stimulation for long-term relief of chronic neuropathic pain: a 10 year experience. Pain. 2006;121:43–52.
15. Saitoh Y, Yoshimine T. Stimulation of primary motor cortex for intractable deafferentation pain. Acta Neurochir Suppl. 2007;97(pt 2):51–6.
16. Schestatsky P, Kumru H, Valls-Solé J, et al. Neurophysiologic study of central pain in patients with Parkinson disease. Neurology. 2007;69:2162–9.
17. Vaney C. Understanding pain mechanisms in multiple sclerosis. MS Manage. 1996;3:11–8.
18. Willoch F, Schindler F, Wester HJ, et al. Central poststroke pain and reduced opioid receptor binding within pain processing circuitries: a [11C]diprenorphine PET study. Pain. 2004;108:213–20.
19. Wolff A, Vanduynhoven E, van Kleef M, Huygen F, Pope JE, Mekhail N. Phantom pain. Pain Pract. 2011;11:403–13.

Part VII

Painful Disease States: Chronic Visceral Pain

Abdominal Pain

29

Leonardo Kapural and Jianguo Cheng

L. Kapural, MD, PhD (✉)
Carolinas Pain Institute, Winston-Salem, NC, USA

Wake Forest University, School of Medicine, Winston-Salem, NC, USA
e-mail: LKaural@ccrpain.com

J. Cheng, MD, PhD
Departments of Pain Management and Neurosciences, Cleveland Clinic Anesthesiology Institute and Lerner Research Institute, Cleveland, OH, USA

Key Concepts

- Approximately two million Americans suffer from severe abdominal pain, which is the most prevalent symptom in any gastrointestinal specialty clinic. The etiology of chronic abdominal pain often remains elusive despite a multitude of imaging studies, and surgical procedures may have been conducted before a patient is referred to a pain specialist.
- Chronic abdominal pain has a negative impact on the patient's socioeconomic status, frequently produces strong affective responses, and is a major burden on the healthcare system.
- General characteristics of abdominal pain include a diffuse pain that may be difficult to localize, a referral/transferal pain to the somatic structures, the presence of enhanced autonomic and/or motor reflexes, and hyperalgesia in the cutaneous and deep tissues. Manifestations of visceral hyperalgesia in chronic abdominal pain may include a viscero-visceral convergence, viscerosomatic convergence, referred visceral hyperalgesia/allodynia, referred cutaneous hyperalgesia/allodynia, or referred muscle hyperalgesia/allodynia.
- Location of the pain may suggest the source of abdominal pathology. Pain in the upper abdominal/epigastric area may be caused by biliary or pancreatic sources or ulcer or dyspepsia. Pain in the mid-abdominal area is suggestive of Crohn's disease, celiac disease, partial intermittent SBO, and/or chronic mesenteric ischemia. Pain in the lower abdomen is often associated with irritable bowel syndrome (IBS) or colitis.
- Several studies have demonstrated a decrease in analgesic intake and pain scores after sympathetic blocks (celiac, splanchnic nerve blocks). These therapies should be considered as parts of a multimodal analgesic strategy.
- Animal studies suggest that spinal cord stimulation suppresses visceral hyperalgesia. Large case series of spinal cord stimulation demonstrated a significant pain relief in patients with various causes of chronic abdominal pain. Given the limitations of conservative and surgical treatments for chronic visceral pain,

J. Cheng, R.W. Rosenquist (eds.), *Fundamentals of Pain Medicine*,
https://doi.org/10.1007/978-3-319-64922-1_29

spinal cord stimulation may be a very useful therapeutic option.

Prevalence and Etiology

The overall prevalence of general, but not specific, chronic abdominal pain is 22.9 per 1000 individual-years. It is one of the most frequent pain complaints with about 25% of adults having it at least one time in their life. Prevalence of abdominal pain does not differ with age, ethnicity, or geographic regions. However, women are more likely to report abdominal pain than men. While inflammatory bowel disease (IBD) is thought to be a disease of adolescents and young adults with a peak incidence from 15 to 35 years of age, a second smaller peak is seen between the ages of 50 and 60. The number of pediatric IBD cases is increasing with more patients being diagnosed with Crohn's disease. Risk factors for persistent abdominal pain include preexisting psychiatric illness, female gender, smoking, and longer duration of disease. Despite clinical remission of IBD, continued use of opioids is seen in about 20% of patients.

Chronic pancreatitis is another frequent cause of chronic abdominal pain. Its incidence is on the rise worldwide, possibly due to increased consumption of alcohol and application of better diagnostic modalities, among other causes. Chronic or intermittent pain is present in about 80–90% of patients.

Postsurgical adhesions may cause chronic abdominal pain in as high as 45–90% of patients. Risk factors of developing adhesions include open procedures, use of various implants (i.e., mesh), and presence of a contaminated surgical field (i.e., gallbladder/bowel contamination). The most common surgical procedures linked to chronic abdominal pain include cholecystectomy, herniorrhaphy, and adhesiolysis. Preexisting psychiatric illness, female gender, and younger age are additional risk factors of developing chronic abdominal pain.

Chronic abdominal wall pain (CAWP) is pain of more than 1 month with fixed location of tenderness of less than 2.5 cm of diameter. About 10–30% of the patients with chronic abdominal pain may have CAWP. The most common cause of abdominal wall pain is the entrapment of the cutaneous abdominal nerve branches (ACNES) as a result of direct surgical trauma or anatomical variations. CAWP is frequently present in association with chronic visceral diseases. In addition to visceral pain and somatic abdominal wall pain, central pain, generated in the spinal cord and/or brain, may also play an important role in this population.

Mechanisms of Chronic Abdominal Pain

Chronic abdominal pain is a complex process involving physical, emotional, and perceptual integration that may no longer play adaptive and protective roles. Hyperalgesia and allodynia may result from maladaptive neuroplastic changes, namely, peripheral and central sensitization, as described in Chap. 4. Nociceptive pain may result from localized inflammation in some abdominal chronic pain syndromes. For example, the degree of inflammation correlates with the severity of the pain in human as well as in animal models of chronic pancreatitis. There are, however, chronic abdominal pain syndromes, where no significant gross tissue injury or structural disease is clinically evident. The presence of visceral hypersensitivity via central and peripheral mechanisms and lack of structural changes are hallmarks of dysmotility disorders such as irritable bowel syndrome (IBS).

Gastrointestinal inflammation has been associated with the development of acute and chronic pain in such diseases as inflammatory bowel disease, celiac disease, and acute infectious gastroenteritis. Intestinal inflammation may cause increased expression of transient receptor potential vanilloid type 1 (TRPV-1) that is also overexpressed in other non-visceral chronic pain syndromes. Importantly, the neuropathic pain component may predominate in some chronic abdominal pain syndromes, such as chronic pancreatitis, possibly mediated through direct changes in nociceptors innervating the pancreas.

Visceral hyperalgesic responses in chronic pancreatitis may perpetuate persistent neuropathic pain.

Clinical Presentations

Clinical presentations vary, depending on the etiology. For example, patients with chronic pancreatitis often complain of epigastric pain that radiates to the back and increases after fatty food ingestion. It is often described as boring, deep, sharp, and penetrating and may be associated with nausea and vomiting. In advanced chronic pancreatitis, steatorrhea may occur when pancreatic lipase secretion is significantly reduced; endocrine insufficiency may result in diabetes mellitus in up to 80% of the patients with chronic pancreatitis. Other signs and symptoms include jaundice, joint pain, abdominal distension, shortness of breath, pleural effusions, pancreatic ascites, significant weight loss, an abdominal mass, and blood in the stool.

Inspection of the abdomen may provide a first clue on possible chronic pain source. For example, surgical scars from previous laparotomies might be present. When associated with localized allodynia and/or hyperalgesia, one should consider possible nerve damage and/or neuroma. CAWP is best diagnosed based on patient's history and physical examination. The pain is usually well localized with point tenderness on palpation. On the contrary, visceral pain is usually poorly localized. Carnett's test is a useful physical examination for abdominal wall pain. In supine position with the knees and hips slightly flexed to decrease abdominal wall tension, the patient is asked to tighten his abdominal muscles by lifting the head and shoulders off the bed. A positive Carnett's test is increased pain on palpation as the patient contracts the abdominal muscles. Positive response to trigger point injections or nerve blocks may confirm the diagnosis and is considered one of most cost-effective procedures in gastroenterology. Limitations to this approach are the high placebo responses to injections especially in chronic pain patients with visceral abdominal disease involving the peritoneum, leading to false-positive Carnett's.

Psychosocial assessment is an essential component of the diagnostic process. Psychometric tests such as depression inventories are useful tools. In addition to history and physical examinations, many physicians suggest ordering additional tests on the basis of objective findings rather than pain severity. Diagnostic procedures are often required to establish appropriate diagnosis.

Diagnosis

Careful history and physical examinations help guide diagnostic testing. Excluding correctable organic diseases is essential, but many times repetitive diagnostic testing is unnecessary to confirm a functional disorder. In general, nerve blocks may be of diagnostic, therapeutic, or even prognostic value. Initial nerve blocks in chronic abdominal pain are often done for diagnostic purposes. The cause of abdominal pain often remains elusive in a significant group of patients despite extensive work-ups to determine the source of the abdominal pain. In such cases, various nerve blocks may have both diagnostic and therapeutic values. There are two types of blocks that are commonly performed for abdominal pain. Sympathetic nerve blocks are used to block the splanchnic nerves, celiac plexus, superior hypogastric nerve plexus, or ganglion impar. Somatic nerve blocks include paravertebral nerve block, intercostal nerve block, transversus abdominis plane (TAP) block, rectus abdominis sheath block, and blocks of the ilioinguinal, iliohypogastric, and genitofemoral nerves. These blocks may help determine visceral vs. somatic pain and guide treatments.

Differential retrograde epidural block (DREB) may be used to help differentiate visceral from non-visceral sources of pain. Studies of case series suggest that responses to DREB may be a useful predictor of treatment responses. The diagnostic value of DREB relies on the sensitivity of various nerve fibers to local anesthetics. Sympathetic fibers and visceral afferent nerves have a higher C to Aδ fiber ratio (10:1) and are more sensitive to local anesthetic blockade than the somatic nociceptive fibers. DREB involves placement of an epidural catheter under fluoroscopy and injection of saline twice (placebo), followed by incremental doses of a local anesthetic under close monitoring of vital signs and frequent neurological examinations. A local anesthetic (usually 2% 3-chloroprocaine or 1% lidocaine 10–30 cc) serves to differentiate between predominantly visceral, somatosensory, and central chronic pain, while the saline injections may help differentiate placebo effects, malingering, and sometimes psychogenic source of pain. However, the validity of DREB remains to be established. Accurate interpretation can be difficult due to the facts that there is a significant overlap between visceral and somatic nociceptive nerves, that visceral pain may coexist with somatic abdominal pain, and that central sensitization may be a significant component of abdominal pain. In addition, contributions from the vagal nerves to abdominal pain cannot be determined by DREB. Furthermore, the sensitivity and specificity of DREB are relatively low. Thus, responses to DREB combined with other clinical information are only suggestive of visceral, somatic, or central source of pain.

TAP block is a newer diagnostic and therapeutic technique for somatic abdominal pain. TAP provides analgesia to the entire anterolateral abdominal wall between the costal margin and the inguinal ligament. Ultrasound guidance for TAP block allows for precise installation of local anesthetics around the anterior branches of the thoracolumbar ventral rami to block most of the anterior abdominal wall. The initial posterior ultrasound-guided approach to TAP block allows visualization of three muscular layers of the lateral abdominal wall, namely, the external oblique, the internal oblique, and the transverse abdominis muscles. The needle is placed between the internal oblique muscle and the transverse abdominis muscles, and a local anesthetic is injected within this wide plane. Although the value of TAP block in determining abdominal wall pain is still debatable, it is believed that TAP block as a single injection or continuous infusion through a catheter can be used to treat various abdominal wall pain syndromes.

Treatment Options

Management of chronic abdominal pain exemplifies the multidisciplinary nature of the pain medicine. Processes of evaluating and treating abdominal pain frequently cross the traditional specialty boundaries. Due to a lack of large-scale clinical trials and investigations, the current decision-making algorithms are based on case reports, case series, and larger retrospective and prospective studies.

Conservative Treatment

Managing the pain, rather than curing disease, is often the objective. Lifestyle changes such as abstinence from alcohol, smoking cessation, nutritional consultation, and regular physical exercise are among the first steps. Acetaminophen is often the first choice of pharmacological management. The use of nonsteroidal anti-inflammatory drugs (NSAIDs) may be justified against the possibility of causing side effects such as dyspepsia, gastric ulcerations, and even renal toxicity. Membrane stabilizers and antidepressants for chronic pain are used predominantly for neuropathic pain but can also be used for chronic abdominal pain. Tricyclic antidepressants, SSRI and SNRI are frequently prescribed. Calcium channel blockers such as pregabalin or gabapentin may be effective in some patients and may provide an opioid-sparing effect. Ketamine, in various doses, has been used for chronic pain. S-ketamine infusion in patients with chronic pancreatitis may reduce hyperalgesia in the short-term and decrease opioid consumption.

Short-acting opioids may be used in short duration for severe breakthrough pain. The use of chronic opioid therapy should be minimized given the known detrimental consequences of opioid tolerance, dependence, opioid-induced hyperalgesia, overdose, abuse, addiction, and deaths. In a subset of properly selected patients, it may be appropriate to use a combination of a short-acting and a long-acting opioid to treat persistent severe abdominal pain as long as the treatment provides improved functions and better pain control without causing significant adverse effects. The common side effects, such as nausea, vomiting, and constipation, can be controlled with low doses of centrally acting antiemetics or laxatives, respectively.

Psychological Interventions

Psychological treatments should be considered in patients with persistent chronic abdominal pain. Biofeedback is the process of gaining greater awareness of many physiological functions primarily using instruments that provide information on the activity of those same systems, with a goal of being able to control them at will. Some of the processes that can be controlled include brainwaves, muscle tone, skin conductance, heart rate, and pain perception. Studies on biofeedback for chronic pain control have been promising, but current clinical evidence is limited for chronic abdominal pain. Thermal biofeedback seems to be an effective tool for patients with chronic abdominal pain. EMG biofeedback appears to be useful in reducing constipation and pain. Patients with IBS may respond to relaxation training with progressive muscle relaxation, thermal biofeedback, cognitive therapy, and education.

Analgesic hypnosis induces relaxed states of focused attention and inner absorption, with a relative suspension of peripheral awareness, and is combined with suggestions for pain control. Hypnotherapy has been used for the treatment of chronic pain from IBS. Studies documented reduction of IBS symptoms, improvement in quality of life, and changing pain perception threshold. Cognitive behavior therapy (CBT) includes various behavioral (e.g., relaxation, coping skills training) and cognitive approaches to reducing chronic pain. Multidisciplinary chronic pain rehabilitation programs may provide both short-term and long-term benefits improving chronic abdominal pain. Such programs typically provide comprehensive patient education, physical therapy, occupational therapy, medication management, individual psychotherapy, group therapy, cognitive therapy, thermal biofeedback, weaning of opioids and habituating substances, substance use education, and progressive muscle relaxation.

Nerve Blocks, Ablation, and Neuromodulation Procedures

These interventional approaches aim at interrupting or modulating neural/pain conduction and/or transmission. Historically, the splanchnic nerves, mainly the greater and lesser, and the celiac plexus were considered as targets for visceral pain control. Sympathetic innervation of the abdominal organs consists of preganglionic fibers of T5 to T12 that merge with the ventral ramus. Together with communicating rami, these fibers course in the direction of the sympathetic chain and then make synaptic contacts with postganglionic neurons at the celiac, aortorenal, and superior mesenteric ganglion. Splanchnic nerves confluence with the vagal preganglionic parasympathetic fibers, sensory fibers of the phrenic nerve, and postganglionic sympathetic fibers to form celiac plexus which is widely spread around the abdominal aorta, especially anteriorly. In contrast, the splanchnic nerves are localized in a relatively narrow space between the lateral border of the vertebra and pleura. Splanchnic and celiac plexus blocks are commonly performed percutaneously under fluoroscopic guidance. Celiac plexus blocks may be performed through a transaortic, retrocrural, or transdiscal approach without clear advantage of using one over another. Classical description of celiac plexus block involves placement of the needle through the paraspinal area of the middle back (L1 vertebral body). Bilateral splanchnic block is performed at T11 to deliver local anesthetic/steroid combination to the paravertebral compartment medial to the pleural cavity and in close proximity to the greater and lesser splanchnic nerves (posterior third of T11 vertebral body) (Fig. 29.1).

Splanchnic nerve blocks may be followed by radiofrequency ablation (RFA) (Fig. 29.2) for

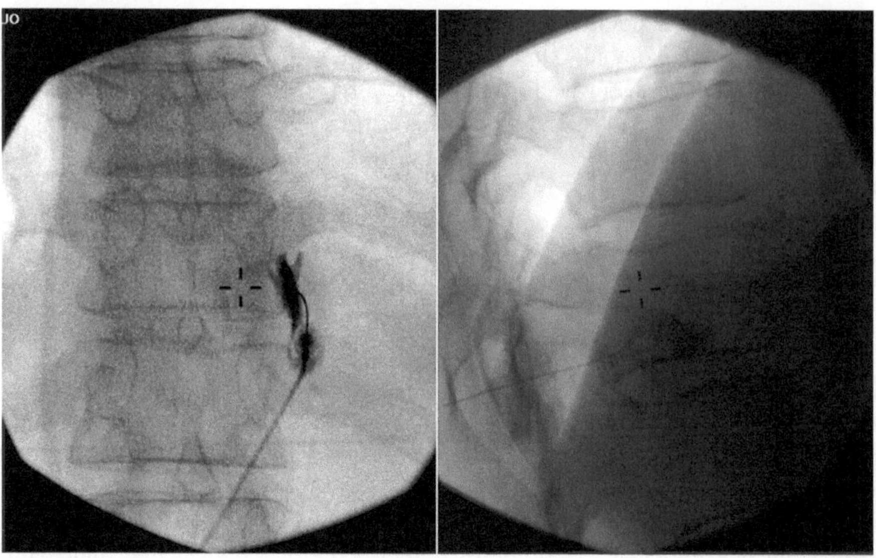

Fig. 29.1 Splanchnic nerve block. Needle placement and contrast spread in anteroposterior (**a**) and lateral (**b**) views. Notice that the needle is kept in contact with the lower one-third of the T11 vertebral body

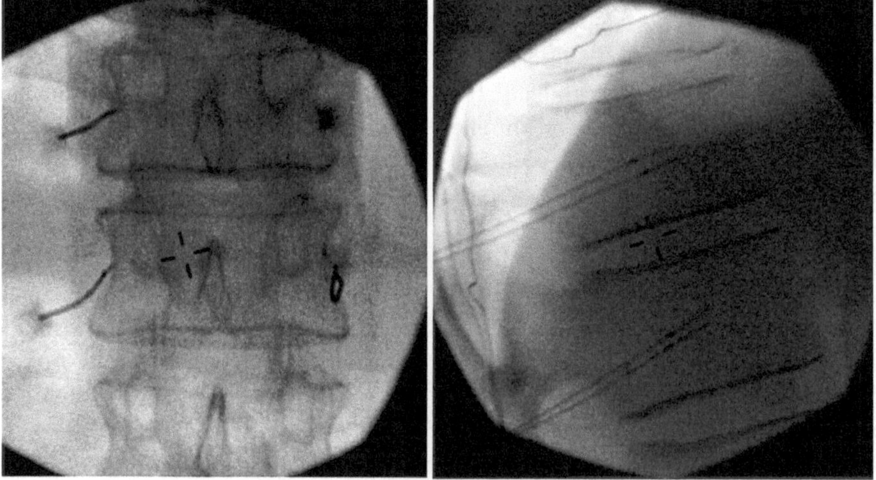

Fig. 29.2 Properly positioned radiofrequency (RF) electrodes at T11 and T12 for splanchnic nerve denervation in anteroposterior and lateral views

prolonged pain relief. The predictable nerve location and a low frequency of serious complications compared to chemical neurolytics are among the advantages of splanchnic RFA. Several case series showed significant improvements in pain scores and reduction of opioid consumption and frequency of hospitalization. Improved pain relief lasted for a mean duration of 45 weeks. Patients with previous positive responses may have repeated denervations with comparable therapeutic effects. Return of abdominal pain may be a result of nerve regeneration. Complications may include pneumothorax, post-procedural neuritis, hypotension, or diarrhea. An alternative approach, through thoracoscopic splanchnicectomy, provided continuous pain relief in only about 25% of the patients at 6-month follow-up. This approach is largely abandoned in light of the low success rate, an extensive dissection of the parietal pleura, and risks of anesthesia with a double-lumen endotracheal tube.

The use of spinal cord stimulation (SCS) to treat chronic abdominal pain in the last10 years has gained support from a few large case series, which provided evidence that SCS is an effective long-term solution for some selected patients. Included in these studies were patients with visceral hyperalgesia caused by dysmotility disorders such as gastroparesis, postsurgical visceral adhesions, and chronic pancreatitis. In the first case series, 30 out of 35 patients (86%) achieved more than 50% pain relief and were advanced to SCS implant. The recipients maintained similar level of pain relief at 1-year follow-up. This study was followed by a comprehensive survey of 76 case reports. Both studies confirmed that the tip of the standard octrode lead is mostly placed near the top of the fifth thoracic vertebral body in the posterior epidural space (Figs. 29.3 and 29.4). Pain relief exceeded 50% in most of the patients, and long-term opioid use decreased by more than two-thirds. The latest case series reported improvements of pain scores in 24 consecutive patients with chronic pancreatitis. At 1-year follow-up, the VAS pain scores and opioid consumption were both significantly reduced. Rare complications of SCS include wound infection and lead migration.

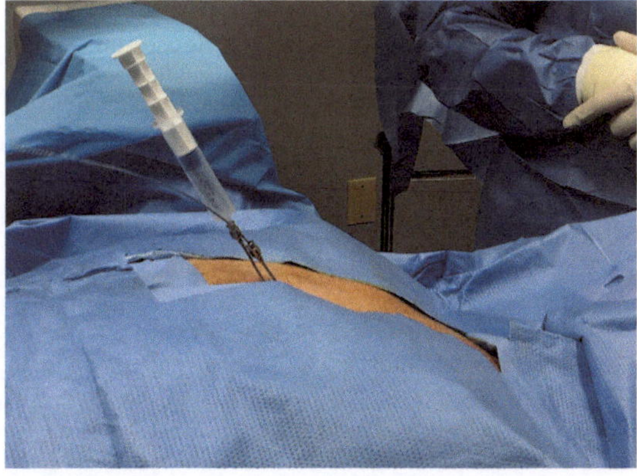

Fig. 29.3 Thoracic placement of the spinal cord stimulation electrodes. Loss of resistance technique in conjunction with lateral fluoroscopy is used

Surgical Interventions

Surgery for chronic abdominal pain relief was mainly studied in chronic pancreatitis to provide pancreatic duct decompression with or without resection. Lateral pancreaticojejunostomy, a Partington-Rochelle modification of the Puestow procedure, is performed to provide persistent ductal drainage. Other ductal drainage procedures are the Frey and DuVal procedures. The Frey procedure includes incomplete resection of the pancreatic head in conjunction with a later longitudinal drainage of the duct as is done in the Puestow procedure. The DuVal procedure includes a short distal pancreatectomy with drainage of the duct into a Roux jejunal limb for ductal decompression. More extensive resections occur in distal or subtotal pancreatectomy, Whipple, Beger, and Berne procedures. Total pancreatectomy is considered the most drastic form of resection and is indicated in some patients with chronic abdominal pain due to chronic pancreatitis. Recent studies suggest that preoperative opioid use is a negative predictor of long-term pain relief after either surgical or endoscopic interventions. It could be a result of central sensitization or opioid dependency. Earlier surgical interventions likely provide better pain relief compared to endoscopic interventions with similar complication rates.

Conclusions

Chronic abdominal pain is a complex clinical problem that requires understanding the physical and psychosocial features of chronic abdominal pain and providing treatment options tailored to the needs of patients. An integrated biopsychosocial treatment strategy may produce better clinical outcomes. When establishing a pharmacological treatment plan, non-opioid drugs should be considered. Membrane stabilizers and antidepressants for pain such as calcium channel blocking agents and norepinephrine reuptake inhibitors seem to be effective in some patients. Although celiac and splanchnic nerve blocks are in the armamentarium, radiofrequency

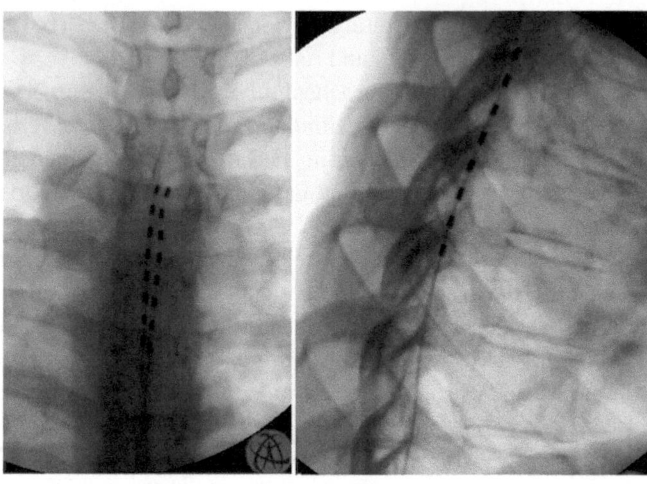

Fig. 29.4 Lateral and anteroposterior views of two epidural electrodes positioned in the midline and at the top of the T5 vertebral body

denervation of the splanchnic nerves deserves further investigation in the form of randomized controlled trials to determine its efficacy and safety for long-term pain relief. Spinal cord stimulation has shown promise as an effective and minimally invasive therapy. Comparative studies between surgery and endoscopic treatment show evidence in favor of early surgery.

Suggested Reading

1. Ahmed Ali U, Nieuwenhuijs VB, van Eijck CH, et al. Clinical outcome in relation to timing of surgery in chronic pancreatitis: a nomogram to predict pain relief. Arch Surg. 2012;147:925–32.
2. Azpiroz F, Bouin M, Camilleri M, et al. Mechanisms of hypersensitivity in IBS and functional disorders. Neurogastroenterol Motil. 2007;19(1 Suppl):62–88.
3. Bassotti G, Chistolini F, Sietchiping-Nzepa F, De Roberto G, Morelli A, Chiarioni G. Biofeedback for pelvic floor dysfunction in constipation. Br Med J. 2004;328(7436):393–6.
4. Bouwense SA, Buscher HC, van Goor H, Wilder-Smith OH. S-ketamine modulates hyperalgesia in patients with chronic pancreatitis pain. Reg Anesth Pain Med. 2011;36:303–7.
5. Cahen DL, Gouma DJ, Nio Y, et al. Endoscopic versus surgical drainage of the pancreatic duct in chronic pancreatitis. New Engl J Med. 2007;356:676–84.
6. Calkins BM, Mendeloff AI. Epidemiology of inflammatory bowel disease. Epidemiol Rev. 1986;8:60–91.
7. Calkins BM, Lilienfeld AM, Garland CF, Mendeloff AI. Trends in incidence rates of ulcerative colitis and Crohn's disease. Dig Dis Sci. 1984;29(10):913–20.
8. Carnett JB. Intercostal neuralgia as a cause of abdominal pain and tenderness. Surg Gynecol Obstet. 1926;42:625–32.
9. Coulter ID, Favreau JT, Hardy ML, Morton SC, Roth EA, Shekelle P. Biofeedback interventions for gastrointestinal conditions: a systematic review. Altern Ther Health Med. 2002;8(3):76–83.
10. Dite P, Ruzicka M, Zboril V, Novotny I. A prospective, randomized trial comparing endoscopic and surgical therapy for chronic pancreatitis. Endoscopy. 2003;35:553–8.
11. Drossman DA, Toner BB, Whitehead WE. Cognitive-behavioral therapy versus education and desipramine versus placebo for moderate to severe functional disorders. Gastroentrology. 2003;125:19–31.
12. Heading RC. Prevalence of upper gastrointestinal symptoms in the general population: a systematic review. Scand J Gastroenterol Suppl. 1999;231:3–8.
13. Jones RC 3rd, Xu L, Gebhart GF. The mechanosensitivity of mouse colon afferent fibers and their sensitization by inflammatory mediators require transient receptor potential vanilloid 1 and acid-sensing ion channel 3. J Neurosci. 2005;25(47):10981–9.
14. Kapural L, Nagem H, Tlucek H, Sessler DI. Spinal cord stimulation for chronic visceral abdominal pain. Pain Med. 2010a;11:347–55.
15. Kapural L, Deer T, Yakovlev A, et al. Technical aspects of spinal cord stimulation for managing chronic visceral abdominal pain: the results from the national survey. Pain Med. 2010b;11:685–91.
16. Kapural L, Cywinski JB, Sparks DA. Spinal cord stimulation for visceral pain from chronic pancreatitis. Neuromodulation. 2011;14:423–6.
17. Lindsetmo R, Stulberg J. Chronic abdominal wall pain—a diagnostic challenge for the surgeon. Am J Surg. 2009;198:129–34.
18. Narouze S. Chronic Abdominal Wall pain: diagnosis and interventional treatment. In: Kapural L, editor. Chronic abdominal pain: an evidence-based,

comprehensive guide to clinical management. New York: Springer; 2015. p. 189–95.
19. Olesen SS, Bouwense SA, Wilder-Smith OH, van Goor H, Drewes AM. Pregabalin reduces pain in patients with chronic pancreatitis in a randomized, controlled trial. Gastroenterology. 2011a;141:536–43.
20. Olesen SS, Graversen C, Olesen AE, et al. Randomised clinical trial: pregabalin attenuates experimental visceral pain through sub-cortical mechanisms in patients with painful chronic pancreatitis. Aliment Pharmacol Ther. 2011b;34:878–87.
21. Palsson OS, Whitehead WE. Psychological treatments in functional gastrointestinal disorders: a primer for the gastroenterologist. Clin Gastroenterol Hepatol. 2013;11(3):208–16.
22. Pasricha PJ. Unraveling the mystery of pain in chronic pancreatitis. Nat Rev Gastroenterol Hepatol. 2012;9:140–51.
23. Puylaert M, Kapural L, van Zundert J, Peek D, Lataster A, Mekhail N, van Kleef M, Keulemans Y. Pain in chronic pancreatitis (chapter 26). In: van Zundert J, Patjin J, Hartrick C, Lataster A, Huygen F, Mekhail N, van Kleff M, editors. Evidence-based interventional pain practice: according to clinical diagnoses. Oxford: Wiley; 2012. p. 202–12.
24. Raj PP, Sahinder B, Lowe M. Radiofrequency lesioning of splanchnic nerves. Pain Pract. 2002;2:241–7.
25. Rathmell JP, Gallant JM, Brown DL. Computed tomography and the anatomy of celiac plexus block. Reg Anesth Pain Med. 2000;25:411–6.
26. Rizk MK, Tolba R, Kapural L, Mitchell J, Lopez R, Mahboobi R, Vrooman B, Mekhail N. Differential epidural block predicts the success of visceral block in patients with chronic visceral abdominal pain. Pain Pract. 2012;12:595–601.
27. Sandler RS, Stewart WF, Liberman JN, Ricci JA, Zorich NL. Abdominal pain, bloating, and diarrhea in the united states: prevalence and impact. Dig Dis Sci. 2000;45(6):1166–71.
28. Tea S. Resection vs drainage in treatment of chronic pancreatitis: long-term results of a randomized trial. Gastroenterol. 2008;134:1406–11.

30 Urogenital and Pelvic Pain

Mercy A. Udoji and Timothy J. Ness

Key Concepts

- Urogenital and pelvic pains may have multiple etiologies including urologic, gastrointestinal, vascular, musculoskeletal, or neurologic origins.
- The prevalence of urogenital and pelvic pain is significantly higher in women than in men, and it is often accompanied by urinary or sexual symptoms.
- In the evaluation and treatment of these pains, it must be kept in mind that these sites of pain generation are private places that are associated with bodily functions with strong emotions: sexual function, defecation, and urination.
- After infection, ischemia, inflammation, obstruction, or neoplasm has been ruled out as likely etiologies, one is often left with simply a descriptive diagnosis coupled to an empiric treatment.
- Diagnosis is made based on thorough history and physical exam with emphasis on multiple organ systems (gynecologic, musculoskeletal, etc.) as well as a sexual and psychosocial history.
- A multimodal approach for treatment is often utilized for optimal pain management. Medications such as antidepressants, anticonvulsants, topical creams, and opiates can aid in symptom control. There is evidence supporting complementary and alternative approaches including yoga, physical therapy, biofeedback, and dietary therapy.
- Interventional options range from nerve blocks, peripheral nerve, and spinal cord stimulation to surgery.

Epidemiology

Urogenital and pelvic pain is defined as pain originating in the pelvis or lower abdominal organs. These pains may be further described as acute or chronic depending on presentation. Acute urogenital and pelvic pain may be due to infectious and inflammatory pain states (such as pelvic inflammatory disease, sexually transmitted disease, or infectious cystitis) as well as cancer, trauma, or injury to external genitalia. Chronic urogenital and pelvic pain is pain in the aforementioned area that has been present for at least 3 months duration. When these pains don't have a clear etiology and other more common diagnoses have been ruled out, patients are given a diagnosis of chronic pelvic pain (CPP) (females) or prostatodynia/chronic prostatitis (males).

M.A. Udoji, MD • T.J. Ness, MD, PhD (✉)
Department of Anesthesiology and Perioperative Medicine, University of Alabama at Birmingham, BMR2-210, 901 19th Street S, Birmingham, AL 35205, USA
e-mail: mudoji@uab.edu; tness@uabmc.edu

J. Cheng, R.W. Rosenquist (eds.), *Fundamentals of Pain Medicine*,
https://doi.org/10.1007/978-3-319-64922-1_30

Overall, chronic urogenital and pelvic pain is three to four times more prevalent in women, and its incidence does not vary significantly among various age groups. In some populations, this disease is as common as asthma or chronic low back pain and carries an estimated annual cost of greater than 800 million dollars to the US health system. This cost grows exponentially when absenteeism and decreased work productivity are taken into consideration. In addition, the emotional toll on patients and providers alike is high as both parties often become frustrated at the lack of a definitive diagnosis, treatment progress, medical cost coverage, or loss of symptom control that is common in the management of this disorder.

Pathophysiology

Numerous structures within the pelvis may be responsible for chronic urogenital and pelvic pain. Diagnosis is further confounded by the complex innervation of the pelvis, as well as the fact that patients often present with dyspareunia and urinary symptoms. Pain in this area of the body can be inflammatory, neuropathic, sympathetic, somatic, or visceral in nature. Additionally, the gastrointestinal (irritable bowel syndrome, Crohn's disease), neurologic (neuropathy, lumbar disc herniation), gynecologic (pelvic inflammatory disease, pelvic congestion syndrome), urologic (prostatitis, urethritis), and musculoskeletal systems (myofascial pain syndrome, abdominal wall pain) may all play a role in pain generation (Table 30.1).

Regarding etiology, there is no universally agreed upon cause of chronic urogenital and pelvic pain. The most widely discussed theories are that chronic urogenital and pelvic pain may be caused by a vascular phenomenon or may be a subtype of complex regional pain syndrome (CRPS). Other considerations include the possibility of coexisting pain syndromes that serve to enhance organ sensitivity to stimuli via cross-sensitization, leading to viscerosomatic or viscero-visceral hyperalgesia.

Clinical Features and Diagnosis

Patient presentation and symptomatology vary and often involve more than one organ system. As such, a comprehensive and chronological history and physical exam (including thorough neurological exam and psychosocial assessment) are essential for accurate diagnosis as well as to establish rapport with the patient. While there is increased incidence of depression, anxiety, and a history of physical or sexual abuse in patients with chronic urogenital and pelvic pain, it is important to understand that there is *not* a proven cause and effect relationship. Additionally, the practitioner must bear in mind that the sites of exam are private and associated with bodily functions (i.e., sexual function, defecation, urination) that elicit strong emotions in patients.

The patient should be asked about onset of pain, its location, associated symptoms, exacerbating or remitting factors, whether the pain is cyclic or present at all times, dyspareunia, increase in symptoms with valsalva maneuvers, history of abdominal surgeries, and other pertinent information as guided by their presenting symptoms (Table 30.2). The physical exam should be conducted in as gentle a manner as possible, recognizing that it is often a painful experience for the patient. A methodical approach to the physical examination is recommended in an attempt to duplicate the pain either by palpation or by positioning. One way to approach this often challenging task is to divide the exam by systems (i.e., neurologic, gynecologic, and gastrointestinal) or by postural components (i.e., standing, sitting, supine, and lithotomy). In addition to a thorough history and physical exam, careful utilization of laboratory and imaging studies to aid diagnosis may include modalities such as ultrasonography, magnetic resonance imaging (MRI), urodynamic testing, urethral cultures, and CA-125. In some cases, surgery (e.g., diagnostic laparoscopy) is necessary for a proper diagnosis as well as to relieve pain.

Table 30.1 Sources of urogenital and pelvic pain

I. **Acute recurrent**
Infectious-inflammatory pain states
Sexually transmitted diseases
Urethritis, epididymitis, prostatitis, genital herpes
Pelvic inflammatory disease
Salpingo-oophoritis-tuberculous salpingitis
Posterior parametritis
Infectious cystitis (bacterial, viral, fungal)
Radiation-induced cystitis
Chemical cystitis
Acute herpes zoster
Urethral caruncle
Secondary to cancer
Kidney, urinary bladder
Prostate, testicular
Ovarian, cervical-uterine, vaginal
Lymphoma
Spinal involvement of metastases
Other metastatic including carcinomatosis
Obstructive – hydronephrosis – urinary bladder distension
Kidney stones – ureteropelvic junction obstruction
Injury of external genitalia
Labor – delivery – postpartum trauma
II. **Chronic**
Urologic
Interstitial cystitis
Polycystic kidney
Loin pain hematuria
Stag horn calculus
Urethral syndrome
Urethral diverticulum or caruncle
Detrusor dyssynergia
Female reproductive (gynecological) pain
Cyclic
Mittelschmerz – other ovarian pain
Primary dysmenorrhea
Secondary dysmenorrhea
Endometriosis
Noncyclic or atypical cyclic
Adhesions
Endometriosis
Pelvic relaxation prolapse
Retroversion of the uterus
Vulvodynia
Ovarian remnant syndrome

(continued)

Table 30.1 (continued)

Dyspareunia without vulvodynia
Pelvic congestion syndrome
Adenomyosis – fibroids
Chronic pelvic pain without obvious pathology
Male reproductive
Orchalgia
Prostatodynia
Penile pain
Neurologic origin
Herniated nucleus pulposus (sacral radiculopathy)
Tarlov cysts
Postherpetic neuralgia
Peripheral neuropathy
Migraine variant
Central pain – poststroke or postspinal cord injury
Postsurgical neuroma – painful scar
Neuralgias/entrapment (i.e., iliohypogastric, ilioinguinal, genitofemoral, pudendal)
Guillain-Barre syndrome
Neurofibromatosis
Gastrointestinal origin
Radiation enterocolitis
Crohn's disease/ulcerative colitis
Other colitis/ulcerations
Diverticular disease of the colon
Irritable bowel syndrome
Chronic constipation – fecal impaction
Proctalgia fugax
Infectious diarrhea
Hernia – recurrent small bowel obstruction
Musculoskeletal origin
Thoracic, lumbar, and sacral spinal disease
Pelvic floor or abdominal muscular spasm
Sacroiliitis
Coccydynia
Fibromyalgia
Other pain states
Chronic pelvic organ ischemia
Acute intermittent porphyria
Familial Mediterranean fever
Systemic lupus erythematosus
Psychogenic pain

Table 30.2 Important questions for history taking in patients with urogenital and pelvic pain

1.	Location of pain
2.	Quality of pain
3.	Pain score (using VAS, VNS, or other similar scale) at rest? With activity?
4.	Pain associated with menstrual periods? Pain worsens with menses or just before menses?
5.	Pattern of pain? Cyclic? Waxes and wanes in intensity?
6.	When did pain begin? Is it getting better or worse?
7.	Things that make the pain better? Things that make the pain worse?
8.	Do you have pain with intercourse? Urination? Bowel movement?
9.	Obstetric history?
10.	History of sexually transmitted disease?
11.	Previous abdominal or pelvic surgeries?
12.	History of psychological diagnosis (including abuse)?

Treatment

There are few monotherapies with proven clinical efficacy for this disorder, mandating a multidisciplinary, multimodal approach to management (Table 30.3). Unfortunately, the diagnosis assigned to this painful condition has often depended on the initial specialist who evaluated the patient and not on the underlying pathophysiology. In general, if the underlying cause of pain is defined, then treatment is focused on that particular etiology; otherwise, a more empiric approach is taken. The UPOINT system is a phenotypic approach to therapy consisting of six components: urinary, psychosocial, organ-specific, infection, neurologic/systemic, and muscle tenderness. This system was originally designed for male urogenital pain; however, it has been extended and modified to include urogenital and pelvic pain in females as well. Physicians utilizing the UPOINT system first classify or assign patients to a specific phenotype based on clinical symptoms and presentation; this phenotypic characteristic is then used to guide therapy.

A trial of oral medication is the most common first step in management. Drugs from multiple

Table 30.3 Therapies for urogenital and pelvic pain

I. *Cancer-related pain*
A. Analgesics and side effect management1
1. Around-the-clock opioids (sustained release)*
2. Breakthough opioids (all others except mixed agonist-antagonists)*
3. Neuraxial opioids, local anesthetics, and/or clonidine (epidural, intrathecal)*
4. Anti-inflammatories (COX nonselective, COX2 selective, corticosteroids)**
5. Antiemetics (antidopaminergic, 5HT-3 inhibitors)
6. Adjuvants
(a) Antidepressants (tricyclics, SSRIs, SNRIs)**
(b) Stimulants (methylphenidate, dextroamphetamine)*
(c) Anticonvulsants (gabapentin, carbamazepine, phenytoin, other)**
(d) Antiarrhythmics (mexiletine, transdermal lidocaine)**
B. Curative surgery**
C. Palliative treatments (surgery, radiotherapy, chemotherapy)*
D. Neurolysis (neurolytic presacral plexus – superior hypogastric plexus; other neuroablative interventions)*
E. Stenting procedures for obstruction**
F. Psychological interventions**
II. *Treatment options for nonmalignant pain*
A. Same as for section I above. Those marked with * controversial, those marked with ** encouraged
B. Additional etiological therapies
1. Antioxidants and micronutrients
2. Other dietary changes (particularly in interstitial cystitis)
3. Cysto-/ureteroscopic management (dilation, stents, stone removal)
4. Hormonal modulation (cyclic gynecological pain)
C. Deafferentation/sympathectomy blocks (local anesthetic blockade)
D. Surgical diversion or resection*
E. Intravesical treatments (interstitial cystitis)
1. Hydrodistention (80 cm H_2O × 30 min)
2. Dimethyl sulfoxide
3. Heparin
4. Corticosteroids
5. Bicarbonate
6. Bacillus Calmette-Guerin
F. Antihistamines (e.g., hydroxyzine)
G. Anti-pelvic floor spasm treatments**
1. Medical (e.g., baclofen, tizanidine, clonidine)

(continued)

Table 30.3 (continued)

2. Pelvic floor physical therapy
H. Immunosuppressants (e.g., methotrexate or cyclosporine)
I. Oral pentosan polysulfate (interstitial cystitis)
J. Botulinum toxin injections*
K. Neurostimulation (sacral nerve root, pudendal nerve, spinal cord, TENS)
L. Other radiofrequency procedures (e.g., neuroablative, pulsed)*
M. Biofeedback – behavioral interventions**
N. Complementary and alternative medicine (e.g., acupuncture, phytotherapy, yoga)**

Curative surgery implies a known etiology for the pain that is amenable to surgical resection/repair and not simply resection of painful part
COX cyclooxygenase, *5-HT* serotonin, *SNRIs* serotonin-norepinephrine reuptake inhibitors, *SSRIs* serotonin specific reuptake inhibitors, *TENS* transcutaneous electrical nerve stimulation

classes (i.e., muscle relaxants, NSAIDS, antidepressants, anticonvulsants, opioids) have all been used with varying efficacy. The following is a list of the most commonly used drug classes as well as examples of medications in each class:

- *Nonsteroidal anti-inflammatory drugs (NSAIDS)*: They reduce prostaglandin production throughout the body, but this class of medications carries the risk of stomach ulcers and bleeding problems, especially in the elderly. Suggested treatments include meloxicam 7.5–15 mg daily or ibuprofen 800 mg Q8 hours for short-term management. Celecoxib, a selective COX2 inhibitor (200–400 mg/day), is also an option due to decreased risk of gastrointestinal issues.
- *Oral contraceptives (OCPs)*: OCPs are used to treat female pelvic pain related to ovulation or mittelschmerz and endometriosis. OCPs are often combined with NSAIDS to increase efficacy.
- *Gonadotropin-releasing hormone analogues (GNRH analogues)*: These are used to treat patients with cyclic pain symptoms usually due to endometriosis. Examples include leuprolide and goserelin.
- *Antidepressants*: The most commonly used medications in this class are agents that decrease the reuptake of norepinephrine, serotonin, or both. Duloxetine and amitriptyline are common choices in this class.
- *Anticonvulsants*: These agents are utilized for neuropathic pelvic pain. Gabapentin and pregabalin are common choices, but others such as carbamazepine, lamotrigine, and topiramate have anecdotal support for use.
- *Topical formulation*: Local anesthetics and capsaicin are commonly employed to help manage allodynia and hyperalgesia. Initial application of capsaicin can be very painful and so may need to be preceded by use of local anesthetics.
- *Opioids:* They are used to decrease overall pain levels, irrespective of etiology. Side effects include respiratory depression, constipation, nausea, and vomiting. Opioids also carry a risk of dependence, tolerance, addiction, and possibly hyperalgesia at higher doses. Regimens include combinations of hydrocodone or oxycodone with or without acetaminophen, fentanyl patches, methadone, or extended release formulations of oxymorphone, hydromorphone, morphine, and oxycodone.

Interventional management of chronic pelvic pain should include consideration of the following:

- *Neuromodulation*: Spinal cord stimulation targeting the S2-S4 nerve roots has been well described in this population. Other, less traditional approaches may include lead placement as high as the T6/7 level or as low as the conus medullaris. Peripheral lead placement including percutaneous posterior tibial nerve stimulation and lead placement in the subcutaneous tissues of the lower abdomen have been described.
- *Fluoroscopically guided pain procedures*: This includes epidural injections, pudendal nerve block, genitofemoral nerve block, lumbar sympathetic, ganglion of impar, and

hypogastric plexus blockade. In some patients, radiofrequency thermocoagulation or neurolysis with alcohol or phenol is an option after repeated successful blocks, but normally this modality is reserved for the most severe cases such as those associated with cancer.
- *Other procedures*: Botulinum toxin injections or trigger point injections are used to manage chronic symptoms or to treat acute flares.

Surgical options commonly utilized in this population include:

- Diagnostic laparoscopy
- Lysis of adhesions
- Exploratory laparotomy

Some complementary and alternative medicine (CAM) approaches to consider are:

- Transcutaneous electrical nerve stimulation (TENS) unit
- Acupuncture
- Physical therapy (including pelvic physical therapy where available)
- Biofeedback
- Dietary therapy

Common Causes of Urogenital and Pelvic Pain in Males and Females

Interstitial Cystitis/Bladder Pain Syndrome (IC/BPS)

IC/BPS is one of the most common causes of pelvic pain in both sexes. IC/BPS is likely not a single disease entity but rather a complex of urological complains including pain that may have a common, but as yet undetermined, etiology. IC/BPS has a female-to-male ratio of 10:1, with an estimated prevalence of 2 in 10000 patients, primarily in young to middle-aged females. It is regularly implicated as a reason for continued pelvic pain after hysterectomy. Diagnosis of IC/BPS in the past was based on criteria that mandated the presence of glomerulations or a Hunner's ulcer on cystoscopic examination as well as bladder pain and urinary urgency or frequency. More recent definitions are surely symptom-based. Urodynamic testing and intravesical potassium sensitivity testing have also been used to support the diagnosis. Therapies unique to the management of IC/BPS include oral pentosan polysulfate, hydrodistention (using dimethyl sulfoxide, heparin, steroids, etc.), and immunosuppressive agents. In general, the least invasive therapies are attempted first prior to trial of more invasive treatment modalities. The prognosis of IC/BPS is mildly favorable with reports that up to 50% of patients experience spontaneous remission within 5–7 years.

Endometriosis

Endometriosis is a gynecologic condition whereby endometrial glandular tissue is found in other areas of the body (i.e., ovaries, bladder, and peritoneal cavity). Pain secondary to endometriosis is often cyclic in nature, worsening during the hormonal cycling associated with menstruation. Pathophysiology of endometriosis is unconfirmed but postulated to be retrograde menstruation from the fallopian tubes into the pelvis and adjacent structures leading to implantation of viable endometrial tissue at these sites. The presentation of endometriosis varies and includes urinary urgency, back pain, leg pain, bladder pain, and dyspareunia. The gold standard of diagnosis is visualization and histologic confirmation of endometrial tissue outside the uterus at the time of laparoscopy. Initial therapy of endometriosis is fairly well defined utilizing hormonal therapy with OCPs or GNRH agonists (see above; Table 30.3) as well as surgical excision of endometriomas.

Vulvodynia

Vulvodynia differs from other chronic urogenital and pelvic pains due to the fact that pain is clearly located outside of the pelvis and in the external genitalia. This disorder is more prevalent in women who are in their reproductive years and is characterized by a stinging, burning discomfort in their vulva. Research has identified at least six subgroups of this disorder. In general, therapeutic intervention begins with a cream or ointment containing local anesthetics before progressing to more systemic and invasive treatment options (Table 30.3). For long-term therapy, there is some evidence that surgical excision or pelvic floor muscle training as well as cognitive behavioral therapies are beneficial.

Male Chronic Pelvic Pain Syndrome (mCPPS)

This disease entity is the equivalent of chronic pelvic pain in females, but there appear to be some unique qualities that differentiate it from the female variety. Despite the numerous urogenital structures that are unique to men, the prostate has been assumed to be the organ generating mCPPS. Diagnosis of mCPPS can be aided by the use of the Chronic Prostatitis Symptom Index (CPSI), a nine-point questionnaire that inquires about the patient's quality of life, pain, as well as the presence of urinary symptoms. Patient presentation is characterized by urinary urgency, poor flow, and perineal discomfort. A complete history and physical exam that includes examination of the external genitalia should be completed. For males with chronic urogenital and pelvic pain, a urine culture should be sent to rule out bacterial prostatitis or a urinary tract infection as a reversible etiology of the patient's pain. If the clinical situation warrants, a PSA may also be checked to rule out prostate cancer. There is some thought that alpha blockers play a unique role in managing pain in patients with chronic prostatitis due to the abundance of alpha receptors in the bladder neck and prostate despite the lack of conclusive clinical evidence of this effect. Anti-inflammatory agents, immunosuppressants, and skeletal muscle relaxants have all been evaluated for management with inconsistent results. Surgery is generally reserved for patients with proven etiology/obstructive symptoms (i.e., bladder neck obstruction). The UPOINT system also provides a practical approach to the management of this patient population. Prognosis is similar to that of chronic urogenital and pelvic pain as discussed above.

Orchialgia

Orchialgia is defined as pain located in the male testes. Pain secondary to orchialgia can be acute or chronic in nature. Etiology of this disorder includes prior surgeries, trauma, chronic inflammation, infection, and neuropathology associated with the lower thoracic spine (e.g., can be a form of T10 radiculopathy). Management is procedural when thoracic pathology is identified, but otherwise is pharmacologic in nature or via CAM methodologies (as described above under "Treatment").

Summary

Urogenital and pelvic pains are common and may have urologic, gynecologic, gastrointestinal, vascular, musculoskeletal, or neurologic origins. In the evaluation and treatment of these pains, it must be kept in mind that these sites of pain generation are private places associated with bodily functions that are associated with strong emotions: sexual function, defecation, and urination. After infection, ischemia, inflammation, obstruction, or neoplasm has been ruled out as likely etiologies, one is often left with simply a descriptive diagnosis coupled to an empiric treatment. Pain types may be generally categorized as neuropathic or as somatic or visceral nociceptive pains. Treatments are similar to those for other parts of the body but due to psychosocial modifiers are often more difficult to assess. Pain management is generally multimodal and commonly includes pharmacotherapy and interventional procedures. Other options include surgery, yoga, biofeedback, and physical therapy.

Suggested Reading

1. Cheong Y, Stones WR. Chronic pelvic pain: aetiology and therapy. Best Pract Res Clin Obstet Gynaecol. 2006;20(5):695–711.
2. Hanno PM, Burks DA, Clemens JQ, Dmochowski RR, Erickson D, FitzGerald MP, et al. American urological association guidelines: diagnosis and treatment of interstitial cystitis/bladder pain syndrome. J Urol 2011; 185(6):2162–70.
3. Howard FM. Chronic pelvic pain. Obstet Gynecol. 2003;101(3):594–611.
4. Konkle KS, Clemens JQ. New paradigms in understanding chronic pelvic pain syndrome. Curr Urol Rep. 2011;12:278–83.
5. Nickel JC, Shoskes D, Irvine-Bird K. Clinical phenotyping of women with intestitial cystitis/painful bladder syndrome: a key to classification and potentially improved management. J Urol. 2009;182: 155–60.

Part VIII

Painful Disease States: Headaches

Primary Headaches

31

Brinder Vij and Stewart J. Tepper

Key Concepts

- A patient seeking help for a headache disorder is likely to have migraine unless proved otherwise.
- The presence of primary headache features never rule out a secondary headache disorder; rather they are comfort signs. Headache disorders are a very common adjunct to other pain syndromes and are often overlooked.
- Always classify headache disorders per the International Classification of Headache Disorders, 3rd Edition beta (ICHD-3). Document headache-related disability using a valid tool such as the headache impact test-6 (HIT-6) or the migraine disability assessment scale (MIDAS) at the initial visit and follow-ups.
- Use migraine-specific medications to treat acute migraine attacks, and start migraine prevention early on to prevent chronification of headache.
- Always pay attention to the associated psychosocial issues, and address them appropriately for optimal outcomes. Patient involvement and headache education are of paramount importance for the success in headache care.
- Interventional pain procedures such as neuromodulation for headache disorders are available in tertiary care centers and becoming more sophisticated but remain without FDA approval, with the exception of transcranial magnetic stimulation for acute treatment of migraine with aura.

Primary Headache Disorders

Primary Headache Disorders, Definitions, and Diagnoses

By definition, primary headache occurs in the absence of those secondary disorders known to cause headache and does not happen in temporal proximity of an underlying disorder. This definition remains true even if the headache has features suggestive of one of the primary headache phenotypes. For example, a new headache having migrainous features such as photophobia, phonophobia, and nausea in the presence of a new space-occupying lesion on brain imaging

B. Vij, MD, FACP, FAHS (✉)
Neurology & Rehabilitation Medicine, University of Cincinnati Medical Center, Cincinnati, OH, USA
e-mail: vijbr@ucmail.uc.edu

S.J. Tepper, MD
Department of Neurology, Dartmouth-Hitchcock Medical Center, Lebanon, NH, USA

J. Cheng, R.W. Rosenquist (eds.), *Fundamentals of Pain Medicine*,
https://doi.org/10.1007/978-3-319-64922-1_31

would be considered a secondary headache and not primary. Both the primary and secondary headache diagnoses should be considered if there is a preexisting primary headache syndrome and a patient develops a new problem, which could potentially cause headache, and then if in the same time frame the previous headache gets worse or the patient develops new headache symptoms.

There are multiple ways headache disorders are classified for management purposes. The validated international classification system, which helps to differentiate headaches into clinically significant categories, is provided by the International Headache Society (IHS) and the International Classification of Headache Disorders, 3rd Edition, Beta version (ICHD-3) [8]. The finalized ICHD-3 is expected by 2016.

According to this ICHD-3 taxonomy, all headache disorders can be grouped as:

- Primary headaches
- Secondary headaches
- Cranial neuralgias, other facial pain, and other headaches

ICHD-3 is a hierarchical and comprehensive classification scheme and is to be used as a reference, especially when a diagnosis of a headache disorder is a challenge. A condensed version of primary headache disorders per ICHD-3 is presented in Table 31.1.

Table 31.1 Primary headache syndromes classification, adapted from ICHD-3

1. Migraine
1.1. Migraine without aura
1.2. Migraine with aura
1.3. Chronic migraine
1.4. Complications of migraine, e.g., status migrainosus, migrainous infarction
1.5. Probable migraine (probable is the ICHD-3 term for meeting all criteria for a diagnosis except one)
1.6. Episodic syndromes associated with migraine e.g., abdominal migraine, cyclical vomiting, benign paroxysmal vertigo
2. Tension-type headache
2.1. Infrequent episodic tension-type headache
2.2. Frequent episodic tension-type headache
2.3. Chronic tension-type headache
2.4. Probable tension-type headache
3. Trigeminal autonomic cephalalgias (TACs)
3.1. Cluster headache (CH)
3.2. Paroxysmal hemicranias (PH)
3.3. Short-lasting unilateral neuralgiform headache attacks (SUNHA)
3.3.1. Short-lasting unilateral neuralgiform headache attacks with conjunctival injection and tearing (SUNCT)
3.3.2. Short-lasting unilateral neuralgiform headache attacks with cranial autonomic symptoms (SUNA)
3.4. Hemicrania continua (HC)
3.5. Probable TACs
4. Other primary headache disorders
4.1. Primary cough headache
4.2. Primary exercise headache
4.3. Primary headache associated with sexual activity
4.4. Primary thunderclap headache
4.5. Cold stimulus headache
4.6. External pressure headache
4.7. Primary stabbing headache
4.8. Nummular headache
4.9. Hypnic headache
4.10. New daily persistent headache (NDPH)

Migraine

Migraine is one of the most common primary headache disorders, accounting for the majority of headache consultations in physician office studies [9, 10]. Diagnosis is a critical part of managing migraine headaches, and it is clinical (see Table 31.2). Patients having recurrent disabling headaches with a normal neurological exam in the absence of secondary causes of headache should be asked about migraine features.

Migraine can be with aura or without aura. Migraine with aura per ICHD-3 is defined as a "Recurrent attack lasting [5–60] minutes of unilateral, fully reversible, visual, sensory, or other nervous system symptoms that usually develops gradually and [is] usually followed by headache and associated migraine symptoms" [8]. Aura typically is considered a reversible neurologic event lasting 5–60 min. It is critical to differentiate aura symptoms from cerebro-

Table 31.2 ICHD-3 migraine diagnostic criteria

At least five attacks fulfilling:
Headache lasting from 4 to 72 h (untreated)
Headache with at least 2 of the following features:
Unilateral
Pulsating
Worsening with routine physical activity
Moderate or severe in intensity
Associated with at least one of the following:
Nausea
Photophobia and phonophobia
Not secondary

vascular events such as transient ischemic attack (TIA) or stroke, especially when the aura has motor, sensory, and other nonvisual symptoms. Migraine with aura is found to double the risk of ischemic stroke, and the risk increases further in females who are smokers and are on oral contraceptive pills [11]. Aura occurs in about 28–38% of those with migraine, [12, 13] and the most common aura is visual [14].

Menstruation and Migraine

Females are more prone to migraine, and 66% of women with migraine have attacks with menstruation. Menstrual migraine is classified as pure menstrual migraine (PMM, A1.1.1) when the migraine attack is documented for at least three consecutive cycles occurring exclusively on days −2 to +3 of menses where the first day of flow is numbered +1 and at no other time of the cycle. Menstrually related migraine (MRM, A1.1.2) is the term used for migraine attacks like those of PMM for at least 2/3 of menstrual cycles but with attacks also occurring at other times of the cycle.

Status Migrainosus

Status migrainosus is a debilitating unremitting headache occurring in a patient with a known diagnosis of migraine, lasting for more than 72 h, and is similar in description to the previous migraines except for duration. If the persistent headache is not debilitating or if there are periods of resolution of headache because of medications or sleep, it should not be diagnosed as status migrainosus. A chronic, daily, or near-daily unrelenting and incapacitating headache occurs with medication overuse, which should be diagnosed as chronic migraine (1.3) and medication overuse headache (8.2) per ICHD-3.

Persistent aura can last up to a week or more. In such cases of "persistent aura without headache" it is critical to rule out stroke or any other acute cerebrovascular event.

Tension-Type Headache

Episodic tension-type headache is a more common headache disorder in the general population than migraine, but tension-type headache and its impact are far less than that of migraine for the individual [15]. Tension-type headache can be infrequent (<1 episode/month or <12 days/year), frequent (1–14 episodes/month or >12 but <180 headache days/year), or chronic (>15 days / month or >180 headache days/year).

Using ICHD-3, tension-type headache should not have migrainous features. Essentially, tension-type headache is a featureless headache best diagnosed as "not migraine." The following features favor a diagnosis of tension-type headache:

- Bilateral headache, that is, not one-sided, so non-migrainous
- Pressing and tightening, that is, not pounding, so non-migrainous
- Mild to moderate in intensity, that is, not severe, so non-migrainous
- Not worsening with routine activity, unlike migraine
- Not associated with nausea and, generally, no photophonophobia, so once again, no migrainous-associated symptoms

Chronic Daily Headache (CDH)

CDH refers to primary headaches occurring at least 15 days per month for more than 4 h per day for at least 3 months. There are four forms of CDH:

1. Chronic migraine is CDH with migraine features for at least 8 days per month.
2. Chronic tension-type headache is low-level featureless CDH without migrainous features.
3. Hemicrania continua (HC) is described under trigeminal autonomic cephalalgias (TACs) and is a continuous one-sided headache with periodic exacerbations, autonomic features, and indomethacin responsiveness.
4. New daily persistent headache (NDPH) is the abrupt onset of a primary CDH with any features beginning on a particular, remembered day of onset. The short daily headaches (<4 h/day) are not classified as CDH.

Trigeminal Autonomic Cephalalgias (TACs)

The trigeminal autonomic cephalalgias (TACs) are a group of headache disorders having some unique features such as:

- The headache is lateralized and generally side locked.
- The headache is generally associated with parasympathetic activation features ipsilateral to the headache, such as conjunctival injection, lacrimation, nasal congestion, eyelid edema, or sweating.
- The headache may be associated with clinical signs of cranial sympathetic dysfunction such as a partial Horner's syndrome.

There are different types of TACs; few of the common ones are detailed in Table 31.3.

Approach to Management of Primary Headache Disorders

Once the diagnosis of the primary headache disorder has been established and the patient's headache-related disability and quality of life documented using well-documented tools such as the headache impact test (HIT-6) or the migraine disability assessment scale (MIDAS), the next step in management should be individualizing headache care. The patient should play an active role in establishing goals and a commitment to achieve them. Some of the common principles to keep in mind while evaluating and treating headache disorders are as follows:

- The diagnosis of headache disorders is essentially clinical; pay close attention to the onset, progression, and features of the headaches.
- Always document all of the pain disorders in the patient, and manage them simultaneously; this is very important for the success of overall pain care. Remember that patients with multiple pain syndromes usually take analgesics (opiates, NSAIDs, etc.) in quantities sufficient to contribute to medication overuse headache (MOH).
- Acute migraine attack treatment should be aimed to achieve at least a 50% reduction in headache intensity in less than 2 h, preferably a pain-free response in that time. Avoid barbiturates and opiates to prevent MOH, as these two categories of medications have the most evidence for transformation to CDH.
- Suboptimal treatment of acute attacks of migraine leads to transformation of the episodic primary headache disorder into the chronic daily one. Always try to use the recommended doses of migraine-specific medications such as triptans or dihydroergotamine (DHE) for episodic migraine unless contraindicated (see Table 31.4).
- About 1/3 of patients with migraine need prophylaxis (see Table 31.5) and should be offered the most effective medications suggested by AAN/AHS guidelines (See Table 31.6).
- OnabotulinumtoxinA (onabot, brand name BOTOX) is the only FDA-approved treatment for chronic migraine at this time. Onabot has been shown to be safe and effective in improving the quality of life in chronic migraine patients, as well as reducing the number of headache days per month [16, 17]. It is critical

Table 31.3 The trigeminal autonomic cephalalgias (TACs)

TAC type	Diagnostic criteria	Comment
Cluster headache (CH) Episodic cluster: cycles or periods of attacks lasting from 7 days to 1 year and separated by remissions of more than1 month Chronic cluster attacks occurring for more than 1 year *without* remission or remissions of at least 1 month (10–15% of cluster patients)	Attacks of unilateral pain involving orbital, supraorbital, or temporal location Duration of each attack 15–180 min (untreated) Ipsilateral autonomic features Sense of restlessness or agitation Frequency of attacks one every other day to 8/day during the cycles	Cluster periods can last from 2 weeks to 3 months In episodic cluster, attack cycles are separated by remission periods lasting from months to years Male: Female incidence 3:1 Cluster usually recurs on the same side Triggered by alcohol or nitroglycerin
Paroxysmal hemicrania (PH) Episodic PH: cycles or periods of attacks lasting from 7 days to 1 year and separated by pain-free periods lasting >1 month Chronic PH: cycles or periods of attacks occurring for >1 year and remission periods <1 month	Attacks are similar to cluster, i.e., strictly unilateral pain involving orbital, supraorbital, or temporal location Duration of attacks 2–30 min, so generally shorter than cluster attacks (mean 13 min) Frequency of attacks must be >5 times per day for more than half of the time during active periods. So PH attacks are generally both shorter and more frequent per day than cluster Absolute response to indomethacin	No male predominance Indomethacin has both diagnostic and therapeutic value for PH Recommended dose is between 150 and 225 mg/day in divided doses for at least 2 weeks as an adequate trial
Hemicrania continua (HC) HC unremitting form: continuous side-locked headache for a least 1 year without remission of >1 day HC remitting form: continuous side-locked headache that is interrupted by periods of at least 1 day	Persistent strictly unilateral headache Ipsilateral autonomic features Present for >3 months Absolute response to therapeutic doses of indomethacin	May have some migrainous features such as usually ipsilateral photophobia or phonophobia
Short-lasting unilateral neuralgiform headache attacks (SUNHA). It has two main subtypes, short-lasting unilateral neuralgiform headaches with conjunctival injection and tearing (SUNCT) and short-lasting unilateral neuralgiform Headache attacks with cranial autonomic symptoms (SUNA) SUNCT (short-lasting neuralgiform headache attacks with conjunctival injection and tearing) SUNA (short-lasting neuralgiform headache attacks with cranial autonomic symptoms)	Moderate to severe unilateral pain in orbital, supraorbital, temporal, and other trigeminal distribution, but the attacks are short Duration of each attack 1–600 s Occur as single stabs or in salvos Frequency of attacks at least one/day for more than half days during active stage but usually hundreds of attacks per day SUNCT has all of the above SUNHA features plus significant ipsilateral conjunctival injection and tearing SUNA has all of the abovementioned SUNHA features and only one or neither tearing and conjunctival injection but other cranial autonomic symptoms	Both SUNCT and SUNA can be either episodic or chronic based on similar criteria, as for cluster and PH SUNHA should suggest posterior fossa or pituitary fossa lesions, and careful work up with MRI without and with contrast and sellar scrutiny is mandatory

Table 31.4 Medications for acute treatment of migraine

Specific antimigraine medications:
Triptans – serotonin (5-HT) 1B/1D agonists that inhibit the release of CGRP (calcitonin gene-related peptide) and vasoconstrict
Sumatriptan (optimal dose 100 mg po ×1, may repeat in after 2 h; max. daily dose is 200 mg po (injectable, nasal, and patch forms available or approved))
Zolmitriptan (2.5–5 mg po ×1, max. daily dose is 10 mg. Nasal form available)
Eletriptan (optimal dose 40 mg po ×1, max. daily dose 80 mg)
Almotriptan (optimal dose12.5 mg po ×1, max. daily dose 25 mg)
Rizatriptan (optimal dose 10 mg po ×1, max. daily dose 30 mg)
Naratriptan (optimal dose 2.5 mg po ×1, max. daily dose 5 mg)
Frovatriptan (2.5 mg po ×1, max. daily dose 7.5 mg)
Ergots – the oldest migraine-specific medication but less specific for receptors. Use limited by side effects such as nausea, vomiting, and cardiovascular side effects
Ergotamine tartrate is available as tablet and suppository
Dihydroergotamine (DHE) is available as parenteral and nasal
Absolutely contraindicated in pregnancy (category X)
Contraindications to triptans and ergots:
Coronary artery disease
Uncontrolled blood pressure
History of stroke or cerebrovascular disease
Brainstem (basilar-type) aura or hemiplegic migraine
Simultaneous use of different triptans and ergot in a 24 h period is prohibited
Pregnancy (ergots FDA category X and triptans category C)
Nonspecific antimigraine medications:
Acetaminophen (Tylenol) is one of the most common used analgesics. Effective dose is usually 1 gm at the onset of headache. Maximum daily dose is 3–4 gm/day and is limited by hepatotoxicity. May be effective for mild to moderate headaches
NSAIDs (nonsteroidal anti-inflammatory drugs) – these cyclooxygenase (COX) inhibitors help reduce migrainous neurogenic inflammation at the peripheral level and trigemino-vascular activation at the central level

(continued)

Table 31.4 (continued)

NSAIDs can be used in combination with triptans for synergistic effect in refractory or prolonged cases of migraine or to prevent migraine recurrence after triptan monotherapy use has failed
NSAIDs can be preferred when migraine is associated with menstrual symptoms, as they can help both headache and menstrual discomfort
NSAIDs alone are indicated for moderate headaches, although solubilized diclofenac potassium is FDA approved for acute treatment of all levels of migraine
The most common side effects of NSAIDs include GI, renal, and hepatic toxicities
Commonly used NSAIDs are:
Solubilized diclofenac potassium (brand name CAMBIA) 50 mg po. This powder sachet is the only FDA-approved prescription NSAID for acute migraine
Ibuprofen 400–800 mg po q 6–8 h prn, max daily dose 3.2 gm
Naproxen – Up to 500–550 mg BID
Indomethacin 25–50 mg po TID, max daily dose rarely >150 mg
Celecoxib 100–200 po mg/day
Mefenamic acid 250 mg po up to QID
Meloxicam 7.5–15 mg po/day
Barbiturates and opiates – the US Headache Consortium recommends against using barbiturates alone or in combinations for migraine treatment because of concerns of MOH. Avoid opiates, which should be considered only for short durations when all other medications are contraindicated, and risk of abuse or addiction has been formally assessed and is minimal
MOH can occur with opiate use as infrequently as 2 times/week and with butalbital use as infrequently as once per week
Steroids: steroids are reserved for status migrainosus or refractory migraine. Commonly used ones are:
Prednisone 60 mg po daily for 3–5 days
Dexamethasone short course:
Day 1, 4 mg po ×3 with meals
Day 2, 4 mg po ×2 with breakfast and lunch
Day 3, 4 mg with breakfast
Injectable dexamethasone 4–10 mg is an option

Table 31.5 Indications for migraine prophylaxis

Recurrent disabling headache attacks affecting quality of life despite abortive therapy
Migraine attacks more than 3–4 times/month
Headache days >10–14/month
Patient's choice
Medication overuse headache
Adverse effects from acute antimigraine medications
Uncommon headache disorders such as hemiplegic migraine, migraine with prolonged aura, and migraine with brainstem aura (formerly basilar-type migraine)

Table 31.6 Medications for prevention of episodic migraine per AAN/AHS guidelines [18]

Medications along with level of evidence for use
Level A: established as effective
Sodium valproate (400–1000 mg/day)
Topiramate (25–200 mg/day)
Propranolol (120–240 mg/day)
Timolol (10–15 mg BID)
Metoprolol (50–200 mg/day)
Petasites (butterbur root extract) 50–75 mg BID
Level B: probably effective
Naproxen sodium (550 mg BID)
Amitriptyline (25–150 mg/day)
Magnesium (trimagnesium dicitrate, 600 mg qd)
Atenolol (100 mg/day)
Venlafaxine XR (150 mg/day)
Riboflavin (400 mg/day)
Ibuprofen (200 mg BID)
Ketoprofen (50 mg TID)
Feverfew (50–300 mg BID)
Fenoprofen (200–600 mg TID)
Histamine (1–10 ng s/q twice/wk)
Level C: possibly effective
Candesartan (16 mg/day) [note: a second randomized controlled trial published online in December 2013 suggests that candesartan 16 mg should be reclassified level B [19]
Lisinopril (10–20 mg/day)
Carbamazepine (600 mg/day)
Pindolol (10 mg/day)
Nebivolol (5 mg/day)
Clonidine (0.15–0.075 mg/day) patch could be used
Flurbiprofen (200 mg/day)
Mefenamic acid (500 mg TID)
Coenzyme Q10 (100 mg TID)
Cyproheptatidine (4 mg/day)
Guanfacine (0.5–1 mg/day)

to inject according to the FDA-approved evidence-based protocol (PREEMPT, Phase III REsearch Evaluating Migraine Prophylaxis Treatment) to get the maximum benefit from this intervention.

- If there is clinical suspicion about possible secondary headache, do not delay the evaluation.
- Generally speaking, non-acute (>6 months duration) headaches with a normal physical examination have a very low probability of abnormality on brain imaging, but it is prudent to remain vigilant about any clue for secondary headache and image as appropriate in the clinical context. For example a patient with a history of malignancy in remission with subacute headache has more likelihood of an abnormality than an otherwise healthy patient.
- The patient should be encouraged to keep a detailed headache diary to monitor disease progression, treatment response, and planning management.
- Refractory chronic migraine patients may need an interdisciplinary headache program and should be assessed for associated psychological and physical deconditioning.
- Consider interventional pain procedures such as greater occipital nerve (GON) blocks and neuromodulation in properly selected patients.
- For all practical purposes, the treatment of chronic tension-type headache should be exactly as for chronic migraine, especially if the headache is disabling even though it may not have other features of migraine.

Treatment of TACs/Cluster Headache

For this chapter, the treatment of TACs will be restricted to cluster headache as the most common among this group of headache disorders.

Acute Treatment of Cluster Headache

The aim of acute treatment is to abolish cluster headache in about 15 min:

- Oxygen 100% (high-flow mask) 12–15 L/min
- Sumatriptan 6 mg subcutaneous (FDA approved)

- Sumatriptan nasal spray 20 mg
- Zolmitriptan nasal spray 5–10 mg
- DHE injection (FDA approved)

Preventive Therapy for Cluster Headache

Cluster periods can last for weeks to months, so preventive therapy is usually indicated. The duration of preventive therapy can be indefinite in chronic cluster headache.

- Verapamil 360–480 mg/day (use only the short-acting form in divided doses; constipation and bradycardia are the common side effects).
- Valproate 500–1000 mg/day (monitor for hepatotoxicity and weight gain. Avoid in woman of childbearing age).
- Lithium 900 mg/day (monitor for cognitive side effects, hyponatremia, and hypothyroidism).
- GON (greater occipital nerve blocks) with local anesthetic and steroid can be tried as an abortive, bridge, and preventive therapy in cluster headache.

Imaging in Primary Headaches

Considerable argument surrounds this issue in clinical practice, but as a rule "when in doubt, image." The American Academy of Neurology evidence-based guidelines for migraine imaging [20] suggested to consider imaging for patients with non-acute headache in the presence of following situations:

- Rapidly increasing headache frequency
- Unexplained abnormal findings on neurological examination
- History of lack of coordination
- History of localized neurological signs such as numbness or tingling, etc.

A history of headache newly causing awakening from sleep, which happens commonly in migraine, is also the grounds for imaging. Recent data from a headache center found the incidence of abnormalities on brain imaging was up to 5.5% in patients suspected to have intracranial pathologies compared to only 2% in all headache patients, suggesting brain imaging in selected patients as described above rather than imaging them all [21]. The imaging study is preferentially MRI without and with contrast (for suspected neoplasm or space-occupying lesions, trauma, headaches suspected to be related to causes in brainstem, posterior fossa lesions, evaluating TACs, or intracranial hypotension-related meningeal enhancement).

Interventional Procedures and New Treatments for Primary Headache Disorders

Once a definitive refractoriness to conservative treatments is ascertained and MOH is excluded, neuromodulation options can be considered in selected headache disorders. Various invasive and noninvasive approaches, such as hypothalamic deep brain stimulation, occipital nerve stimulation, stimulation of the sphenopalatine ganglion, cervical spinal cord stimulation, noninvasive handheld vagus nerve stimulation, transcranial direct current stimulation, transcranial magnetic stimulation, and transcutaneous electrical nerve stimulation, have all been tried, although proper evidence, depending on the form of neuromodulation, is often limited. A position statement from the European Headache Federation states that until randomized controlled studies are available, any neurostimulation device should only be used in patients with medically intractable syndromes at tertiary headache centers either as part of a valid study or have shown to be effective in such controlled studies with an acceptable side effect profile [22].

Greater occipital nerve blocks (GONB) are a simple office-based procedure involving injection of local anesthetic with or without steroids in the area of the greater occipital nerve in the occipital groove. The rationale of performing a GONB for the treatment of chronic headache is based on the anatomical connections between the trigeminal and upper cervical sensory fibers at the level of the trigeminal nucleus caudalis. GONBs have been found to be effective in different refractory headache syndromes such as chronic migraine and chronic cluster to yield temporary relief and could be an option to consider especially when there is significant suboccipital tenderness [23, 24].

Summary and Conclusion

Evaluating and diagnosing primary headache syndromes should involve a very structured and scientific approach using the latest standard international classification criteria. The ICHD-3 is hierarchical and has a specific code for each headache disorder and should be used for consistency and proper diagnoses. Headache disorders require categorization as episodic or chronic, and this has significant treatment implications. Chronic primary headache disorders with normal neurological examinations do not generally require brain imaging, but TACs are the exception to this rule. All TACs and other atypical headaches should be worked up with an MRI of the brain with and without contrast to rule out posterior fossa or brainstem lesions. Use migraine-specific medications unless contraindicated, and use them in recommended dosage. Always remember that a headache disorder can be just one of the pain syndromes a patient is suffering from and addressing all the pain issues comprehensively in an interdisciplinary fashion is often a recommended approach for successful outcomes.

References

1. Kolodner K, Lipton RB, Lafata JE, Leotta C, Liberman JN, Chee E, et al. Pharmacy and medical claims data identified migraine sufferers with high specificity but modest sensitivity. J Clin Epidemiol. 2004;57(9):962–72.
2. Lipton RB, Diamond S, Reed M, Diamond ML, Stewart WF. Migraine diagnosis and treatment: results from the American migraine study II. Headache. 2001;41(7):638–45.
3. Lipton RB, Bigal ME, Diamond M, Freitag F, Reed ML, Stewart WF, et al. Migraine prevalence, disease burden, and the need for preventive therapy. Neurology. 2007;68(5):343–9.
4. Kucuksen S, Genc E, Yilmaz H, Salli A, Gezer IA, Karahan AY, et al. The prevalence of fibromyalgia and its relation with headache characteristics in episodic migraine. Clin Rheumatol. 2013;32(7):983–90.
5. Park JW, Cho YS, Lee SY, Kim ES, Cho H, Shin HE, et al. Concomitant functional gastrointestinal symptoms influence psychological status in Korean migraine patients. Gut Liver. 2013;7(6):668–74.
6. Igarashi H. Societal impact of migraine chronification. Rinsho shinkeigaku. Clin Neurol. 2013;53(11):1225–7.
7. Arslantas D, Tozun M, Unsal A, Ozbek Z. Headache and its effects on health-related quality of life among adults. Turk Neurosurg. 2013;23(4):498–504.
8. Headache Classification Committee of the International Headache Society (IHS). The international classification of headache disorder, 3rd edition, Beta version. Cephalalgia. 2013;33:629–808.
9. Tepper SJ, Dahlof CG, Dowson A, Newman L, Mansbach H, Jones M, et al. Prevalence and diagnosis of migraine in patients consulting their physician with a complaint of headache: data from the landmark study. Headache. 2004;44(9):856–64.
10. Kaniecki R, Ruoff G, Smith T, Barrett PS, Ames MH, Byrd S, et al. Prevalence of migraine and response to sumatriptan in patients self-reporting tension/stress headache. Curr Med Res Opin. 2006;22(8):1535–44.
11. Schurks M, Rist PM, Bigal ME, Buring JE, Lipton RB, Kurth T. Migraine and cardiovascular disease: systematic review and meta-analysis. Br Med J. 2009;339:b3914.
12. Russell MB, Rasmussen BK, Thorvaldsen P, Olesen J. Prevalence and sex-ratio of the subtypes of migraine. Int J Epidemiol. 1995;24(3):612–8.
13. Kelman L. The aura: a tertiary care study of 952 migraine patients. Cephalalgia. 2004;24(9):728–34.
14. Russell MB, Olesen J. A nosographic analysis of the migraine aura in a general population. Brain. 1996;119(Pt 2):355–61.
15. Schwartz BS, Stewart WF, Simon D, Lipton RB. Epidemiology of tension-type headache. JAMA. 1998;279(5):381–3.
16. Aurora SK, Dodick DW, Diener HC, Degryse RE, Turkel CC, Lipton RB, et al. OnabotulinumtoxinA for chronic migraine: efficacy, safety, and tolerability in patients who received all five treatment cycles in the PREEMPT clinical program. Acta Neurol Scand. 2014;129(1):61–70.
17. Aurora SK, Winner P, Freeman MC, Spierings EL, Heiring JO, DeGryse RE, et al. OnabotulinumtoxinA for treatment of chronic migraine: pooled analyses of the 56-week PREEMPT clinical program. Headache. 2011;51(9):1358–73.
18. Loder E, Burch R, Rizzoli P. The 2012 AHS/AAN guidelines for prevention of episodic migraine: a summary and comparison with other recent clinical practice guidelines. Headache. 2012;52(6):930–45.

19. Stovner LJ, Linde M, Gravdahl GB, Tronvik E, Aamolt AH, Sand T, Hagen K. A comparative study of candesartan versus propranolol for migraine prophylaxis: a randomised, triple-blind, placebo-controlled, double cross-over study. Cephalalgia 2013.; Published online before print December 11, 2013, doi:https://doi.org/10.1177/0333102413515348.
20. Silberstein SD. Practice parameter: evidence-based guidelines for migraine headache (an evidence-based review): report of the Quality Standards Subcommittee of the American Academy of Neurology. Neurology. 2000;55(6):754–62.
21. Clarke CE, Edwards J, Nicholl DJ, Sivaguru A. Imaging results in a consecutive series of 530 new patients in the Birmingham Headache Service. J Neurol. 2010;257(8):1274–8.
22. Martelletti P, Jensen RH, Antal A, Arcioni R, Brighina F, de Tommaso M, et al. Neuromodulation of chronic headaches: position statement from the European Headache Federation. J Headache Pain. 2013;14(1):86.
23. Saracco MG, Valfre W, Cavallini M, Aguggia M. Greater occipital nerve block in chronic migraine. Neurol Sci. 2010;31(Suppl 1):S179–80.
24. Baron EP, Tepper SJ, Mays M, Cherian N. Acute treatment of basilar-type migraine with greater occipital nerve blockade. Headache. 2010;50(6):1057–9.

Secondary Headaches

32

Brinder Vij and Stewart J. Tepper

Key Concepts

- Any new headache or subacute headache (<3–6 months) occurring in close temporal relation to a disorder known to cause headache should be considered secondary unless proved otherwise.
- Any change in character, frequency, and intensity of a primary headache should raise suspicion for a secondary cause.
- Never hesitate to evaluate if there is clinical doubt for the cause of a given headache.
- Overtreatment of a primary headache such as migraine or treatment of another pain syndrome such as back pain is a very common cause of a secondary or transformed headache disorder, medication overuse headache (MOH).
- When treating multiple pain syndromes, always plan a comprehensive pain management strategy addressing headache along with the other pertinent pain issues.
- Psychosocial factors can be very important in patients with multiple pain problems, including headache.
- Referral to the appropriate specialty should be made early based on a suspected cause of headache. For example, refer to neuro-oncologist for brain lesions, to a neurovascular specialist for brain aneurysm, etc.

Diagnostic Criteria for Secondary Headaches

The general diagnostic criteria for secondary headaches in the ICHD-3 are as follows:

A. Any headache fulfilling criterion C.
B. Another disorder scientifically documented to be able to cause headache has been diagnosed.
C. Evidence of causation demonstrated by at least two of the following:
  (a) Headache has developed in temporal relation to the onset of the presumed causative disorder.
  (b) One or both of the following:
    (i) Headache has significantly worsened in parallel with worsening of the presumed causative disorder.
    (ii) Headache has significantly improved in parallel with improvement of the presumed causative disorder.

B. Vij, MD, FACP, FAHS (✉)
Neurology & Rehabilitation Medicine, University of Cincinnati Medical Center, Cincinnati, OH, USA
e-mail: vijbr@ucmail.uc.edu

S.J. Tepper, MD
Department of Neurology, Dartmouth-Hitchcock Medical Center, Lebanon, NH, USA

J. Cheng, R.W. Rosenquist (eds.), *Fundamentals of Pain Medicine*,
https://doi.org/10.1007/978-3-319-64922-1_32

(c) Headache has characteristics typical for the causative disorder.
(d) Other evidence exists for causation.

The ICHD-3 criteria often suggest a direction for workup rather than an obvious cause. The temporal association with a cause is most important. It is essential to rule out a secondary cause of a headache before assuming it is primary in nature. Missing a secondary headache may have serious implications for both the patient and the healthcare provider. Dr. David Dodick in 2003 recommended a clinical guide to look for "red flags" for a "dangerous" headache in the form of the mnemonic SNOOP (see Table 32.1).

Classification of Secondary Headache Disorders

Secondary headache disorders are classified into eight categories in the ICHD-3, and each diagnosis is associated with specific numeric codes and is hierarchical, as with primary headaches (Table 32.2).

Medication Overuse Headache (MOH)

This term refers to the development of a new headache or worsening of a previous primary headache in the context of overuse of the medications used for acute headache relief or other pain conditions (see Table 32.3 for diagnostic criteria). Other terms used for this headache type are "rebound headache," "transformed headache," "drug-induced headache," and "medicine misuse headache." MOH is extremely common in primary settings [3] and even more common in specialized headache and pain management settings [4, 5].

Table 32.1 SNOOP mnemonic for secondary causes of headache

Systemic features (weight loss, fever, night sweats, etc.)
Secondary risk factors – immune deficiency, cancer, systemic disease, infectious and noninfectious diseases
Neurological symptoms and signs (focal neurological deficit, confusion, seizures, etc.)
Older age of onset (new headache after age of 50 years)
Onset of headache: acute, sudden, abrupt
Pattern change: progressive headache without headache-free intervals, change in previous headache history (new distribution pattern, change in intensity, and frequency of headache)

Adapted from Dodick [2]

Chronic migraine is defined by the ICHD-3 as a *primary* headache occurring ≥15 days per month ≥4 h/day. MOH is a *secondary* headache ≥15 days per month ≥4 h per day, with acute medication overuse in a patient with a previous history of episodic migraine or headache. From a clinical standpoint, the phenotype of these patients (chronic migraine and MOH) is the same, so it is impossible to tell them apart until after weaning the overused medication. In the ICHD-3, the instruction is to diagnose both until after the wean makes the previous diagnosis clear. It is important to be mindful that a patient with MOH might be taking analgesics for some other pain syndrome such as chronic back pain or fibromyalgia. In an episodic migraine patient, MOH can be precipitated by different acute medications (regardless of what condition for which they are used), but their ability to transform to chronic daily headache is variable. Opiate use in a migraineur at 8 days/month or butalbital at 5 days/month is the most likely medications to convert episodic migraine to chronic migraine/MOH [6]. Other acute headache medications such as triptans, combination analgesics, and NSAIDs are likely to contribute to MOH if taken more than 10–15 days/month [6]. As a general rule, a patient should be instructed to avoid using any acute headache medication more than 2 days per week to prevent MOH.

Mechanism of MOH Development

MOH develops as a result of the interaction of acute analgesic and anti-migraine medications and a predisposed primary headache patient. There are multiple mechanisms proposed for the transformation of episodic headache to chronic

Table 32.2 Secondary headaches as classified by ICHD-3 [1]

5. Headache attributed to trauma or injury to the head and/or neck
5.1. Acute headache attributed to traumatic injury to the head
5.2. Persistent headache attributed to traumatic injury to the head
5.3. Acute headache attributed to whiplash
5.4. Persistent headache attributed to whiplash
5.5. Acute headache attributed to craniotomy
5.6. Persistent headache attributed to craniotomy
6. Headache attributed to cranial or cervical vascular disorders
6.1. Headache attributed to ischemic stroke or transient ischemic attack
6.2. Headache attributed to non-traumatic intracranial hemorrhage
6.3. Headache attributed to unruptured vascular malformation
6.4. Headache attributed to arteritis
6.5. Headache attributed to cervical carotid or vertebral artery disorder
6.6. Headache attributed to cerebral venous thrombosis (CVT)
6.7. Headache attributed to other acute intracranial arterial disorder
6.8. Headache attributed to genetic vasculopathy
6.9. Headache attributed to pituitary apoplexy
7. Headache attributed to nonvascular intracranial disorder
7.1. Headache attributed to increased cerebrospinal fluid pressure
7.2. Headache attributed to low cerebrospinal fluid pressure
7.3. Headache attributed to noninfectious inflammatory disease
7.4. Headache attributed to intracranial neoplasia
7.5. Headache attributed to intrathecal injection
7.6. Headache attributed to epileptic seizure
7.7. Headache attributed to Chiari malformation type I (CM1)
7.8. Headache attributed to other nonvascular intracranial disorder
8. Headache attributed to a substance or its withdrawal
8.1. Headache attributed to the use of or exposure to a substance
8.2. Medication overuse headache (MOH)
8.3. Headache attributed to substance withdrawal
9. Headache attributed to infection
9.1. Headache attributed to intracranial infection
9.2. Headache attributed to systemic infection
10. Headache attributed to disorders of homoeostasis
10.1. Headache attributed to hypoxia and/or hypercapnia
10.2. Dialysis headache
10.3. Headache attributed to arterial hypertension
10.4. Headache attributed to hypothyroidism
10.5. Headache attributed to fasting
10.6. Cardiac cephalalgia
10.7. Headache attributed to other disorder of homoeostasis
11. Headache or facial pain attributed to disorders of the cranium, neck, eyes, nose, sinuses, or cervical structures
11.1. Headache attributed to disorder of the cranial bone
11.2. Headache attributed to disorder of the neck
11.3. Headache attributed to disorder of the eyes
11.4. Headache attributed to disorder of the ears
11.5. Headache attributed to disorder of the nose or paranasal sinuses
11.6. Headache attributed to disorder of the teeth or jaw
11.7. Headache attributed to temporomandibular disorder (TMD)
11.8. Head or facial pain attributed to inflammation of the stylohyoid ligament
11.9. Headache or facial pain attributed to other disorder of the cranium, neck, eyes, ears, nose, sinuses, teeth, mouth, or other facial or cervical structure
12. Headache attributed to psychiatric disorder
12.1. Headache attributed to somatization disorder
12.2. Headache attributed to psychotic disorder

Table 32.3 Diagnostic criteria for MOH by ICHD-3 [1]

Headache occurring on ≥15 days per month in a patient with a pre-existing primary headache disorder
Consistent overuse for >3 months of ≥ one medication that can be taken for acute treatment of headache

headache, but a few hypothesized theories [7] include central sensitization [8, 9], cortical hyperexcitability [10], kindling, withdrawal, habituation, and basement membrane leakage [11]. Opiates in particular have been shown to cause persistent pro-nociceptive neural adaptation at trigeminal neurons by increased excitatory neurotransmission at the level of the dorsal horn and

Table 32.4 Medication overuse headache (MOH) by ICHD-3 criteria [1]

8.2.1. Ergotamine overuse headache
8.2.2. Triptan overuse headache
8.2.3. Simple analgesic overuse headache
8.2.3.1. Acetaminophen overuse headache
8.2.3.2. Acetylsalicylic acid overuse headache
8.2.3.3. Other NSAID overuse headache
8.2.4. Opioid overuse headache
8.2.5. Combination analgesic overuse headache
8.2.6. MOH attributed to unverified multiple drug classes not individually overused
8.2.7. MOH attributed to other medications

nucleus caudalis [12]. Opioids also lead to hyperalgesia by increasing expression of calcitonin gene-related peptide (CGRP) in trigeminal primary afferent neurons [12].

MOH is subclassified per ICHD-3 based on the type of medication overused, and the following table gives an overview of this classification (Table 32.4).

Treatment of MOH

Treatment of MOH requires weaning and completely stopping the overuse of the acute medication in question. It is of course always best to prevent MOH from developing. The common cause for development of MOH is suboptimal treatment of acute attacks of disabling migraine. Most of the time, a lack of good response to acute treatment of migraine is the result of not using migraine-specific medications or prescribing subtherapeutic doses of such medications. Specific anti-migraine medications such as DHE and triptans should be the first choice for migraine acute treatment, followed by NSAIDs if vasoactive medications are contraindicated. As noted above, a general rule of thumb is to limit acute treatment days to no more than 2 days per week. If a patient is using different acute treatments on different days, then for practical purposes these days are additive. For example, 6 days of NSAIDs, 6 days of triptans, and 4 days of opiates count as 16 total acute treatment days. The aim should be to have a patient use less than 10 acute treatment days per month, less for opiates (<8) and butalbital (<5), to prevent development of MOH. However, the recommendation is that barbiturates and opiates should not be used at all for acute treatment of migraine. Absolute elimination of a culprit medication in overuse is usually possible in an outpatient setting, but occasionally the offending medication cannot be weaned safely outpatient, such as the case with high-dose barbiturates, where an inpatient wean may be required. Sometimes bridge therapy with antimigraine intravenous infusions (DHE, valproate, magnesium, steroids, ondansetron, neuroleptics) is necessary for the patient to have a successful outcome. An outpatient short course of oral steroid (prednisone 60 mg po × 3–5 days) or intravenous steroid (dexamethasone 12 mg, 8 mg, or 4 mg) can also be used as a bridge in these patients to tide over the bump of the weaning period.

Another major factor after overuse of acute medications implicated in transformation of episodic migraine to chronic daily headache is the number of headache days per month. If a patient starts a year with 6–10 headache days/month, the odds of developing chronic daily headache over a 1-year period is about six times that compared with lower frequency of headache, and these odds go up to 20 times if the baseline frequency is between 11 and 14 headache days/month at the beginning of the year [13]. Therefore, it is important to start daily preventive therapy for migraine to limit the number of headache days and thus to prevent transformation to chronic migraine. OnabotulinumtoxinA (onabot, brand name BOTOX) is another option which can be used for prevention of chronic migraine and can work in prophylaxis started on day 1 of weaning and is the only FDA-approved medication for chronic migraine. General principles of MOH management are outlined in Table 32.5

Headache Attributed to Increased CSF Pressure

Raised intracranial CSF pressure can lead to a prominent secondary headache. Increased intracranial pressure can happen in the absence of an identifiable cause. Also known as idiopathic intracranial hypertension (IIH), benign intracra-

Table 32.5 General principles to follow for MOH treatment/management

Prevention of development of MOH is the best policy
Patient education about the concept of MOH and building a therapeutic alliance are keys early in the course of management of MOH. Patience on the part of both care provider and patient is important because treatment of MOH might take up to 3–6 months before clear clinical benefits become obvious
Always use migraine-specific medications in therapeutically recommended doses for optimal treatment of acute attacks of migraine to prevent overuse in partially treated headaches
In established cases of MOH, start preventive medication or onabot early on to reduce the number of headache days per month and at the same time wean completely the use of overused medication
Absolute discontinuation of offending overused medications is necessary to obtain successful results
Aim to limit the use of acute analgesics for whatever purpose and anti-migraine medication to less than 2 days per week
As with any chronic headache and pain disorder, never hesitate to involve other disciplines such as psychology, psychiatry, and PT/OT when necessary for MOH treatment
Always have a follow-up plan, as these patients can fall back again to a cycle of medication overuse and chronification of headache

Table 32.6 Common secondary causes of raised intracranial CSF pressure

Intracranial mass or edema
Meningitis
Vitamin A intoxication
Intracranial sinus venous thrombosis
Hypothyroidism/parahypothyroidism
Obesity
Renal disease
Encephalopathy secondary to toxins, drugs, or disturbance of homeostasis such as hypertensive and metabolic encephalopathy
Neck dissection causing obstruction of mediastinal and jugular veins
Obstruction to CSF flow by disease at the base of the brain such as Arnold-Chiari malformation

nial hypertension (BIH), and pseudotumor cerebri, elevated intracranial pressure can be due to multiple secondary causes (Table 32.6). Normal CSF pressure is between 70 and 250 mm of H_20. When intracranial pressure is raised and is associated with headache, papilledema and other

Table 32.7 Diagnostic criteria for idiopathic intracranial hypertension, by ICHD-3 criteria [1]

CSF pressure > 250 mm CSF (measured by lumbar puncture performed in the lateral decubitus position, without sedative medications, or by epidural or intraventricular monitoring)
Causation demonstrated by at least two of the following:
Headache developed in temporal relation to IIH or led to its discovery
Headache is relieved by decreasing intracranial hypertension
Headache is aggravated in temporal relation to the increase in intracranial pressure

signs and symptoms of raised intracranial pressure (bradycardia, elevated blood pressure, ventricular size change) in the absence of secondary causes, it can be categorized as IIH (see Table 32.7 for ICHD-3 diagnostic criteria). Lumbar puncture (LP) is necessary to make the diagnosis of pseudotumor cerebri. The typical patient is an obese middle-aged (20–50 years) female.

Treatment of Idiopathic Intracranial Hypertension

- Patients with IIH are at risk of visual loss and development of cranial nerve palsies (especially sixth nerve palsy) because of raised intracranial pressure.
- The aim of treatment should be to reduce intracranial pressure, which can be achieved by medications or by LP, which can be both diagnostic and, at least temporarily, therapeutic.
- The commonly used medications to treat IIH are the following:
  - Acetazolamide (carbonic anhydrase inhibitor) 1–4 gm/day
  - Furosemide (brand name Lasix) 40–120 mg/day
  - Topiramate (brand name Topamax) 100–200 mg/day
- Weight reduction is recommended in all obese patients with IIH.
- Neurosurgical and neuro-ophthalmic consultations are recommended in most cases to establish a multidisciplinary team approach in this complex secondary headache disorder.

Optic nerve fenestration can be used to preserve vision in some cases, but this procedure does not help headache.
- Ventriculoperitoneal or lumbo-peritoneal shunting can be used for both headache and for vision preservation in refractory cases of IIH.

Headache Attributed to Intracranial Hypotension

Low cerebrospinal fluid (CSF) pressure is also associated with headache. Low CSF pressure headache can occur post-LP, because of CSF fistula, or can develop in the context of a spontaneous leak resulting in low CSF pressure (see Table 32.8 for diagnostic criteria). Low CSF pressure headache is classically orthostatic and is worse when the patient stands up in the morning and improves with lying down.

Low CSF pressure headache is a relatively common situation in interventional pain practices especially after accidental dural punctures while doing epidural injections (see Table 32.9 for features and treatment of low CSF pressure headache).

Headache Attributed to Intracranial Neoplasm

Intracranial masses or cancer may present as headache, seizures, neurological deficit, or confusion via increasing intracranial pressure. Most of the headache patients with intracranial lesions have metastases rather than a primary nervous system tumor (see Table 32.10 for diagnostic criteria of headache attributed to intracranial neoplasms). Traction on pain-sensitive structures in the brain is the proposed explanation for headache due to intracranial neoplasms. Common phenotypes of headache with brain neoplasm include tension-type headache, followed by migraine and TACs such as cluster headache [16].

Table 32.8 Diagnostic criteria for low CSF pressure headache

Low CSF pressure (<60 mm CSF) and/or evidence of CSF leakage on imaging (brain sag on imaging, pachymeningeal enhancement after intravenous contrast)
Headache has developed in temporal relation to the low CSF pressure or CSF leakage or led to its discovery

Table 32.9 Other features of low CSF pressure headache [14]

Headache is bilateral either bifrontal or bi-occipital in location
Usually throbbing quality and may have photophobia
Tinnitus and decreased hearing
Vertigo, dizziness, and gait disturbance
Nausea and vomiting
Multiple cranial nerve palsies presenting with horizontal diplopia
The headache gets worse within 15 min of getting up or standing from a sitting or lying position and improves upon lying supine
Neuroimaging in low CSF pressure headaches has a specific role. Most reliable is MRI with and without gadolinium, which usually demonstrates pachymeningeal enhancement, sagging of the brain (crowding of the posterior fossa, cerebellar tonsil herniation), flattening of the optic chiasm, collapse of the ventricles, and sometimes subdural hematomas or hygromas
MRI or CT myelogram can demonstrate extradural and extra-arachnoid fluid collection or leak, meningeal diverticula, or dilated nerve root sleeves
A fat suppression MRI of the entire spine can often identify the site of the leak
Treatment of low CSF pressure headache [15]
The first step in the treatment of low CSF pressure is identifying the low CSF pressure. If the headache occurs just after an LP, then improvement can occur spontaneously within 1 week
Initial conservative treatment involves bed rest, IV hydration, caffeine (300 mg po), simple analgesics, steroids, theophylline (282 mg po TID), and even an abdominal binder
An epidural blood patch and epidural saline infusion can be helpful
On rare occasions, a surgical correction of the leak or fistula may be required
Post-LP headache can be prevented by using a small, non-cutting LP needle, replacing the stylet before removal of the needle, and inserting the needle bevel parallel to dural fibers

Table 32.10 Diagnostic criteria for headache attributed to intracranial neoplasms, ICHD-3 [1]

A space-occupying intracranial neoplasm has been demonstrated
Causation of headache demonstrated by at least two of the following:
Headache developed in temporal relation to the development of the neoplasm or led to its discovery
Either or both of the following:
Headache worsened with worsening of neoplasm
Headache improved with successful treatment of neoplasm
Headache has at least one of the following:
Progressive in nature
Aggravated by Valsalva-like maneuvers
Worse in the morning or after daytime napping

Table 32.11 Diagnostic criteria of cervicogenic headaches by ICHD-3 [1]

Clinical, laboratory, and/or imaging evidence of a disorder or lesion within the cervical spine or soft tissues of the neck, known to cause headache
Causation evidenced by at least two of the following:
Headache developed in temporal relation to the onset of the cervical disorder or appearance of the lesion
Headache has improved or resolved simultaneously with improvement in or resolution of the cervical disorder or lesion
Cervical range of motion is reduced, and headache is made significantly worse by provoking movements
Headache is abolished following diagnostic blockade of a cervical structure or its nerve supply

Treatment of Headache Attributed to Intracranial Neoplasms

Treatment of the neoplasm headache is primarily limited to using high-dose steroids, particularly dexamethasone 10 mg IV × 8–12 h per day until symptomatic relief is achieved. Further therapy should focus on treatment of the tumor with radiation therapy or with chemotherapy as appropriate. Patients who are very advanced in their illness should be treated in palliative care settings in which the main focus of treatment can be symptomatic relief. Unlike other headache disorders, it is appropriate to use opiates if they are effective to treat headaches in advanced cancer patients.

Cervicogenic Headache

In the ICHD-3, cervicogenic headaches are classified under headaches attributed to disorders of the neck (see Table 32.11). Cervicogenic headache is the result of pathology of the cervical spine and its components such as the bone, discs, and soft tissue and is invariably accompanied by neck pain. Patients at risk of developing such headaches are the ones with a history of neck trauma, cervical spondylosis, degenerative disc disease, and facet arthritis. The pain of true cervicogenic headache is usually unilateral with occipitofrontal distribution of spread. The proposed mechanism of cervicogenic headache is activation of the trigeminal nucleus caudalis via stimulation from upper cervical nerve roots particularly C1 and C2. Neck stiffness and pain occur in up to 75% of patients with migraine. The key to diagnosis is that the patient does not meet criteria for chronic migraine, MOH, or hemicrania continua. The headache should not appear clinically as one of the other ICHD-3 primary or secondary headaches.

Treatment of Cervicogenic Headache

Initial management of cervicogenic headaches includes simple analgesics (NSAIDs, acetaminophen) and muscle relaxants. Sometimes, a GON block can be helpful to provide temporary relief. Generally, however, interventional procedures such as a cervical facet/median branch block/radio-frequency ablation (C2–4) can be diagnostic and/or therapeutic. Unless contraindicated, physical therapy should be recommended in most of these patients to address associated physical/myofascial deconditioning.

Headache Attributed to Cranial or Cervical Vascular Disorder

Intracranial vessels, both arteries and veins, are pain-sensitive structures. Disorders of the intracranial and cervical vasculature are typically associated with abrupt onset of headache (see Table 32.12 for diagnostic criteria). Sometimes the intensity of such headaches can reach peak within a few seconds to minutes, and these are referred as thunderclap headaches. Establishing causality in vascular headaches is relatively easy, as they generally occur acutely and usually have some associated neurological deficit. Common vascular causes of headache are listed in Table 32.13. These headaches can improve rapidly in temporal relation to the vascular event.

Principles for Treatment and Management of Vascular Headaches

- Headache associated with vascular disorders such as stroke and hemorrhage is typically self-limiting and generally does not require long-term treatment.
- Sometimes, however, these headaches do require medical management for prolonged duration. Commonly used medications include acetaminophen (1 gm po every 6 or 8 h) or tramadol (50–200 mg/day in divided doses). Only short courses of opiates should be considered in properly selected patients who have low risk of abuse, dependence, and addiction.
- Giant cell arteritis is a large vessel vasculitis, usually affects females above 50, and presents with headache, jaw claudication, early morning stiffness, and axial pain. Diagnosis is by temporal artery biopsy after demonstrated of an elevated sedimentation rate. Specific treatments for temporal arteritis (giant cell arteritis, GCA) headache include high-dose steroids (60–80 mg/day) sometime accompanied by other immunosuppression for up to 2 years and then a very slow taper [17]. Treatment can

Table 32.12 Diagnostic criteria of headaches attributed to cranial or cervical vascular disorders by ICHD-3 criteria [1]

Usually an acute new headache previously unknown to patient
Demonstration of cranial or cervical vascular disorder known to be able to cause headache
Evidence of causation established by at least two of the following:
Headache developed in temporal relation to development of the cervical or cranial vascular disorder
Either or both of the following:
Headache worsened with worsening of cervical or cranial vascular disease
Headache improved in parallel to improvement with cranial or cervical vascular disease
Headache has features typical of vascular headache
Presence of other evidence of causation

Table 32.13 Common causes of vascular headaches

Intracranial hemorrhage
Subarachnoid hemorrhage
Intracerebral hemorrhage (hypertensive, traumatic)
Intracerebral ischemic events
Thrombotic stroke
Transient ischemic attack (TIA)
Arteritis
Primary CNS angiitis
Giant cell arteritis
Venous thrombosis
Cerebral venous thrombosis
Unruptured vascular malformation
Arteriovenous malformation and fistula
Intracranial saccular aneurysm
Cavernous hemangioma
Vertebral or carotid artery-related pain
Post-carotid endarterectomy headache
Post-angioplasty headache
Cervical artery dissection
Post-aneurysm clipping headache
Post-stenting headache
Other vascular causes
Reversible cerebral vasoconstriction syndrome (RCVS)
Mitochondrial encephalopathy, lactic acidosis and stroke-like episodes (MELAS)
Cerebral autosomal dominant arteriopathy with subcortical infarcts and leukoencephalopathy (CADASIL)

be monitored and guided by inflammatory parameters such as the sedimentation rate.

- Reversible cerebral vascular syndrome (RCVS) should be distinguished from primary CNS angiitis, as the latter is an autoimmune vasculopathy and requires long-term immunosuppression, similar to GCA. RCVS is a transient vasospasm, presents as an acute abrupt thunderclap headache [18], and should be treated with a calcium channel blocker such as verapamil 240 mg po daily or nimodipine 60 mg po 6–8 h for 8–12 weeks. Total duration of therapy is not clearly defined and may be prolonged based on clinical context. RCVS can recur with repeated episodes of thunderclap headache over time.
- Certain medications such as triptans and ergots should be avoided in vascular-related headaches, because of the risk of worsening of neurovascular pathology such as the spasm of RCVS or further narrowing of blood vessels in GCA, ischemic stroke, or aneurysm. NSAIDs and aspirin should be avoided in headaches associated with intracranial hemorrhage.

Conclusions and Summary

Secondary headache evaluation should be carried out by keeping focus on potentially painful anatomical structures such as vessels, meninges, bony structures, cranial and peripheral nerves, myofascial structures around the head and neck, and their possible pathophysiologies. No age group is immune to developing secondary headaches, but older age groups are more likely to have a sinister etiology of headache such as neoplasm and vascular events including hemorrhage, GCA, stroke, and TIA.

Any new headache or change in pattern of headache in immunocompromised states such as HIV infection, post-chemotherapy, or malignancy should be considered as secondary and investigated. Use the SNOOP mnemonic to screen for secondary causes of headaches. MRI with and without contrast is a superior investigation to CT to look for any intracranial pathology. MR or CT angiogram is a specific investigation when suspecting an arterial disorder, and MR venography is the investigation of choice for cortical venous thrombosis. Successful management of secondary headaches may involve multiple medical specialties including neurology, neurosurgery, neurovascular surgery, neuro-oncology, pain management, and headache medicine.

References

1. Headache Classification Committee of the International Headache Society (IHS). The international classification of headache disorder, 3rd edition, Beta version. Cephalalgia. 2013;33:629–808.
2. Dodick DW. Clinical clues and clinical rules: primary versus secondary headache. Adv Stud Med. 2003;3:S550–5.
3. Rapoport A, Stang P, Gutterman DL, Cady R, Markley H, Weeks R, et al. Analgesic rebound headache in clinical practice: data from a physician survey. Headache. 1996;36(1):14–9.
4. Mathew NT. Transformed migraine, analgesic rebound, and other chronic daily headaches. Neurol Clin. 1997;15(1):167–86.
5. Bigal ME, Sheftell FD, Rapoport AM, Tepper SJ, Lipton RB. Chronic daily headache: identification of factors associated with induction and transformation. Headache. 2002;42(7):575–81.
6. Bigal ME, Serrano D, Buse D, Scher A, Stewart WF, Lipton RB. Acute migraine medications and evolution from episodic to chronic migraine: a longitudinal population-based study. Headache. 2008;48(8):1157–68.
7. Bigal ME, Lipton RB. Concepts and mechanisms of migraine chronification. Headache. 2008;48(1):7–15.
8. Srikiatkhachorn A. Chronic daily headache: a scientist's perspective. Headache. 2002;42(6):532–7.
9. Srikiatkhachorn A, Tarasub N, Govitrapong P. Effect of chronic analgesic exposure on the central serotonin system: a possible mechanism of analgesic abuse headache. Headache. 2000;40(5):343–50.
10. Srikiatkhachorn A, le Grand SM, Supornsilpchai W, Storer RJ. Pathophysiology of medication overuse headache-an update. Headache. 2014;54(1):204–10.
11. Moskowitz MA. Neurogenic versus vascular mechanisms of sumatriptan and ergot alkaloids in migraine. Trends Pharmacol Sci. 1992;13(8):307–11.
12. De Felice M, Porreca F. Opiate-induced persistent pronociceptive trigeminal neural adaptations: potential relevance to opiate-induced medication overuse headache. Cephalalgia. 2009;29(12):1277–84.
13. Katsarava Z, Schneeweiss S, Kurth T, et al. Incidence and predictors for chronicity of headache in patients with episodic migraine. Neurology. 2004;62:788–90.
14. Mokri B. Low cerebrospinal fluid pressure syndromes. Neurol Clin. 2004;22(1):55–74. vi.

15. Schievink WI. Spontaneous spinal cerebrospinal fluid leaks. Cephalalgia. 2008;28(12):1345–56.
16. Forsyth PA, Posner JB. Headaches in patients with brain tumors: a study of 111 patients. Neurology. 1993;43(9): 1678–83.
17. Weyand CM, Goronzy JJ. Giant-cell arteritis and polymyalgia rheumatica. Ann Intern Med. 2003; 139(6):505–15.
18. Calabrese LH, Dodick DW, Schwedt TJ, Singhal AB. Narrative review: reversible cerebral vasoconstriction syndromes. Ann Intern Med. 2007;146(1):34–44.

Orofacial Pain Syndromes (Trigeminal Neuralgia Excluded)

33

Ying (Amy) Ye and Jennifer S. Kriegler

Definitions

In the ICHD-3, *classical* describes pain when the cause is unknown. *Secondary* refers to pain when the cause is due to a specific lesion or abnormality. *Neuropathy* is defined as "A disturbance in function or pathological change in a nerve or nerves (in one nerve: **mononeuropathy,** several nerves: **mononeuritis multiplex**: when diffuse and bilateral: **polyneuropathy**). The term *neuropathy* is not intended to cover neurapraxia, neurotmesis, section of a nerve, disturbances of a nerve such as a result of transient impact such as a blow, stretching or epileptic discharge (the term ***neurogenic*** applies to pain attributed to such perturbations)." Neuralgia is simply defined as "pain in the distribution of the nerve or nerves" and is not reserved for paroxysmal pain.

Most diagnoses are categorized in Chap. 13 of the International Classification of Headache Disorders, painful cranial neuropathies and other facial pains; however, a few are discussed in Chap. 11.

Ying (Amy) Ye, MD, MPH • J.S. Kriegler, MD (✉)
Department of Neurology, Center for Neurological Restoration, Headache and Facial Pain, Clevelanad Clinic, Cleveland, OH, USA
e-mail: eimiie@gmail.com

Key Concepts

- Afferent fibers from the trigeminal nerve, glossopharyngeal and vagus nerves, and nervus intermedius mediate pain in the face, mouth and head. Lesions in the central or peripheral nervous system or perturbations of these nerves caused by temperature or compression result in head and face pain.
- Anticonvulsants, tricyclic antidepressants, serotonin/norepinephrine reuptake inhibitors, selective serotonin reuptake inhibitors, and muscle relaxants are all used either alone or in combination to treat face, mouth, and head pain. None are FDA approved for management of these conditions, except for the pain in Ramsay Hunt syndrome where the pain is caused by a herpes zoster infection.
- Glossopharyngeal neuralgia is severe, stabbing unilateral pain in the ear, beneath the angle of the jaw, tonsillar fossa, or base of the tongue. Swallowing, talking, and coughing may provoke the pain.
- Nervus intermedius neuralgia presents as brief paroxysms of pain deep in the internal auditory canal. It may be idiopathic or caused by herpes zoster infection. When caused by zoster, it is known as Ramsay Hunt syndrome.

J. Cheng, R.W. Rosenquist (eds.), *Fundamentals of Pain Medicine*,
https://doi.org/10.1007/978-3-319-64922-1_33

- Optic neuritis caused by demyelination of the optic nerve presents as severe retro-orbital pain increased with eye movement. Vision, predominantly central vision, is diminished. Severe head pain is seen in approximately 90% of individuals.
- Unilateral frontal or orbital pain may be due to ischemia of the oculomotor nerves which results in ipsilateral weakness of the third, fourth, or sixth cranial nerves causing diplopia.
- Tolosa-Hunt syndrome is caused by a granulomatous inflammation of the cavernous sinus, superior orbital fissure, or orbit and presents as unilateral orbital pain and diplopia caused by weakness of the third, fourth, or sixth cranial nerves.
- Raeder's syndrome (paratrigeminal oculosympathetic syndrome), a disorder of the middle cranial fossa or carotid artery, produces constant and unilateral pain in the first division (occasional spread to the second division) of the trigeminal nerve. It is associated with a Horner's syndrome.
- Painful ophthalmoplegic neuropathy presents in childhood and is characterized by repeated attacks of weakness of the oculomotor nerves, primarily cranial nerve III. Preceding the weakness or occurring concurrently with it is an ipsilateral headache.
- Burning mouth syndrome, previously known as glossodynia or stomatodynia, presents with burning mouth or tongue pain. It is most often seen in middle-aged women.
- Persistent idiopathic facial pain, also known as atypical facial pain, presents as facial or oral pain that occurs without a neurological deficit or abnormality on imaging.
- Lesions of the central nervous system particularly in the ascending connections of the trigeminal nerve or thalamus caused by multiple sclerosis or poststroke can produce unilateral facial pain.
- Temporomandibular joint dysfunction may produce headache which is provoked by manipulations of the affected mandible.

Glossopharyngeal Neuralgia

Epidemiology

Glossopharyngeal neuralgia is rarer than trigeminal neuralgia despite presenting with similar pain symptoms. In a 39-year retrospective study from 1945 to 1984 on the population of Rochester, Minnesota, it was found that the incidence of glossopharyngeal neuralgia in this population was 0.7/100,000 population/year.

Pathophysiology

Similar to trigeminal neuralgia, glossopharyngeal neuralgia can be idiopathic or due to secondary causes. Pain in glossopharyngeal neuralgia results when there is compression or injury to the cranial nerves IX and X by vascular structures such as carotid aneurysms, space-occupying lesions such as cerebellopontine angle tumors or peritonsillar abscess, or trauma. Glossopharyngeal neuralgia is more commonly associated with Paget's disease and Sjogren's syndrome than multiple sclerosis. *Eagle's syndrome* which presents with unilateral headache, neck pain, and pharyngeal or facial pain may occur if an ossified stylohyoid ligament compresses cranial nerve IX.

Clinical Features and Diagnosis (Table 33.1)

Patients with glossopharyngeal neuralgia present with short severe episodes of pain of around 30 s in duration. In between episodes of pain, patients may experience a dull aching sensation. The pain generally localizes to the left. Contrary to trigeminal neuralgia, a small portion of patients with glossopharyngeal neuralgia may have pain bilaterally. The pain most commonly affects the throat, but can also affect the mandible, ears, and tongue. Around 30% of patients will also experience radiation to the temples, neck, or shoulders. Most patients identify swallowing to be a trigger action. Some may also find talking, chewing, and sneezing to trigger episodes of pain. Diagnosis of glossopharyngeal neuralgia is primarily clinical. However, all patients should receive MRI/MRA to rule out tumors or vascular pathologies. AP skull films to evaluate the styloid process should be done as part of the evaluation.

Table 33.1 Glossopharyngeal neuralgia diagnostic criteria

A. Three attacks of unilateral pain described in B and C
B. Located in the posterior part of the tongue, tonsillar fossa, pharynx, beneath the angle of the lower jaw, and/or in the ear
C. Pain has three of the four characteristics:
1. Recurs in paroxysmal attacks that last from a few seconds to 2 min
2. Severe
3. Sharp, shooting, or stabbing quality
4. Precipitated by swallowing, coughing, talking, or yawning
D. No neurological deficit on exam or imaging
E. Not better accounted for by another ICHD-3 diagnosis

Table 33.2 Classical nervus intermedius neuralgia diagnostic criteria

A. Three attacks of unilateral pain described in B and C
B. Located in the auditory canal, sometimes pain radiates to the parieto-occipital region
C. Pain has three of four characteristics:
1. Recurs in paroxysmal attacks lasting from a few seconds to minutes
2. Severe
3. Stabbing, shooting, or sharping
4. Provoked by stimulation of a trigger area in the posterior wall of the auditory canal and/or periauricular region
D. No neurological deficit on exam or imaging
E. Not better accounted for by another ICHD-3 diagnosis

Treatment and Prevention

Glossopharyngeal neuralgia is typically treated with anticonvulsants as first line therapy.

- Carbamazepine, oxcarbazepine, and gabapentin are generally tried first.
  - Carbamazepine: start with a low dose at bedtime and increase slowly every 3 days to benefit or a total of 1200 mg in two divided doses. Monitor drug levels, CBC, and LFTs.
  - Oxcarbazepine: titrate doses to benefit or maximum dose of 1200 mg bid.
    - Monitor drug levels, CBC, and LFTs
  - Gabapentin: 300 mg per day (usually a bedtime dose) and increase to benefit or 3600 mg per day in three to four divided doses. Use caution in individuals with renal impairment.
  - Pregabalin: begin with 50 mg at night and gradually increase to benefit or 150 mg three times per day. Use caution in individuals with renal impairment
- Other antiepileptic medications
- Muscle relaxants such as baclofen either alone or in combination with an antiepileptic.
  - Baclofen 10 mg at bedtime and increase every 3 days by 10 mg to a maximum dose of 120 mg in three divided doses daily. Addition of baclofen to an anticonvulsant may increase efficacy of the anticonvulsant.
- Surgery may be recommended when a defined lesion is discovered. During the surgery, it is recommended to confirm this diagnosis with nerve stimulation.

Nervus Intermedius (Facial Nerve) Neuralgia

Classical Nervus Intermedius Neuralgia

Epidemiology

Classical nervus intermedius neuralgia, also known as geniculate neuralgia, is a rare disorder with little known about its incidence or prevalence. This disorder most commonly affects middle aged women, with a median age of onset of 41 years.

Pathophysiology

The pathophysiology behind classical nervus intermedius neuralgia is not well understood. One current theory is that nervus intermedius neuralgia is caused by compression of a small branch of the facial nerve, the intermediate nerve of Wrisberg, by a blood vessel.

Clinical Features and Diagnosis (Table 33.2)

Patients with classical nervus intermedius neuralgia present with unilateral electrical shock-like sensations in the inner ear. The duration of the pain usually lasts for several seconds, but some patients report pain lasting up to 2 min. Most patients also report a trigger zone in the posterior area of the ear canal, and will avoid contact to this area. In general, patients are pain-free in between episodes of pain. Some patients will describe changes in lacrimation or salivation and occasionally taste may be altered. Diagnosis of classical nervus intermedius neuralgia is based on clinical presentation. MRI should be done to rule out lesions or tumors of the posterior fossa or brain stem. MRA can also be done to confirm compression of the nervus intermedius by nearby blood vessels. Care should also be taken to rule out herpes zoster, which may also cause similar symptoms.

Treatment and Prevention

First-line treatment for classical nervus intermedius neuralgia:

- Carbamazepine: start with a low dose at bedtime and increase slowly every 3 days to benefit or a total of 1200 mg in two divided doses.
- Monitor drug levels, CBC, and LFTs.
- Oxcarbazepine: titrate doses to benefit or maximum dose of 1200 mg bid. Monitor drug levels, CBC, and LFTs.
- Gabapentin: 300 mg per day (usually a bedtime dose) and increase to benefit or 3600 mg per day in three to four divided doses. Use caution in individuals with renal impairment.
- Pregabalin: begin with 50 mg at night and gradually increase to benefit or 150 mg three times per day. Use caution in individuals with renal impairment.
- Baclofen 10 mg at bedtime and increase every 3 days by 10 mg to a maximum dose of 120 mg in three divided doses daily. Addition of baclofen to an anticonvulsant may increase efficacy of the anticonvulsant.
- Surgical options include excision of the nervus intermedius or decompression of the cranial nerves; however, this is rarely a satisfactory resolution to the problem.

Nervus Intermedius (Facial Nerve) Neuralgia Attributed to Herpes Zoster (Ramsay Hunt)

Epidemiology

Secondary nervus intermedius neuropathy, also known as Ramsay Hunt, or herpes zoster oticus, is the second most common cause of facial palsies unrelated to trauma. Of children with facial palsies, 16% are to have been caused by this disease. Herpes zoster oticus is also responsible for 18% of adult cases of facial palsies. There is an increase in incidence of this disease with age. It is rare to occur in children younger than 6 years of age. There have been no associations found with gender. Mean age of onset is around 50 years for both men and women.

Pathophysiology

Previous infection by the varicella zoster virus results in dormant virus in the dorsal root ganglia. Reactivation of this virus can result in herpes zoster. Herpes zoster oticus can develop as a result of viral infection of cranial nerve VII, specifically the geniculate ganglion.

Clinical Features and Diagnosis (Table 33.3)

Patients with acute herpes zoster experience a sharp, tingling, itching, and often painful sensation 2–3 days prior to development of a macular/papular rash. Both the sensation and the rash are dermatomal, and do not cross the midline. The rash will then develop into vesicles and pustules,

Table 33.3 Nervus intermedius (facial nerve) neuralgia attributed to herpes zoster (Ramsay Hunt) diagnostic criteria

A.	Unilateral facial pain fulfilling criterion C
B.	Herpetic eruption in the ear and/or oral mucosa, in the distribution of the nervus intermedius
C.	Evidence of causation includes both of the following:
1.	Pain precedes the herpetic eruption by <7 days
2.	Pain localized to the distribution of the nervus intermedius
D.	Peripheral facial weakness
E.	Not better accounted for by another ICHD-3 diagnosis

with new lesions appearing in 3–5 days and crusting in 7–10 days. Herpes zoster oticus develops in patients who experience reactivation of the varicella zoster virus in the geniculate ganglion. These patients will present with ipsilateral facial paralysis and ear pain, along with vesicles in the same ear, along the pinna, and in the external auditory canal. Many individuals also complain of altered taste and hearing perception. Some patients may also have increased lacrimation as well. Vertigo is another common complaint. Diagnosis of herpes zoster oticus is based on clinical presentation and the presence of herpes vesicles around the ear. Confirmation may be done using direct immunofluorescence assay or polymerase chain reaction (PCR) for detection of the varicella zoster virus.

Treatment

Acute herpes zoster and associated herpes zoster oticus can be treated with antiviral therapies. Indications for use of these agents include:

- Age >50 years old
- Moderate to severe pain
- Severe rash
- Facial or eye involvement
- Increased risk for complications of herpes zoster
- Immunocompromised patients

For non-immunocompromised patients, the following antiviral therapies are recommended.

- Acyclovir: 800 mg PO five times a day for 7–10 days
- Famiciclovir: 500 mg PO three times a day for 7 days
- Valcyclovir: 1 g PO three times a day for 7 days
- Brivudin: 125 mg PO one time a day for 7 days

Immunocompromised patients may require intravenous antiviral therapy:

- Acyclovir 10 mg/kg IV every 8 h for 7–10 days

Pain Control

Patients with herpes zoster oticus also benefit with immediate treatment of prednisone which can dramatically improve pain.

- Prednisone 60 mg × 2 days followed by a taper over 10 days.
- Gabapentin (300–3600 mg daily).
- Carbamazepine or oxcarbazepine.
- Opioids can be used, but for short-term pain control only.
- Sympathetic neural blockades in the stellate ganglion.
- Ice packs.
- Skin application of aluminum sulfate.

Prevention

To prevent herpes zoster and post-herpetic neuralgia, the herpes zoster vaccine may be given to individuals 50 years or older as part of the routine medical care. The vaccine contains almost 14 times the concentration as the chickenpox vaccine. As this vaccine is a live attenuated vaccine, it should not be administered to immunocompromised patients. To control spread of herpes zoster, it is advised that patients avoid touching the affected skin areas. Airborne precautions should also be used for immunocompromised individuals.

Optic Neuritis

Epidemiology

There are approximately 6.4 new cases of optic neuritis per 100,000 persons per year. Optic neuritis is usually seen in patients with multiple sclerosis. Of patients with multiple sclerosis, 15–20% experience optic neuritis as their first presenting symptom. About 50% of these patients will have optic neuritis in their lifetime. Optic neuritis affects more women than men and usually patients between ages of 20 and 50 years of age. Caucasians are at higher risk for developing optic neuritis.

Pathophysiology

Inflammatory demyelination of the optic nerve results in optic neuritis. The process of inflammation and demyelination leading to axonal loss and gliosis that occurs in multiple sclerosis is also seen in the development of optic neuritis. While most cases of optic neuritis are secondary to multiple sclerosis, optic neuritis can also develop from infections and mitochondrial disorders as well.

Clinical Features and Diagnosis (Table 33.4)

Patients with acute onset of optic neuritis will experience a rapid loss of vision over a period of a few hours to days, progressing no further than 1 to 2 weeks. Most patients lose color and central visual acuity and can present with a central scotoma. Over 90% of patients experience pain that is exacerbated by eye movement. Symptoms are unilateral, although some patients may have bilateral optic neuritis. Pain resolves after 1 week, and vision returns after 2–4 weeks in 75% of patients. Some patients may have chronic optic neuritis, in which they continue to experience visual and color perception loss.

Diagnosis is made by clinical presentation and funduscopic exam showing optic disk swelling. It is suggested that patients also receive an MRI to rule out multiple sclerosis. In atypical cases, such as in patients presenting with bilateral vision loss and pain, a lumbar puncture should be considered to rule out any infectious processes.

Table 33.4 Optic neuritis diagnostic criteria

A. Unilateral or bilateral headache fulfilling criterion C
B. Clinical, electrophysiological, imaging, and/or laboratory evidence confirming optic neuritis
C. Evidence of causation demonstrated by both of the following:
1. Headache occurs in temporal relationship to optic neuritis.
2. Headache has one or both of the following features:
(a) Localized in retro-orbital, orbital, frontal, and/or temporal regions
(b) Worsened by eye movement
D. Not better accounted for by another ICHD-3 diagnosis

Treatment and Prevention

For acute optic neuritis, patients should be treated with methylprednisolone 1 g IV daily for 3 days along with 1 mg/kg of oral prednisone for 11 days followed by 4 days of tapering. For patients who do not respond to steroid therapy, plasma exchange may be used. Those experiencing chronic optic neuritis can undergo interferon treatment, which may also help in delaying or preventing symptoms of multiple sclerosis.

Tolosa-Hunt Syndrome

Epidemiology

Tolosa-Hunt syndrome is a rare disorder that affects one per million persons per year. There is no association with age or gender.

Pathophysiology

Tolosa-Hunt syndrome is an idiopathic inflammatory condition of the cavernous sinus. Formation of granulomas along with infiltration of lymphocytes, plasma cells, and fibroblasts along the walls of the cavernous sinus are part of the inflammatory process. The result of the inflammation is a buildup of pressure against the structures inside the cavernous sinus. Cranial nerves III, IV, and VI and the maxillary branch of cranial nerve V can be affected. In some patients, the inflammation can extend intracranially and can also affect structures in the orbit.

Clinical Features and Diagnosis (Table 33.5)

Patients with Tolosa-Hunt syndrome present with episodes of unilateral orbital pain. If untreated, pain can last for approximately 8 weeks, after which, it will spontaneously resolve. In most cases, the pain is unilateral; for 4–5% of patients, the pain may be bilateral. Quality of the pain can range from dull and boring to intense and stabbing. Along with orbital pain, patients may also experience cranial nerve paralysis depending on the extent of inflammation. Paralysis occurs 2 weeks after development of the initial pain. Cranial nerves III, VI, V, and IV are affected in 85%, 70%, 30%, and 29% of patients, respectively. Half of the patients affected with Tolosa-

Table 33.5 Tolosa-Hunt syndrome diagnostic criteria

A. Unilateral headache fulfilling criterion C
B. Both of the following:
1. Granulomatous inflammation of the cavernous sinus, superior orbital fissure, or orbit, demonstrated by MRI or biopsy
2. Weakness of one or more of the ipsilateral cranial nerves III, IV, and/or VI
C. Evidence of causation demonstrated by both of the following:
1. Headache precedes weakness of the nerves III, IV, and/or VI by 2 weeks or develops concurrently with it
2. Headache involves the ipsilateral brow and eye
D. Not better accounted for by another ICHD-3 diagnosis

Hunt syndrome will have recurrent episodes of pain throughout their lifetime. Diagnosis is made by the clinical presentation of headache preceding paralysis of any of the cranial nerves traversing the cavernous sinus, as well as MRI. MRI is necessary to exclude other causes of painful ophthalmoplegias such as diabetes mellitus, basal meningitis, sarcoidosis, or tumors. Biopsy will confirm granulomatous inflammation of the cavernous sinus or orbit.

Treatment and Prevention

- Prednisone 1 mg/kg × 3 days. Taper dose for 2 weeks. If unresponsive to prednisone:
  - Low-dose radiotherapy
  - Immunosuppressive agents: cyclosporine or methotrexate

Follow-up with MRI every 1–2 months until findings normalize, and then MRIs should be performed every 6 months for 2 years.

Paratrigeminal Oculosympathetic (Raeder's) Syndrome

Epidemiology

Raeder's syndrome is a rare disorder affecting men between the ages of 18 to 65. Onset of Raeder's syndrome usually occurs in middle to old age. The exact incidence of this disorder is unknown.

Table 33.6 Paratrigeminal oculosympathetic (Raeder's) syndrome diagnostic criteria

A. Constant, unilateral headache fulfilling criterion C
B. Evidence on imaging of underlying disease of either the middle cranial fossa or the ipsilateral carotid artery
C. Evidence of causation demonstrated by both of the following:
1. Headache develops in temporal relation to the onset of the underlying disorder
2. Headache has one or both of the following:
(a) Localized to the distribution of the ophthalmic division of the trigeminal nerve, with or without spread to the maxillary division
(b) Worsened by eye movement
D. Ipsilateral Horner's syndrome
E. Not better accounted for by another ICHD-3 diagnosis

Pathophysiology

Raeder's syndrome is caused by a space occupying lesion in the middle cranial fossa at the area where the oculosympathetic nerves intersect the internal carotid artery. Raeder's syndrome is similar to Horner's syndrome with the exception of anhidrosis; the lesion in Raeder's syndrome is thus distal to the carotid bifurcation. Carotid dissections, carotid artery disease, and inflammatory conditions can affect this area and produce Raeder's syndrome.

Clinical Features and Diagnosis (Table 33.6)

The presentation of Raeder's syndrome is similar to that of Horner's syndrome with the exception of preserved sweating in Raeder's syndrome. Patients present with severe unilateral facial pain and headache due to involvement of the ophthalmic division of the trigeminal nerve. Most patients experience spontaneous resolution of pain and paresis within 2 months. Some patients may experience recurrent episodes. Diagnosis is made with MRI to detect lesions in the middle cranial fossa and with MRA to evaluate for carotid artery dissection.

Treatment and Prevention

There is limited data on effective treatment for Raeder's syndrome. Some patients have reported effective pain relief with tricyclic antidepressants such as amitriptyline or nortriptyline and antiepileptic medications like carbamazepine, oxcarbazepine, or gabapentin.

Recurrent Painful Ophthalmoplegic Neuropathy

Epidemiology

Recurrent painful ophthalmoplegic neuropathy, also previously known as ophthalmoplegic migraine, is a rare disorder affecting 0.7 per million patients per year. This disorder commonly begins in childhood during the first decade. In rare cases, patients may develop this condition during adulthood.

Pathophysiology

The exact pathophysiology of recurrent painful ophthalmoplegic neuropathy is unknown. There are currently two proposed theories of how this condition develops. One idea is that recurrent painful ophthalmoplegic neuropathy is a result of demyelinating neuropathy of the oculomotor nerve. Some individuals may have an anatomy in which they are prone to leakage of neuropeptides from the cerebral vessels in the area where the oculomotor nerve exits the brain stem; this in turn causes the sterile inflammation that eventually leads to demyelination of the oculomotor nerve. Another theory is that uncontrolled migraines may cause the symptoms experienced by patients with recurrent painful ophthalmoplegic neuropathy. The prominence of these two theories is why this condition has been known either as recurrent painful ophthalmoplegic neuropathy or ophthalmoplegic migraine.

Clinical Features and Diagnosis (Table 33.7)

The classic presentation of recurrent painful ophthalmoplegic neuropathy is a child with a severe unilateral headache lasting for several days up to 2 weeks. Following the headache, the child will experience ipsilateral mydriasis, ptosis, and diplopia as a result of oculomotor nerve involvement. These episodes are often recurrent. Recurrent painful ophthalmoplegic neuropathy is a diagnosis of exclusion. Patients must also fit the diagnostic criteria of having at least two attacks of the above described symptoms. Many patients have been found to have gadolinium enhancement of the cisternal segment of the oculomotor nerve on MRI, although in some, primarily adult patients, there are no abnormalities found on MRI.

Table 33.7 Recurrent painful ophthalmoplegic neuropathy diagnostic criteria

A.	Two attacks fulfilling criterion B
B.	Unilateral headache accompanied by ipsilateral weakness of one, two, or all three ocular motor nerves
C.	Orbital, parasellar, or posterior fossa lesion is excluded
D.	Not better accounted for by another ICHD-3

Treatment and Prevention

There is limited data on treatment of recurrent painful ophthalmoplegic neuropathy. Corticosteroids, calcium channel blockers, and beta-blockers have been shown to alleviate symptoms in small trials and case reports.

Burning Mouth Syndrome

Epidemiology

Burning mouth syndrome is found most commonly in postmenopausal women; 10–40% of women report symptoms of a burning pain sensation in the tongue or oral mucosal membranes. It is rare to find this in younger women or men. Many patients with burning mouth syndrome also have sleep dysfunction, psychosocial, or psychiatric disorders.

Pathophysiology

The pathophysiology of burning mouth syndrome is complex. Currently, burning mouth syndrome can be divided into three subclasses of different pathophysiology. Of patients with burning mouth syndrome, 50–65% belong to the first group, in which pain sensation is caused by peripheral small diameter fiber neuropathy in the intraoral mucosa. Twenty to Twenty-five percentage of patients are affected by dysfunctional lingual, mandibular, or trigeminal nerves. The third group, consisting of 20–40% of patients with burning mouth syndrome, experience symptoms due to

Table 33.8 Burning mouth syndrome diagnostic criteria

A. Oral pain that fulfills criteria B and C
B. Recurs daily for >2 h per day for >3 months
C. Pain characteristics include both:
1. Burning quality
2. Felt superficially in the oral mucosa
D. Oral mucosa is of normal appearance, and clinical examination including sensory testing is normal
E. Not better accounted for by another ICHD-3 diagnosis

hypofunctioning dopaminergic neurons in the basal ganglia which can then cause central pain.

Clinical Features and Diagnosis (Table 33.8)

Patients with burning mouth syndrome present with superficial burning sensation of the oral mucosa; the anterior two-thirds of the tongue, hard palate, and the lower lip are frequently affected. Many patients experience pain bilaterally and symmetrically. The pain begins mid-morning and increases through the day, but will alleviate at night time. Duration of pain lasts for more than 2 h per day for over 3 months. Many patients also experience changes in taste as well. Onset of burning mouth syndrome is usually spontaneous, although some patients report a preceding dental procedure or trauma. In two-thirds of the patients, spontaneous recovery from burning mouth syndrome occurs within 6–7 months of the initial start of symptoms. Diagnosis is done based on clinical symptoms and exclusion. It is important to rule out other causes of oral burning including local causes such as candidal infections, lichen planus, or hyposalivation and systemic causes such as medications including chemotherapeutic agents, anemia, deficiencies of vitamin B12 or folic acid, or Sjogren's syndrome.

Treatment and Prevention

Multimodal treatment for burning mouth syndrome has been found to be the most successful. If a cause is found, treatment for the primary disorder as well as pain control is necessary. Recommended pharmacological treatment for burning mouth syndrome includes tricyclic antidepressants, benzodiazepines, and anticonvulsants. Successful dosages vary between patients. Pain relief has also been found with use of capsaicin mouth rinse, tongue protectors with aloe vera, and acupuncture.

Table 33.9 Persistent idiopathic facial pain (PIFP) diagnostic criteria

A. Facial and/or oral pain that fulfills criteria B and C
B. Recurs daily for >2 h per day for >3 months
C. Pain has both characteristics:
1. Poorly localized and does not follow the distribution of a peripheral nerve
2. Dull, aching, or nagging quality
D. Clinical neurological examination is normal
E. A dental cause is excluded by appropriate investigations
F. Not better accounted for by another ICHD-3 diagnosis

Persistent Idiopathic Facial Pain (PIFP)

This was previously known as atypical facial pain.

Epidemiology

Persistent idiopathic facial pain is a rare disorder affecting 0.03–1% of the general population, and 3–12% of patients who have undergone endodontic procedures. More women than men are affected. Often other comorbid pain conditions such as fibromyalgia or irritable bowel syndrome are present. Psychiatric diagnosis is also commonly seen and there is a high level of psychosocial disability in these patients.

Pathophysiology

The pathophysiology behind persistent idiopathic facial pain is currently unknown. One proposed theory is that persistent idiopathic facial pain is due to peripheral nerve injury or demyelination. Another theory is that the persistent pain sensation is caused by increased dopamine transmission and increased nociceptor sensitivity.

Clinical Features and Diagnosis (Table 33.9)

Patients present with unilateral facial pain that involves any of the areas from the forehead to the lower jaw. Unlike trigeminal neuralgia, the pain is consistent and persistent, occurring daily for at least 3 months. Patients do not typically experience paroxysmal episodes of pain. Patients variably describe the pain as deep and intense or dull, aching, or nagging. Some patients may be able to identify a specific incident such as minor facial trauma or dental procedure preceding developing symptoms of persistent facial pain; however, the majority of patients report spontaneous development of facial pain. Diagnosis is made by exclusion. It is important to rule out other causes of facial pain including migraine, trigeminal neuralgia, and head and neck malignancies. Patients with persistent idiopathic facial pain have no abnormalities on clinical exam or imaging.

Treatment and Prevention

Patients with persistent idiopathic facial pain benefit from a multidisciplinary treatment approach.

- Therapy:
  - Tricyclic antidepressants: amitriptyline at 25–100 mg daily. Begin with 10 mg at bedtime and increase slowly by 10 mg once a week to benefit or 100 mg.
  - Antiepileptics: gabapentin and pregabalin.
  - Serotonin/norepinephrine reuptake inhibitors (SNRI): venlafaxine, desvenlafaxine, and duloxetine.
  - Selective serotonin reuptake inhibitors (SSRI): fluoxetine, citalopram, escitalopram.
  - Lamotrigine 200–400 mg daily plus venlafaxine 150–225 mg daily.
  - Behavioral therapy including cognitive behavioral therapy, hypnosis, and stress-coping management.
  - It is important to relay to patients that surgery and other invasive treatments may be of more harm than help in treating persistent idiopathic facial pain.

Central Neuropathic Pain Attributed to Multiple Sclerosis (MS)

Epidemiology

The prevalence of patients with central neuropathic pain attributed to multiple sclerosis is approximately 50%. The prevalence of central neuropathic pain increases with age and duration of disease, peaking at 40–60 years of age and 10–20 years of disease. However, there is no increase in risk associated with these factors. There is no association with severity of disability caused by multiple sclerosis.

Pathophysiology

Central neuropathic pain attributed to MS is currently thought to be caused by damage to nerves in the central nervous system that are involved in the perception of pain. Damage to these nerves is a result of the demyelination inherent in multiple sclerosis. The generation of pain may be triggered by either ectopic impulses along the demyelinated nerve or develop from uninhibited pain pathways.

Clinical Features and Diagnosis (Table 33.10)

Patients with central neuropathic pain due to MS often experience altered temperature and pain sensations due to the involvement of the spinothalamic tract. Patients may experience brief episodes of sporadic pain sensation; the majority of patients will experience chronic and constant pain. Patients often describe central neuropathic pain as burning and intense. Individuals with multiple sclerosis can experience acute and intermittent neuropathic pain leading to the development of trigeminal neuralgia, L'Hermitte's sign, optic neuritis, and glossopharyngeal neuralgia. Constant central pain experienced by patients with MS is most commonly felt in the legs and feet bilaterally; this is a condition known as central dysesthetic neuropathic pain. Of those with central neuropathic pain to the limbs, 66–95% of these patients also have accompanied loss of temperature sensation. Diagnosis of central

Table 33.10 Central neuropathic pain attributed to multiple sclerosis (MS) diagnostic criteria

A.	Facial and/or head pain that fulfills criterion C
B.	Multiple sclerosis (MS) has been diagnosed. MRI demonstrates a demyelinating lesion in the brain stem or ascending projections of the trigeminal nuclei
C.	Pain developed in temporal relation to the demyelinating lesion, or led to its discovery
D.	Not better accounted for by another ICHD-3 diagnosis

neuropathic pain attributed to MS is made based on clinical presentation, diagnosis of multiple sclerosis, and MRI results demonstrating lesions in the central nervous system.

Treatment and Prevention

- Tricyclic antidepressants, such as amitriptyline, nortriptyline, or clomipramine.
- In patients who do not respond to these medications, antiepileptic medications such as carbamazepine or lamotrigine may be used.
- Some patients respond positively to intrathecally administered baclofen.
- Multidisciplinary pain program including medications, cognitive behavioral strategies, and physical therapy.

Central Poststroke Pain (CPSP)

Epidemiology

Of patients with stroke, 8–46% develop central poststroke pain. This disorder appears most commonly in patients with stroke to the lateral medulla or to the ventroposterior aspect of the thalamus. There is no established risk of developing central poststroke pain with gender, age, or side of lesion. While most patients will develop central poststroke pain within the first 6 months of the initial stroke, central poststroke pain can appear anytime within the first 10 years. Time of onset is dependent on the area of the lesion.

Pathophysiology

There are several theories on the mechanism behind central poststroke pain. It is thought that this pain disorder will occur due to damage to structures involved in the somatosensory pathway from stroke. Interruptions in this somatosensory pathway may then result in abnormal perceptions of sensation, leading to pain. Below are four of several predominating theories on the pathophysiology behind central poststroke pain:

1. Central sensitization theory: Lesions from the stroke may result in increased excitability of nociceptive neurons leading to increased pain perception.
2. Central disinhibition theory: A stroke may lead to damage to structures that normally inhibit the pain response. Absence of the inhibitory system can then result in heightened perception of pain.
3. Thalamic dysfunction theory: The thalamus is an important structure in the pain pathway, and disruption to it from stroke may lead to altered processing of pain.
4. Dynamic reverberation theory: There may be an oscillatory pattern operating between the thalamus and cortex, which, when disrupted by a stroke, can produce altered body sensations, ultimately leading to central poststroke pain.

Table 33.11 Central poststroke pain (CPSP) diagnostic criteria

A. Facial and/or head pain that fulfills criterion C
B. Ischemic or hemorrhagic stroke has occurred
C. Evidence of causation demonstrated by both of the following:
1. Pain develops within 6 months of the stroke
2. Imaging (usually MRI) demonstrates a vascular lesion in an appropriate site
D. Not better accounted for by another ICHD-3 diagnosis

Clinical Features and Diagnosis (Table 33.11)

Central poststroke pain presents similarly to other central neuropathic pain syndromes. Generally, patients will complain of hemi-pain, localized to either the face or upper or lower extremity. The right side is more commonly affected than the left. The location of pain often correlates to the site of the stroke, though it is also possible for patients to complain of diffuse pain that wanders from one location to another. Most individuals describe their pain as burning or aching; the pain is often spontaneous or constant. Diagnosis of central poststroke pain is dependent on the clinical presentation, and MRI results documenting site of lesion. For many patients, the neurological exam should also show increased sensitivity to touch in areas of pain.

Treatment and Prevention

Treatment for central poststroke pain is similar to that of other central neuropathic syndromes.

- Tricyclic antidepressants.
- Tricyclic antidepressants plus gabapentin or pregabalin.
- Carbamazepine or oxcarbazepine.
- Selective serotonin or norepinephrine reuptake inhibitors.
- Psychological or behavioral therapy.
- Invasive treatment options include spinal cord or deep brain stimulation; these options have yet to be shown to be effective in large clinical trials.

Headache Due to Retropharyngeal Tendinitis

Epidemiology

Retropharyngeal tendinitis is considered to be a rare disease, and little is known on incidence or prevalence of this disorder. Recent studies have shown, however, that it may be more common than once thought. The benign course of this disease and symptoms similar to other disorders contribute to under diagnosis of retropharyngeal tendinitis.

Pathophysiology

The pathophysiology behind retropharyngeal tendinitis is not well understood. Some patients may develop this disease due to abnormally increased calcium hydroxyapatite deposition in the musculotendinous areas around the attachment at the C1–C2 level of the spine. It may also result from damage to the longus colli muscle from repetitive use or trauma. All of these causes may lead to inflammation of the muscle and cause the painful syndrome.

Clinical Features and Diagnosis (Table 33.12)

Patients with retropharyngeal tendinitis present with spontaneous onset of neck pain radiating up the neck and up to the back of the head. The pain is usually intense and can range from being sharp and pulsating to dull and aching. Most patients also report pain in the neck and head with neck movement. Low-grade fever and dysphagia may also accompany these symptoms. Usually, patients recover within 1–2 weeks. Diagnosis is made by X-ray or CT imaging showing calcifications in the C1–C2 region with prevertebral soft tissue swelling in the C1–C4 region.

Table 33.12 Headache due to retropharyngeal tendinitis diagnostic criteria

A. Any headache that fulfills criterion C
B. Retropharyngeal tendonitis is demonstrated by imaging evidence of abnormal swelling of prevertebral soft tissues at upper cervical spine levels
C. Evidence of causation is demonstrated by two or more of the following:
1. Headache develops in temporal relation to the onset of the retropharyngeal tendonitis
2. Either or both of the following:
(a) Headache significantly worsens in parallel with progression of the retropharyngeal tendonitis
(b) Headache significantly improves or resolves in parallel with improvement in or resolution of the retropharyngeal tendonitis
3. Headache is significantly aggravated by extension of the neck, rotation of the head, and/or swallowing
4. There is tenderness over the spinous processes of the upper three cervical vertebrae
D. Not better accounted for by another ICHD-3 diagnosis

Treatment and Prevention

Retropharyngeal tendinitis spontaneously remits in 1–2 weeks.

- NSAIDs for pain and inflammation control
- Corticosteroids
- Limit neck movement

Chronic cases of retropharyngeal tendinitis are rare.

Headache Attributed to Temporomandibular Joint Dysfunction (TMD)

Epidemiology

In the United States, the prevalence of TMD in adults with at least one sign or symptom is between 33% and 75%. Women and individuals between 20 and 50 years of age are at a higher risk for developing TMD.

Pathophysiology

TMD syndrome has a wide range of causes. This disorder can result from congenital malformations, infections, or trauma to the temporomandibular joint. Other causes include inflammation or displacement of the joint. Sometimes TMD can result from hypermobility or hypomobility of the joint, such as in cases of post-radiation fibrosis. Muscular pathologies can also cause TMD. These causes include myositis and myospasms. While much is understood about the etiology behind TMD, the exact pathophysiology of how pain is produced is still unclear. In many patients, there is no definite tissue damage to explain the sensations of pain felt among these individuals. One prevailing theory is that pain felt in patients with TMD is due to altered pain processing systems in the central nervous system resulting from multifactorial causes.

Clinical Features and Diagnosis (Table 33.13)

Patients with TMD present most commonly with unilateral facial pain localized around the ear, temporal and periorbital regions, near the mandible or the posterior neck. This pain is usually constant, dull, and aching; the pain worsens with jaw movement. Many patients may experience episodes of pain, and remain pain-free in between episodes. Other common symptoms reported are ear pain or discomfort, unilateral morning headaches, and neck pain. Patients also frequently experience locking of the jaws, most commonly in the closed position. Many individuals will also feel clicking or popping in the temporomandibular joint region with jaw movement. Diagnosis is made based on clinical presentation and physical exam findings of pain or clicking noise with jaw movement or limited jaw motion. Physical exam should also reveal normal cranial nerve function. Imaging is currently controversial in the diagnosis of TMD. However, plain radiographs may sometimes be useful in confirming suspected TMD.

Table 33.13 Headache attributed to temporomandibular joint dysfunction (TMD) diagnostic criteria

A. Any headache that fulfills criterion C
B. Clinical and/or imaging evidence of a pathological process affecting the temporomandibular joint (TMJ), muscles of mastication, and/or associated structures
C. Evidence of causation demonstrated by at least two of the following:
1. Headache develops in a proximal relationship to the onset of the temporomandibular disorder
2. Either or both of the following:
(a) Headache significantly worsens with progression of the temporomandibular disorder
(b) Headache significantly improves or resolves simultaneously with improvement or resolution of the temporomandibular disorder
3. The headache is produced or worsened by active jaw movements, passive movements through the range of motion of the jaw, and/or provocative maneuver of temporomandibular structures such as pressure on the TMJ and surrounding muscles of mastication
4. Headache, when unilateral, is ipsilateral to affected temporomandibular joint
D. Not better accounted for by another ICHD-3 diagnosis

Treatment and Prevention

Acute pain from TMD syndrome is largely managed with NSAIDS.

- Naproxen 250–500 mg twice a day for 10–14 days.
- In patients with pain on palpation over the temporomandibular joint: cyclobenzaprine 10 mg at bedtime or other musculoskeletal relaxants such as baclofen or tizanidine.
- Severe, acute pain: diazepam 2.5–5 mg or clonazepam 0.5 mg for 2–3 weeks. This should not be used as long-term therapy.
- Individuals refractory to these medications:
  - Add a tricyclic antidepressant.

Non-pharmacological Treatment

- Adequate patient education. Learning about how to avoid triggers is key to preventing further pain episodes.

- Behavioral management, including both psychosocial and physical (such as positional changes in sleeping or sitting) have also helped reduce pain in TMD syndrome.
- Massaging the area of the temporomandibular joint.
- Splints or bite blocks.
- Physical therapy.

In Cases of Refractory TMD

- Botulinum toxin injections
- Intra-articular injections
- Trigger point injections

Surgery is reserved for patients who have structural pathologies causing this disorder, or are refractory to more than 6 months of nonsurgical management. For the majority of patients, medical management alone is effective. Forty percent of patients report resolution of symptoms spontaneously. Only 5% of adults develop chronic pain from TMD syndrome.

Suggested Reading

1. Acute calcific tendinitis of the longus colli muscle: case report and review of the literature. Springer. [cited 2014 Jan 3]. Available from http://link.springer.com/article/10.1007%2Fs00586-012-2584-5/fulltext.html.
2. Balcer LJ. Optic neuritis. N Engl J Med. 2006;354(12):1273–80.
3. Cairns BE. Pathophysiology of TMD pain–basic mechanisms and their implications for pharmacotherapy. J Oral Rehabil. 2010 May;37(6):391–410.
4. Charleston L 4th. Burning mouth syndrome: a review of recent literature. Curr Pain Headache Rep. 2013;17(6):336.
5. Chung T, Rebello R, Gooden EA. Retropharyngeal calcific tendinitis: case report and review of literature. Emerg Radiol. 2005;11(6):375–80.
6. Didier H, Marchetti C, Borromeo G, Tullo V, Bussone G, Santoro F. Persistent idiopathic facial pain: multidisciplinary approach and assumption of comorbidity. Neurol Sci. 2010;31(1):189–95.
7. Erman AB, Kejner AE, Hogikyan ND, Feldman EL. Disorders of cranial nerves IX and X. Semin Neurol. 2009;29(1):85–92.
8. Evans RW, Agostoni E. Persistent idiopathic facial pain. Headache J Head Face Pain. 2006;46(8):1298–300.
9. Gelfand AA, Gelfand JM, Prabakhar P, Goadsby PJ. Ophthalmoplegic "migraine" or recurrent ophthalmoplegic cranial neuropathy: new cases and a systematic review. J Child Neurol. 2012;27(6):759–66.
10. Goadsby PJ. "Paratrigeminal" paralysis of the oculopupillary sympathetic system. J Neurol Neurosurg Psychiatry. 2002;72(3):297–9.
11. Harnier S, Kuhn J, Harzheim A, Bewermeyer H, Limmroth V. Retropharyngeal tendinitis: a rare differential diagnosis of severe headaches and neck pain. Headache J Head Face Pain. 2008;48(1):158–61.
12. http://www.ihs-classification.org/_downloads/mixed/International-Headache-Classification-III-ICHD-III-2013-Beta.pdf.
13. Jääskeläinen SK. Pathophysiology of primary burning mouth syndrome. Clin Neurophysiol Off J Int Fed Clin Neurophysiol. 2012;123(1):71–7.
14. Jensen DR, Mitsikostas DDD, Wöber DC. Persistent idiopathic facial pain. In: Martelletti P, Steiner TJ, editors. Handbook of headache. Milan: Springer; 2011. p. 505–13. [Cited 2013 Dec 18]. Available from http://link.springer.com/referenceworkentry/10.1007/978-88-470-1700-9_40.
15. Kline LB, Hoyt WF. The Tolosa-hunt syndrome. J Neurol Neurosurg Psychiatry. 2001;71(5):577–82.
16. Klit H, Finnerup NB, Jensen TS. Central post-stroke pain: clinical characteristics, pathophysiology, and management. Lancet Neurol. 2009;8(9):857–68.
17. La Mantia L, Curone M, Rappaport AM, Bussone G. Tolosa-hunt syndrome: critical literature review based on HIS 2004criteria. Cephalalgia. 2006;26:772–81.
18. Margari L, Legrottaglie AR, Craig F, Petruzzelli MG, Procoli U, Dicuonzo F. Ophthalmoplegic migraine: migraine or oculomotor neuropathy? Cephalalgia Int J Headache. 2012;32(16):1208–15.
19. Multiple sclerosis-related central pain disorders. Springer. [Cited 2013 Dec 30]. Available from http://link.springer.com/article/10.1007%2Fs11916-010-0108-8/fulltext.html.
20. Nanda A, Khan IS. Nervus intermedius and geniculate neuralgia. World Neurosurg. 2013;79(5–6):651–2.
21. Rozen TD. Trigeminal neuralgia andglossopharyngeal neuralgia. Neurol Clin. 2004;22(1):185–206.
22. Sardella A, Demarosi F, Barbieri C, Lodi G. An up-to-date view on persistent idiopathic facial pain. Minerva Stomatol. 2009;58(6):289–99.
23. Scrivani SJ, Keith DA, Kaban LB. Temporomandibular disorders. N Engl J Med. 2008;359(25):2693–705.
24. Smith JH, Robertson CE, Garza I, Cutrer FM. Triggerless neuralgic otalgia: a case series and systematic literature review. Cephalalgia Int J Headache. 2013;33(11):914–23.
25. Solaro C, Trabucco E, Messmer UM. Pain and multiple sclerosis: pathophysiology and treatment. Curr Neurol Neurosci Rep. 2013;13(1):320.
26. Solomon S. Raeder syndrome. Arch Neurol. 2001;58(4):661–2.
27. Sweeney CJ, Gilden DH. Ramsay hunt syndrome. J Neurol Neurosurg Psychiatry. 2001;71(2):149–54.

28. Teixeira MJ, de Siqueira SRDT, Bor-Seng-Shu E. Glossopharyngeal neuralgia: neurosurgical treatment and differential diagnosis. Acta Neurochir. 2008;150(5):471–5. discussion 475.
29. Waldman SD. Atlas of common pain syndromes. St. Louis: Elsevier/Saunders; 2012.
30. Waldman SD. Chapter 17 Nervus intermedius neuralgia. In: Waldman SD, editor. Atlas of uncommon pain syndromes. Third ed. Philadelphia: W.B. Saunders; 2014. p. 43–5. [Cited 2013 Dec 31]. Available from http://www.sciencedirect.com/science/article/pii/B9781455709991000174.

Part IX

Painful Disease States in Special Populations

34 Pediatric Pain

Douglas Henry

Key Concepts

- Assessment of pain in children should be developmentally appropriate and should include information from both the child and parents. There are numerous pediatric-specific pain assessment tools available to quantify pain and follow the effectiveness of treatment.
- Diagnostic considerations in painful conditions are often much different in children than in adults.
- A multidisciplinary, pediatric-based approach is critical for successful treatment of chronic pain conditions in children and adolescents. Simply prescribing a medication will rarely lead to significant improvement.
- Cognitive-behavioral therapy (CBT) is important for virtually any child with a chronic pain problem to improve coping, maximize function, and reduce stress.
- In children with chronic pain, functioning in daily activities such as school attendance and social participation should be assessed and promoted at each visit.
- Many medications used in adults for pain are not approved by the Food and Drug Administration (FDA) nor have good scientific backing for use in children with pain. They are however widely used in the pediatric population.

Introduction

Many topics in this chapter are discussed in more detail elsewhere in this book. The focus of this chapter is to emphasize the differences in assessing and managing pain in children compared to adults.

Successful management of pain in children differs from that in adults in many domains.

There are physiologic and developmental differences between children and adults. For example, infants have a higher body water content which can lead to a higher volume of distribution of water-soluble medications. They also have smaller fat and muscle stores and therefore less drug uptake by these pharmacologically inactive tissues, resulting in higher plasma concentrations of many medications. Children heal more completely and quickly from injury and surgery than adults. With various levels of cognitive ability and emotional maturity, clinicians need to interview, examine, and explain their findings and recommendations in a way that is appropriate for each child. There are also social differences. While returning to work is usually a key goal in treating adults with pain, a child's "job" is school

D. Henry, MD (✉)
Department of Developmental and Rehabilitative Pediatrics, Cleveland Clinic Children's, Cleveland, OH, USA
e-mail: henryd@ccf.org

J. Cheng, R.W. Rosenquist (eds.), *Fundamentals of Pain Medicine*, https://doi.org/10.1007/978-3-319-64922-1_34

and play. Adults are responsible for themselves, whereas children are dependent on their caregivers to direct and care for them. Children tend to be less set in their ways and beliefs and to be more open to instruction and guidance. In addition to pediatric-specific medical knowledge, it takes a little more creativity and patience to take good care of children. So the saying "children should not be treated as little adults" should be taken seriously.

Acute Pain in Children

Pain Assessment

Assessing pain in infants and young children can be quite challenging. The infant who is fussy or incessantly crying may not actually have any pain. The infant may instead be hungry or experience emotional distress such as separation or stranger anxiety. Infants and toddlers are generally unable to localize their pain and certainly cannot describe it. Teenagers on the other hand will generally give a good history. Pain assessment therefore must be developmentally appropriate.

The clinician must depend on the following:

- Knowledge of the condition or situation (acute injury, post procedure, sickle cell disease).
- The family members know their children best and can usually be certain when pain is affecting their young child.
- General observation and physical examination (does moving a limb or palpating the abdomen consistently lead to apparent painful reaction?).

There are also standardized pain measures that are helpful in quantifying and following pain intensity in young children. The following are a few commonly used measures.

Face, legs, activity, cry, and consolability scale (FLACC) (Table 34.1) – an observational scale for children between the ages of 2 months and 7 years or those who are unable to communicate their pain. Often used postoperatively.

Wong-Baker FACES pain rating scale – for children 3–12 years old. A self-reported is six point scale as pictured below (Fig. 34.1).

Visual analog scale – for children ≥7 years. A self-reported 11-point scale where zero equals no pain and 10 equals worst possible pain.

Diagnostic Considerations

As in adults, the clinician must determine, if possible, the etiology of the pain in a child in order to best treat the pain and the underlying condition. Clinicians who primarily treat adults need to be aware that the diagnostic considerations in painful conditions can be much different in children than in adults. For example, in children with back pain, many unusual and serious conditions must be considered. These include leukemia and solid tumors, tethered cord, discitis, spondylolysis/spondylolisthesis, Scheuermann's disease, and rheumatologic conditions such as ankylosing spondylitis. On the other hand, disc herniation and radiculopathy are rare in children. Active growth plates in children can be a source of pain in overuse injuries, and the management of these injuries can be somewhat different than in adults with similar musculoskeletal complaints. Pediatric specialists should be involved in diagnosing the etiology of pain when it is not readily apparent.

Treatment

Nonpharmacologic Management

Nonpharmacologic interventions should not be overlooked in children. In fact they are likely more successful in children than adults. Soothing, distraction techniques, explanations, and reassurance are helpful. In the hospital setting, child life therapy or the equivalent can facilitate this, especially in preparing a child for a painful procedure.

Topical anesthetic creams and sprays and/or local vibration should be used whenever possible for procedures. Icing or freezing sprays can be used for superficial pain though they are sometimes not well tolerated by children.

Table 34.1 Face, legs, activity, cry, and consolability scale (FLACC)

Category	Scoring		
	0	1	2
Face	No particular expression or smile	Occasional grimace or frown, withdrawn disinterested	Frequent to constant quivering chin, clenched jaw
Legs	Normal position or relaxed	Uneasy, restless, tense	Kicking or legs drawn up
Activity	Lying quietly, normal position moves easily	Squirming, tense shifting back and forth	Arched, rigid, or jerking
Cry	No cry (awake or sleep)	Moans or whimpers, occasional complaint	Crying steadily, screams or sobs, frequent complaints
Consolability	Content, relaxed	Reassured by occasional touching, hugging, or being talked to; distractable	Difficult to console

Each of the five categories is scoring from 0 to 2, resulting in total range of 0–10
FLACC face, leg, activity, cry, consolability

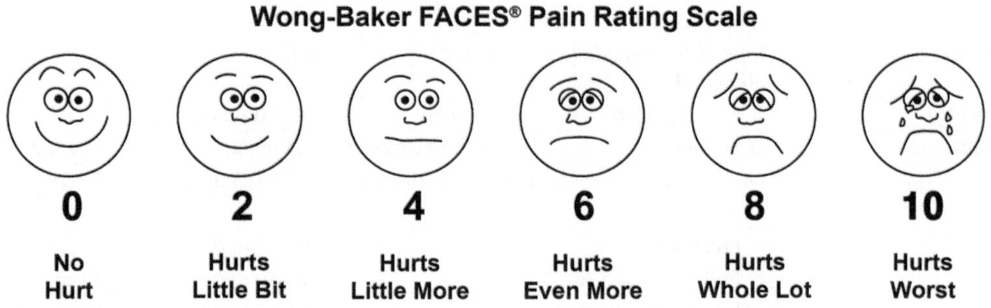

Wong-Baker FACES® Pain Rating Scale

0 No Hurt; 2 Hurts Little Bit; 4 Hurts Little More; 6 Hurts Even More; 8 Hurts Whole Lot; 10 Hurts Worst

Fig. 34.1 Wong-Baker FACES pain rating scale (©1983 Wong-Baker FACES Foundation. www.WongBakerFACES.org. Used with permission. Originally published in *Whaley & Wong's Nursing Care of Infants and Children*. ©Elsevier Inc.)

Pharmacologic Management

The vast majority of acute pain in children is treated medically with acetaminophen, ibuprofen, and codeine. However, codeine should be replaced with another short-acting opioid; some children are ultrafast metabolizers and some very slow metabolizers of codeine into morphine. Combination codeine/acetaminophen medications should be avoided to reduce risk of acetaminophen overdosage, as acetaminophen by itself may also be given. Although aspirin is the treatment of choice in a few pediatric conditions such as Kawasaki syndrome, it should otherwise be avoided in children due to its association with Reye Syndrome. Gabapentin is frequently used for neuropathic pain in children, though it is not FDA approved for pain in children. Beginning at about age 5 or 6 years, many children can appropriately use patient-controlled analgesia.

Pediatric dosages of common pain medications (Table 34.2).

Chronic Pain in Children

Chronic Pain Syndromes

Chronic pain is estimated to occur in 15–30% of school-aged children. The most common chronic pain syndromes are listed below. Prevalence rates for these conditions are extremely variable, due to differences in populations sampled and inclusion criteria. A 2011 review by King, et al. provides the following prevalence rates for the most

Table 34.2 Pediatric dosages of common pain medications

Drug	Preparation	Dose	Interval	
Acetaminophen	Tabs: 325 mg, 500 mg	PO: 10–15 mg/kg	PO: 4 h	
	Chewable tabs: 80 mg, 160 mg	Rectal (single dose): 35–45 mg/kg	Rectal: 6 h	
	Elixir: 160 mg/5 mL	Rectal (repeated dose): 20 mg/kg	Rectal: (premature, newborns): 12 h	
	Drops: 80 mg/0.8 mL			
	Suppositories: 80 mg, 120 mg, 325 mg, 650 mg			
Ibuprofen	Tabs: 200 mg, 400 mg, 600 mg, 800 mg	PO: 6–10 mg/kg	4–6 h	
	Chewable tabs: 50 mg, 100 mg			
	Elixir: 100 mg/5 mL			
	Drops: 50 mg/1.25 mL			
Naproxen	Tabs: 220 mg, 250 mg, 375 mg, 500 mg	PO: 5–10 mg/kg	12 h	
	Elixir: 25 mg/mL			
Ketorolac	Injectable: 15 mg/mL, 30 mg/mL	IV: 0.5 mg/kg	6 h	
Tramadol	1–2 mg/kg/dose	2–4×/day	Max dose 800 mg	
Morphine	Oral, immediate release: infants and children		0.3 mg/kg	Every 3–4 h
	Oral, sustained release: infants and children		0.25–0.5 mg/kg	Every 8–12 h
	IV bolus:			
	Preterm neonate		10–25 μg/kg	Every 2–4 h
	Full-term neonate		25–50 μg/kg	Every 3–4 h
	Infants and children		50–100 μg/kg	Every 3 h
	IV infusion:			
	Preterm neonate		2–5 μg/kg/h	
	Full-term neonate		5–10 μg/kg/h	
	Infants and children		15–30 μg/kg/h	
Hydromorphone	Oral: infants and children		40–80 μg/kg	Every 4 h
	IV bolus: infants and children		10–20 μg/kg	Every 3–4 h
	IV infusion: infants and children		3–5 μg/kg/h	
Fentanyl	Oral transmucosal		10–15 μg/kg	(Oralet)
	Intranasal		1–2 μg/kg	
	Transdermal		12.5, 25, 50, 75, 100 μg/h patches	
	IV bolus		0.5–1 μg/kg	Every 1–2 h
	IV infusion		0.5 μg/kg/h	
Codeine	Oral		0.5–1 mg/kg	Every 4 h
Oxycodone	Oral		0.1–0.15 mg/kg	Every 4 h
Hydrocodone	Oral		0.1–0.2 mg/kg	Every 4 h

common conditions. In each category, the prevalence is higher in females than in males.

Musculoskeletal/limb pain	3.9–40%
Abdominal pain	3.8–53.4%
Back pain	13.5–24%
Multiple pains	3.6–48.8%
Headache	8–82.9%

By the time the pain has been present for months, an extensive diagnostic evaluation has typically been done, and often no specific pathology is identified. The chronic pain problems then are classified by symptom complexes, and several are discussed below. But perhaps compared to adults, classification of chronic pain syndromes in children is less distinct and more clinician dependent. In the above list, complex regional pain syndrome (CRPS) makes up much of limb pain, and multiple pains include what many would call fibromyalgia (FMS), pain amplification syndrome, or central pain sensitivity syndrome.

Children who have pain tend to avoid physical activity as this increases the pain. They are frightened of what is causing the pain and the prospect of having this pain forever. They therefore become sedentary, deconditioned, and socially isolated. They develop more dependent tendencies and parents, trying to be sympathetic and helpful, often promote a more sedentary life. The child stops participating in athletic activities, social and recreational activities, and attending school. A child may become comfortable and even relish the sick role, consciously or subconsciously, using the pain as a means to avoid stress, such as school or family pressures. Underlying anxiety is common and may exacerbate the pain perception and its manifestations. The child and parents often remain focused on finding an organic cause for the pain and a treatment to alleviate the pain, which prevents them from fully embracing a treatment program of acceptance and functional restoration. The needs and limitations of the child also limit their siblings' activities and cause parents to miss work or even quit their job. So while every effort should be made to reduce the pain, just as much attention should be placed on maintaining or improving a child's level of functioning.

Treatment of Chronic Pain

Nonpharmacologic Management

The most common pediatric chronic pain syndromes will be described briefly below. But because their nonpharmacologic management is similar, this will be discussed as a group before the descriptions.

Management of chronic pain in children is not just about trying to eliminate pain but also about maintaining a normal active life. At every outpatient visit, even the initial visit, a child's physical functioning should be addressed and the child should be encouraged to maintain normal functioning in spite of the pain. A multidisciplinary program that includes physical, psychological, and education interventions should be used whenever possible. Intensive 2–3 week therapeutic programs are usually quite successful. As the duration of inactivity and disability increases, it gets harder to get a child back to normal functioning. Physical activity can be in the form of physical or occupational therapy, but activities such as soccer, dance, aquatics, yoga, hiking, etc. can improve their motor abilities and endurance while also returning them to more social interaction with peers and family. School accommodations, such as allowing half days or taking the elevator instead of the stairs, should be minimized. While all of these activities and physical treatments may initially increase pain, it is theorized that they will help to correct the central nervous system's altered processing of stimuli and decrease the perceived pain.

Distraction and encouragement are very important for increasing the child's functional abilities and exercise tolerance. Explaining that while movement may increase pain, it will not cause physical damage can help take away the child's fear of increasing activity. The parents' response to their child's pain, such as constantly asking about pain levels, providing excessive accommodations, and endless searching for the "real" cause of the pain or the treatment that will finally take the pain away, must also be dealt with, instructing them to instead focus on coping strategies and functional gain.

It is important that patients and their parents understand that increased functional use of the affected area is the primary goal of treatment. Parents, and even schools, need to be instructed to minimize accommodations and encourage the patient to be as active as possible. Patients and parents need to be assured that, although increased activity will initially increase pain, the activity will not cause physiologic damage.

Medications and procedures will not cure these problems, but they may allow the patient to better tolerate and participate in a program of functional restoration and reduce the comorbidities.

Pharmacologic Management

For children with CRPS, pain amplification syndrome (fibromyalgia) and chronic functional abdominal pain, medications will seldom lead to a significant improvement in pain levels. Headaches have a relatively better response to medications overall. By the time the pain condition is considered chronic, several of the most appropriate medications have usually been tried.

It is important to note that most medications used for chronic pain conditions in adults are not Food and Drug Administration (FDA) approved for patients under 18 years of age for the indication of pain. This includes gabapentin, pregabalin, duloxetine, onabotulinum toxin A, and many others. Topiramate, gabapentin, oxcarbazepine, and carbamazepine are FDA approved in children only for seizures. This lack of FDA approval prohibits marketing these medications for pediatric use but does not prohibit prescribing the medications to children. In fact many medications used in adult chronic pain are quite commonly used in adolescents with chronic pain syndromes.

Only one medication change (starting a new medication or making dose adjustment) should be made at a time in order to be clear what the effects of that change are. If the medication is not helpful after an adequate trial, it should be discontinued rather than simply adding another medication.

Opioids should not be used for chronic nonmalignant pain in children.

Children with chronic pain almost universally say that NSAIDs and acetaminophen are not helpful. Opioids sometimes relieve pain at this stage but should not be used long term.

Several antianxiety/antidepressant medications are use in chronic pain states in adults as well as in children. Anxiety, and to a lesser extent depression, is common in children with chronic pain disorders. Treating these comorbidities can significantly improve pain complaints, activity levels, and quality of life. Selective serotonin reuptake inhibitors (SSRIs) may be the better medications for anxiety and depression. However with a coexisting chronic pain problem, especially a pain amplification problem such as fibromyalgia, a selective noradrenergic reuptake inhibitor (SNRI) may treat the anxiety or depression, as well as the pain. A tricyclic antidepressant (TCA) may help alleviate central or neuropathic pain and assist with sleep initiation problems. Confirmation of a normal ECG is commonly recommended before starting a TCA in a pediatric patient. Medications in all of the above antidepressant classes carry the black box warning that they may increase suicidal thoughts or actions in some children, teenagers, or young adults within the first few months of treatment or when the dose is changed.

Complex Regional Pain Syndrome (CRPS)

CRPS in adults is described in more detail in Chap. 23. Patients typically present with severe pain in one or more extremities, disproportionate in intensity and duration to an inciting event, such as an ankle sprain or a wrist fracture. The main differential diagnoses include missed fracture, osteomyelitis, cellulitis, and juvenile idiopathic arthritis. Most clinicians use standard adult diagnostic criteria in children. However, there are some differences in presentation and treatment.

Characteristics of CRPS in children compared to adults:

- Lower extremity more commonly affected.
- Inciting event tends to be less traumatic (e.g., sprain vs. fracture)
- More likely to spread to other limbs.
- Better response to noninvasive treatments.
- Psychosocial factors play a greater role.
- Autonomic abnormalities less prominent in general and may be absent.
- Complete resolution of symptoms is more common.

Treatment

Nonpharmacologic Management

In children, CRPS is ideally treated by a multidisciplinary team experienced with the disorder. Furthermore, the primary goals of treatment should be functional restoration of the affected limb and return to a normal lifestyle. Resolution of the pain is a secondary goal. In fact, increased movement of the limb and emotional adjustment/coping are felt to be ultimately helpful for improvement of the pain itself.

Therefore, the initial and primary treatment is physical and/or occupational therapy (PT/OT) and psychological intervention. Physical treatment involves progressive, but fairly aggressive, forced use of the affected limb, range of motion, and tactile desensitization. Since these treatments contrast with the rest and immobilization prescribed after an initial injury, the importance of early diagnosis is important. Cognitive-behavioral therapy (CBT) in conjunction with PT/OT is also helpful. Psychologists can identify and address the stressors and teach the child to cope with their chronic pain and the resultant decrease in their activities of daily living, social interactions, and recreational experiences. They can also identify and help manage common comorbidities such as anxiety and depression.

Pharmacologic Management

There is considerable debate over when to use medications or procedures to treat pediatric CRPS. Some clinicians avoid them completely. Some combine them with the PT/OT and CBT or add them if PT/OT show little improvement. Others use medications or procedures as first line interventions. They include:

- Medications: gabapentin or pregabalin (especially if a nerve lesion or structural defect such as a fracture is present), SNRIs (if pain amplification is prominent), amitriptyline or nortriptyline (helpful for sleep initiation as well), corticosteroids (if early in course), terazosin (if autonomic features are prominent), nifedipine (for a cold, poorly perfused distal limb), and vitamin C. Topical anesthetic patches can be applied but may be painful to apply and remove.
- Procedures: sympathetic ganglion blocks, temporary epidural catheters, or spinal stimulators (very rarely permanently implanted in children).

Amplified Musculoskeletal Pain Syndrome/Fibromyalgia

There are many children who experience diffuse idiopathic chronic pain. They often have increased sensitivity to tactile (trigger points), auditory and visual stimuli, fatigue, and poor sleep initiation and maintenance. In addition, many experience postural light-headedness which may be diagnosed as postural orthostatic tachycardia syndrome (POTS). The main criteria for POTS is an increase in heart rate of over 30 beats/min when going from lying to standing, after 4 min and the postural light-headedness. Some clinicians are hesitant to give children a diagnosis of fibromyalgia and instead prefer the more general terms pain amplification syndrome or central pain sensitivity syndrome. However, many children meet the American College of Rheumatology criteria of 1990 (which requires 11 of 18 painful trigger points) or the criteria for children set forth by Yunus and Masi in 1985 (Yunis). Studies that look at the prevalence of fibromyalgia or diffuse chronic pain in children report prevalence anywhere from 1% to 7.5%.

Yunus and Masi Criteria for Fibromyalgia in Children

Major Criteria

Generalized musculoskeletal aching at three or more sites for 3 or more months
Absence of underlying condition or cause
Normal laboratory tests
Five or more typical tender points (as opposed to the 11 required in adults)

Minor Criteria

Poor sleep
Fatigue
Chronic anxiety or tension
Chronic headaches
Irritable bowel syndrome
Subjective soft tissue swelling
Numbness
Pain modulation by physical activities
Pain modulation by other factors
Pain modulation by anxiety/stress

(Fibromyalgia is defined as present if the subject has all for major criteria and three minor criteria or the first three major criteria, four tender points, and a five minor criteria)

Nonpharmacologic Management

Management is similar to that of fibromyalgia in adults, though with a pediatric perspective. As discussed above, a multidisciplinary biopsychosocial approach to treatment is most appropriate.

Aquatic activities are especially helpful for strengthening, conditioning, and flexibility. Behavioral recommendations for the sleep disturbance include prohibiting television and texting after bedtime. Increased fluid and salt intake, as well as exercise, may reduce POTS symptoms.

Pharmacologic Management

Medication recommendations are also similar to adult practice. This includes NSAIDs, amitriptyline, gabapentin, pregabalin, and the SNRIs. Medications to assist with sleep include melatonin, trazadone, amitriptyline and zolpidem.

Chronic Functional Abdominal Pain

Chronic or recurrent abdominal pain with no identifiable cause is common in children, occurring more frequently in girls. It is necessary to rule out organic problems including Crohn's disease, ulcerative colitis, celiac disease, gastritis/peptic ulcer disease, constipation, gallbladder disease, kidney disease, and neoplastic disease.

The criteria for chronic functional abdominal pain (FAP) are:

- Episodic or continuous abdominal pain
- Insufficient criteria for other functional gastrointestinal disorders
- No evidence of an inflammatory, anatomic, metabolic, or neoplastic process that explains the patient's symptoms

The Rome III criteria further classify this problem into four entities: functional dyspepsia, irritable bowel syndrome (IBS), abdominal migraine, and childhood functional abdominal pain.

Strong contractions and distension of the gastrointestinal tract often play a role in this disorder. But hypersensitivity to pain, and perhaps to otherwise normal visceral sensation, is believed to be a key feature of FAP. And many of these children have hypersensitivity elsewhere, such as trigger points. It is not clear to what extent this hypersensitivity is central versus peripheral. Psychological factors including current or past stress, anxiety, and depression also seem to play a role. Caregiver anxiety can amplify the problem.

Treatment

Nonpharmacologic Management

Again, a multidisciplinary approach to treatment, including PT/OT and psychology is optimal. This includes education/reassurance for child and parents, coping strategies, and maintenance of normal life activities, including school attendance, in spite of the pain.

Identifying and eliminating dietary triggers, even in the absence of a specific disorder, may be helpful. Maintaining normal bowel movements will minimize visceral activity and distension.

Pharmacologic Management

Antispasmodics such as dicyclomine and acid suppression medications should generally be given a trial. Probiotics are helpful, but the mechanism is not known. Peppermint oil is beneficial in many with IBS.

There is currently no good scientific evidence that antidepressant medications are effective for functional abdominal pain in adolescents. Nonetheless, there is anecdotal evidence of benefit, and they are frequently tried. TCAs are usually the first antidepressants tried for FAP. But SSRIs and SNRIs are also used, depending on the comorbidities, such as sleep disturbance and anxiety.

Cyproheptadine and propranolol are used for abdominal migraines.

Headache

Headaches are common in children and can be disabling. They can be classified as primary (with no known underlying pathology) and secondary (due to a medical condition such as concussion or sinusitis). Primary headaches are further classified as migraine, chronic daily headache, tension, and cluster headaches. Cluster headaches are uncommon in adolescents. It is important not only to determine or rule out a medical cause for the headaches but to classify the headaches appropriately in order to guide treatment.

Treatment

For children with disabling headaches, a program that encourages normal functioning with the principles outlined above is recommended. In addition to educating the family about headaches, treatment is largely dietary modification and pharmacologic. To a great extent, pharmacologic management follows the adult guidelines and practice. Treatment of pediatric headache is complex and depends strongly on classification and so is beyond the scope of this chapter.

Suggested Reading

1. Berde CB, Sethna NF. Analgesics for the treatment of pain in children. N Engl J Med. 2002;347:1094–103. October 3
2. Chronic abdominal pain in children: 2012 a technical report of the American Academy of Pediatrics and the North American Society for Pediatric Gastroenterology, Hepatology and Nutrition. AAP Subcommittee and NASPGHAN Committee on Chronic Abdominal Pain.
3. Gladstein J, Rothner AD. Chronic Daily Headache in Children and Adolescents.
4. King S, et al. Guideline for the Management of Fibromyalgia Syndrome Pain in adults and children. American pain society, 2005 the epidemiology of chronic pain in children and adolescents revisited: a systematic review. Pain. 2011;152:2729–38.
5. Slover R, Coy J, Davids HR. Advances in Pediatrics advances in the Management of Pain in children: acute pain. Adv Pediatr. 2009;56(1):341–58.
6. Yunus MB, Masi AT. Juvenile primary fibromyalgia syndrome. A clinical study of thirty-three patients and matched normal controls. Arthritis Rheum. 1985;28(2):138–45.

35 Geriatric Pain

Kenneth D. Candido

Key Concepts

- Pain in the elderly is often associated with barriers to succeed in providing relief, due to multiplicity of pain complaints, multiplicity of medical problems, communication difficulties, poor tolerance of tests and procedures, depression, insomnia, anxiety and fatigue, poor nutrition, lack of family support systems, and ethical concerns including informed consent issues.
- Pain threshold increases with age, while tolerance for pain decreases.
- Pain behaviors in the elderly with dementia often include assessing facial expressions, verbalization, body movements, changes in interpersonal interactions, changes in activity patterns or routine, and mental status changes.
- Pain assessment in the elderly with dementia often relies upon specialized tests including the ADD (Assessment of Discomfort in Dementia), CNPI (Checklist of Nonverbal Pain Indicators), Dolophus 2, PACSLAC (Pain Assessment Scale for Seniors with Severe Dementia), PAINAD (Pain Assessment in Advanced Dementia), and NOPAIN (nursing assistant-administered instrument to assess pain in demented individuals).
- Physiologic changes in aging which may affect treatment choices include decreased renal function, decreased hepatic function, decreased serum protein levels, decreased functional binding to protein, decreased cardiac index, loss of total body water and blood volume, and a higher fat-to-lean body mass ratio.
- Decreased nerve conduction velocity affects response to local anesthetic nerve blocks.
- Vitamin deficiencies can result in metabolic derangements affecting therapeutic options in the elderly. Wernicke's encephalopathy due to thiamine deficiency can be associated with ataxia, confusion, short-term memory loss, and ophthalmoplegia.
- Elimination half-lives of opioids may increase in the elderly due to alterations in cytochrome function.
- Antidepressant use in the elderly as pain adjuvants often is associated with prohibitive side effects including drowsiness, memory loss and cognitive impairment, anticholinergic effects, anxiety, psychosis, psychomotor agitation, Parkinsonism, postural hypotension

K.D. Candido, MD (✉)
Department of Anesthesiology, Advocate Illinois Masonic Medical Center, University of Illinois College of Medicine, 836 West Wellington Avenue; Suite 4815, Chicago, IL 60657, USA
e-mail: kdcandido@yahoo.com

J. Cheng, R.W. Rosenquist (eds.), *Fundamentals of Pain Medicine*,
https://doi.org/10.1007/978-3-319-64922-1_35

and dizziness, extrapyramidal side effects, and dystonia and tardive dyskinesia.

- There are approximately 700,000 new vertebral compression fractures per year in the USA; 20% of women aged 65 or older have at least one fracture.
- Herpes-zoster-related pain is secondary only to painful diabetic peripheral neuropathy as a cause of neuropathic pain in the elderly.
- Trigeminal neuralgia is a condition commonly seen in the elderly with treatment options available including medical, surgical (microvascular decompression/Jannetta procedure), and interventional (CT scan or fluoroscopically guided nerve blocks).

Geriatric Pain

Aging is a progressive, generalized impairment of function resulting in a loss of adaptive response to stress (loss of biologic reserve) and in a growing risk of age-related disease. The percentage of individuals living beyond age 65 is ever increasing. By the year 2050, it is estimated that up to 16% of the world's population or 1.43 billion people will be above that age. 25–50% of elders are thought to suffer from chronic pain, and up to 80% of residents in nursing homes may be so affected. The multiplicity of medical problems in this age group often confounds clinicians in terms of being able to sort out organic pain issues from psychological complaints and those problems due strictly to limitations in cognition and communication. There are considerable barriers to providing adequate pain management while minimizing the trespass attendant to the use of analgesics and advanced interventional pain therapies. Furthermore, while pain thresholds may increase with age, tolerance for pain may decline, which adds to the challenges and constraints on care providers to implement timely and effective pain-relieving strategies in this special needs category of patients.

Pain in elderly patients represents a distinct challenge due to a myriad of factors that include medical comorbidities, cognitive decline, loss of autonomy and self-care, physiologic effects of aging, and altered pharmacodynamics of commonly administered analgesic agents, among others. This chapter presents some of those challenges and also describes common pain scenarios in the geriatric patient as well as remedies that have been shown to be effective for treating those conditions.

Scope of the Problem

The world's population is aging. By some estimates, the percentage of adults older than 65 years will increase as a percentage of the total population will double from 8% presently to up to 16% (Fig. 35.1). As expected, this dramatic increase comes in light of expert predictions that the world population will increase from 7.2 to 9.6 billion by the year 2050 [1].

With this dramatic increase in the aging population, the expectation is that the need to provide competent pain management for this segment of the population will concomitantly be forthcoming. In that regard, it is essential that pain management physicians arm themselves with sufficient knowledge of the unique challenges imposed by the physiological changes associated with aging and furthermore appreciate the specific disease entities that afflict this special needs group. This chapter provides an overview of many of those challenges and also describes some of the established techniques of pain medicine that will be uniquely suited for treating those disease entities.

In a cross-sectional, prospective survey conducted in an age-stratified sample of 4093 people aged 75–105 years old, it was found that 40.4% of the elderly reported having chronic pain [2]. The factors that predicted pain included higher age, as was a lower quality of life (QOL). Pain was found to be associated with functional limitations, fatigue, sleep problems, depressed mood, and reduced QOL. In nursing home residents, pain is often associated with the presence of osteoarthritis, osteoporosis, peripheral neuropathy, fibromyalgia, and cancer [3]. Depression, anxiety, fear, and sleep disturbances characterize this population of pain sufferers.

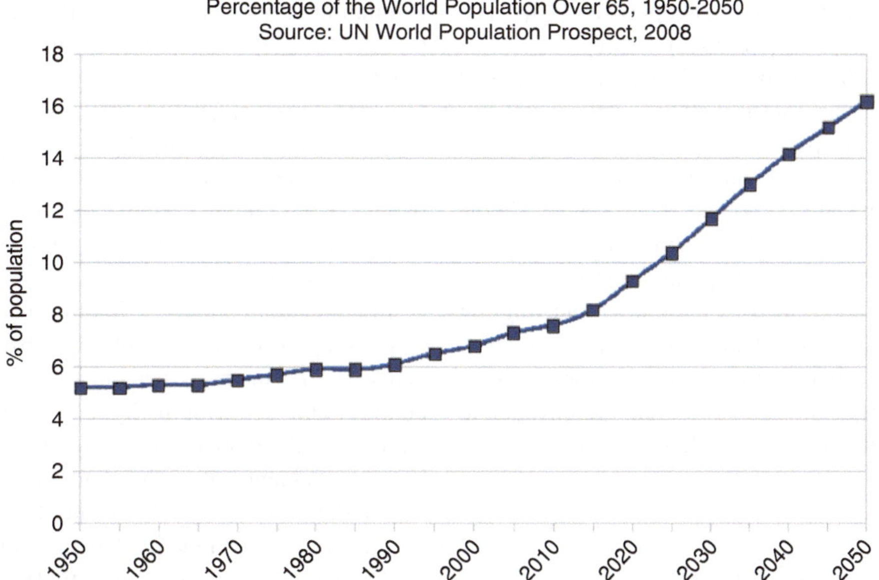

Fig. 35.1 Percentage of the world population over 65 (Adapted from the United Nations, Department of Economic and Social Affairs, Population Division [1])

Physiologic Changes Associated with Aging

Advancing age is associated with declines in renal function, including number of glomeruli and renal blood flow and decreases in renal excretion due to a lowered glomerular filtration rate, lower tubular resorption, and higher serum drug concentrations [4]. Hepatic function is associated with reductions in first-pass metabolism, which may affect many drugs administered as analgesics. There is decreased microsomal oxidation by the hepatic P-450 system, which can lead to higher serum concentrations of drugs administered using standard doses for adults. Serum protein levels decline, including albumin (acidic binding) and alpha-1-acid glycoprotein (basic binding), which also lead to higher serum concentrations of drugs used as analgesics. There is less binding of drugs, leading to greater passage through membranes and enhanced central nervous system (CNS) effects [5].

Cardiac index declines about 1% per year after the age of 30. This means that drugs administered intravenously have a longer circulation time and also a longer time to reach effective analgesic concentrations in the serum. A loss of total body water and reduction in circulating blood volume are also encountered in the elderly. Each of these factors affects drug distribution and clinical effectiveness [6].

Cognitive decline in aging is well described. As well, there are reductions in nerve conduction velocity and axonal loss of myelin, with a decrease in axonal numbers and synapses. Elderly patients rely more upon C-fiber input when reporting pain than do their younger counterparts, versus A-delta fiber input [6–9].

The elderly may have metabolic and nutritional deficiencies largely due to inadequate dietary intake of vital nutrients. Lack of vitamin A consumption can lead to night blindness and corneal damage. Thiamine (vitamin B-1) deficiency can cause beriberi or Wernicke's encephalopathy, which is associated with ataxia, confusion, short-term memory loss, and ophthalmoplegia. Niacin (vitamin B-3) deficiency can cause pellagra, while folate loss leads to diarrhea, weight loss, palpitations, anemia, and behavioral disorders. Untreated niacin deficiency is associated with glossitis, light sensitivity, aggression, weakness, ataxia, and osteoporosis [10]. The treatment is with replacement therapy.

Cobalamin (vitamin B-12) deficiency can lead to pernicious anemia as well as to mania, psychosis, and sleep disturbances. Sensory-motor changes can occur due to demyelination. If severe, subacute combined degeneration of the spinal cord occurs, where there is patchy myelin loss in the dorsolateral spinal columns which is clinically represented as numbness and tingling and vibration sense changes that can lead to spasticity [10]. Vitamin replacement therapy may be useful except in cases of irreversible changes to the nerve membrane, which are resistant to such treatment.

Diagnosis Considerations

The elderly patient in pain often experience pain that persists longer than younger patients who have the same, or similar underlying pathophysiology responsible for that pain [11]. Pain severity also tends to be greater for any degree of trespass. The level of pain and the duration of that pain are directly correlated with a reduction in activity level and functionality. Furthermore, the degree of pathology as assessed using standardized objectified measurements and analyses, such as that determined by CT scans or MRI, does not correlate with the level of pain and disability in this age group [11]. The use of pain questionnaires such as the McGill short form is a useful adjunct to evaluating pain and supplement the verbal pain rating scale [12]. Neuropsychological testing can be useful to assess levels of cognitive functioning. Such tests may include the Repeatable Battery for the Assessment of Neuropsychological Status, Trail Making Test, and the Grooved Pegboard Test. Physical performances (gait speed, functional reach, chair rise, trunk rotation, and static/dynamic lifting) are useful measures to corroborate the degree of expressed dysfunction by these patients [12]. Psychosocial disruption is a major influence on the expression of pain in the elderly and can be assessed using the Geriatric Depression Scale, the Short-Form-36 Mental Health, and the Role Limitations-Emotional Composite Scale. Self-reported disability can be determined using the Functional Status Index, the Short-Form-36 Physical Functioning/Role-Physical Composite Scale, and others and should be employed when evaluating the degree of pain in the geriatric patient [12]. Often pain impairs neuropsychological performance as compared with a group of pain-free cohorts [12–15].

In demented patients, it is often necessary to rely not upon the findings of standardized interactive testing methods but rather on the patient conduct and behavior in light of their chronic pain. Facial expressions, verbalizations, and body movements often need to be scrutinized before determining whether or not to implement a given treatment modality. Changes in interpersonal interactions, changes in activity patterns or routines, and gross mental status changes often herald worsening cognitive functioning, which may prove to be impediments and barriers to providing effective therapies aimed at pain control [15–18]. Standardized tools that are not contingent on patient interaction, per se, for making the assessment of dementia include the Assessment of Discomfort in Dementia protocol (ADD), the Checklist of Nonverbal Pain Indicators (CNPI), Dolophus 2, the Pain Assessment Scale for Seniors with Severe Dementia (PACSLAC), the Pain Assessment in Advanced Dementia scale (PAINAD), and the nursing assistant-administered instrument to assess pain in demented individuals (NOPAIN) [14–27].

Treatment Considerations

It remains true that there exist barriers to effective treatment in nursing home residents, which include both patient factors and staff factors. Among the patient factors include unrealistic fears of addiction, worsening dependence, and the immutable nature of persistent pain [28]. Residents often believe that chronic pain does not or cannot be changed. Staff may often believe in external pathology over pain reports and hence provide inadequate analgesia [28]. Complaints may be minimized by some certified nursing assistants, who cite lack of time constraints as the rationale for why they occasionally or not infrequently ignore or undervalue pain complaints by the elderly [28].

- Using the World Health Organization stepladder approach to pain management has been suggested as being the most efficient way to approach the analgesic needs of these patients, while keeping in mind the constraints imposed by physiologic limitations in this age group [3].
- Nonopioid analgesics should be the cornerstone of pharmacotherapy as a starting point.
- Short-acting or mild opioids can be added during ascent from mild type pain (rated from 1–3/10 on a numeric pain rating scale) to moderate type pain (4–7/10) while reserving stronger, more potent, and longer lasting extended duration opioids for only those individuals suffering from severe type pain (8–10/10).
- Tricyclic antidepressants need to be cautiously used due to their anticholinergic side effects, which are often times pronounced in the elderly.
- Prevention of disease progression and exacerbation is a key element of any proposed treatment plan.
- The success (or failure) of any treatment approach needs to be measured not merely by assessing pain levels but also objectively by the evaluation of activity levels and improvements in psychosocial and cognitive functioning [3].

Specific Pain Conditions and Their Treatment

Pain conditions that are unique to the geriatric population are too numerous to delineate as a complete or comprehensive list. Osteoarthritis, painful osteoporotic vertebral compression fracture, trigeminal neuralgia, and Herpes Zoster pain and postherpetic neuralgia are some of the commonly encountered pain entities. The remainder of this chapter focuses on osteoporosis and painful osteoporotic vertebral compression fracture as other relevant conditions are discussed elsewhere in this book. The interested reader is encouraged to review the suggested references at the completion of this chapter for a greater in-depth appreciation of these respective conditions and concerns in the geriatric pain population.

Osteoporosis and Painful Vertebral Compression Fracture

Osteoporosis is a progressive bone disease, typically of the elderly, which is characterized by a decrease in bone mass and density which can lead to an increased risk of fracture, particularly of the hip but also of the spinal vertebrae [10]. In osteoporosis, the bone mineral density (BMD) is reduced, bone microarchitecture deteriorates, and the amount and variety of proteins in bone are altered. According to the WHO, osteoporosis is defined as a bone mineral density of 2.5 standard deviations or more below the mean peak bone mass seen in health, as measured by dual-energy X-ray absorptiometry. Osteoporosis may be classified as primary or secondary. Primary type 1 or postmenopausal osteoporosis is commonly encountered in postmenopausal women. Primary type 2 osteoporosis also known as senile osteoporosis occurs after age 75 with a female to male ratio of 2:1. Secondary osteoporosis may arise at any age and affect men and women equally. This form results from chronic predisposing medical problems or disease or prolonged use of medications such as glucocorticoids, when the disease is called steroid- or glucocorticoid-induced osteoporosis.

Painful spinal vertebral compression fractures (VCFs) occur due to trauma or osteoporosis. The prevalence in women aged 50 and over has been estimated at 26% when defined as a reduction in vertebral height >15% [29]. Retrospective reviews have shown a clinical detection rate of VCF in white women of 153/100,000 person years. Approximately 1.5 million new VCFs occur per year in the USA. Of these clinically detected VCFs, 84% were associated with pain [29]. VCF may be defined as a clinical event characterized by loss of height and acute pain. The pain of acute fracture usually lasts 4–6 weeks with intense pain at the site of fracture. Chronic pain may also occur in patients with multiple compression fractures, height loss, and low bone density but is probably due to structural changes or osteoarthritis [29]. Multiple adjacent VCFs can lead to progressive kyphosis, loss of appetite, progressive pulmonary dysfunction, and failure to thrive [29]. The aggregate estimated cost of treating comorbidities associated with VCFs in the USA is upward of $750 million dollars per year [29]. Treatment of VCF-related pain may be conservative, using analgesic medication, or may be more aggressive, by implementation of vertebral augmentation procedures (Figs. 35.2, 35.3, 35.4, and 35.5).

The use of vertebral augmentation procedures is a well-established, if somewhat controversial, therapeutic option for managing pain of VCFs [30–32]. Percutaneous vertebroplasty (PVP) and balloon kyphoplasty (BKP) are the two most commonly employed interventional pain management approaches to reducing pain and at times providing some modest restoration in vertebral body height. Results of reducing pain appear to be somewhat similar despite the selection of either PVP or BKP procedures [31]. A recent meta-analysis of 1787 patients (887 PVP; 900 BKP) found no significant difference between the two, both for adjacent fractures as well as for non-adjacent fractures. There was also no significant difference between the two in terms of cement extravasation into the intervertebral disc; however, extravasation into the paravertebral space was higher with PVP than with BKP ($P < 0.01$) [31]. One conclusion that might be drawn from this review is that individuals with marginal pulmonary function might be better candidates for BKP procedures than for PVP procedures due to the high rate of embolization associated with cement injection into the bony trabeculae of the vertebra treated. With PVP, the incidence of cement leakage appears to be doubled when a uni-pedicular (i.e., single needle) is used, compared to a bi-pedicular approach (52.7% vs. 28.1%) [32].

Technique: Figs. 35.2, 35.3, 35.4, and 35.5 demonstrate vertebral augmentation using the PVP approach in an individual with a painful vertebral compression fracture which occurred following a fall, in the segment (L-2) immediately cephalad to a previously performed fusion procedure at L3-L4.

Patient selection determines the efficacy of whether or not someone will respond favorably to vertebral augmentation. Contraindications to these procedures include patient refusal; inability to comprehend written or spoken language, even using translator services, due to cognitive

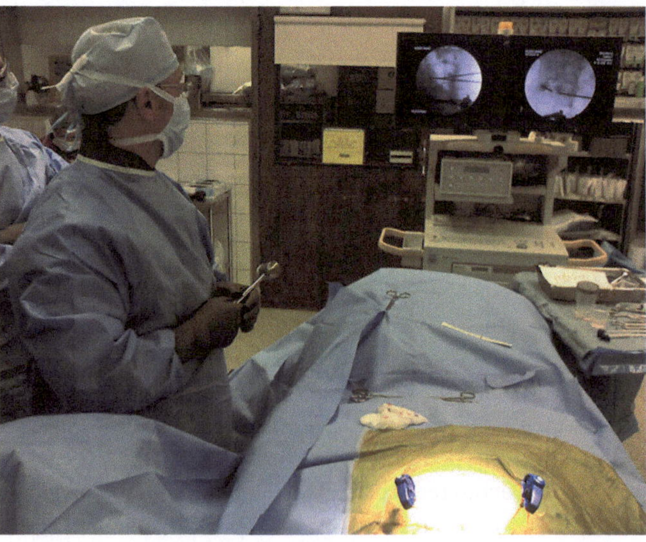

Fig. 35.2 Bi-pedicular vertebral augmentation for osteoporotic compression fracture at L-2; trocars in place (Photo courtesy of Kenneth D. Candido, M.D.)

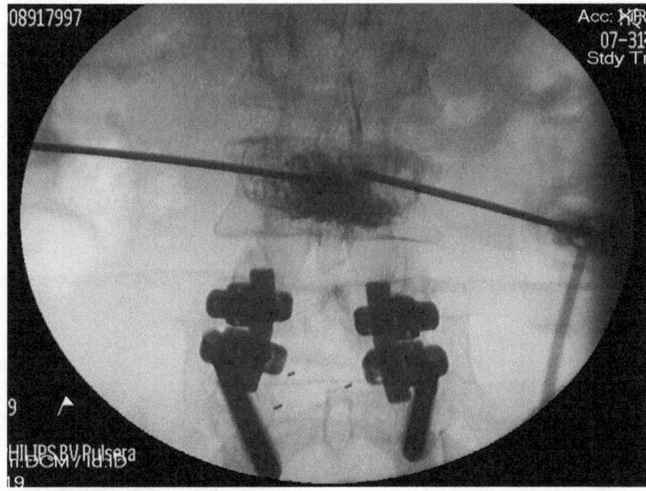

Fig. 35.3 Methyl methacrylate and barium injection using bi-pedicular approach seen under PA fluoroscopy (Photo courtesy of Kenneth D. Candido, M.D.)

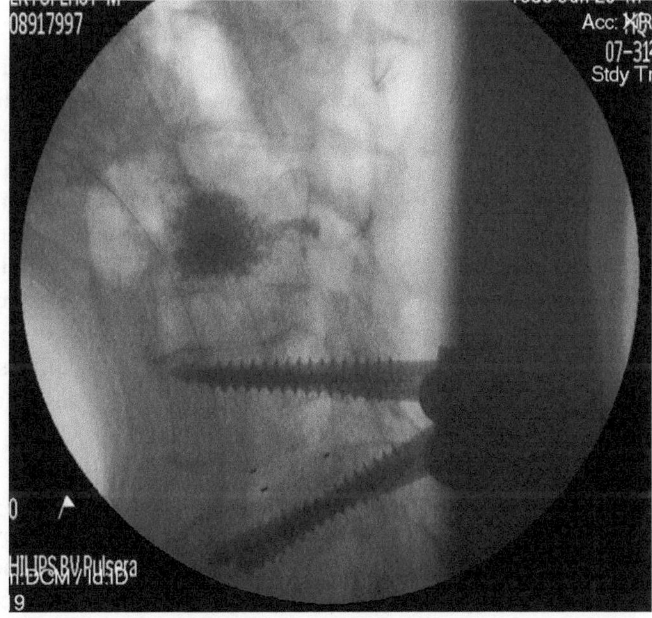

Fig. 35.4 Lateral fluoroscopic view of cement vertebroplasty (Photo courtesy of Kenneth D. Candido, M.D.)

impairment issues; bleeding diatheses or the use of anticoagulation which cannot be duly suspended for the required interval perioperatively; localized infection at the site of needle entry; and vertebral height of the targeted level <30% of neighboring contiguous segments. Additional probable contraindications include the presence of retropulsed bony fragments, which could likely rupture posteriorly into the vertebral canal with the potential for grave consequences. There is ongoing debate as to whether or not the acuity of the fracture, as determined by symptom duration and the presence of edema noted on STIR-sequenced MRI scanning, limits the utility of these therapies for individuals only in the acute phase of injury and healing.

The techniques are as follows:

- Informed consent is attained, detailing all potential risks, benefits, and alternatives to the procedure. Particular care and attention is paid to describing and defining the potential for extravasation of cement into the spinal canal

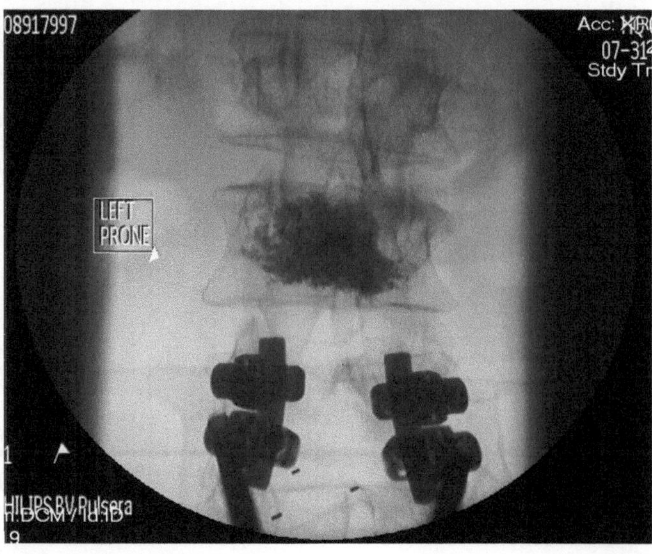

Fig. 35.5 Final PA fluoroscopic image; vertebroplasty procedure completed (Photo courtesy of Kenneth D. Candido, M.D.)

with the possibility of causing paralysis or death.

- Intravenous access is assured for providing monitored anesthesia care and for the administration of perioperative antibiotics, if indicated.
- Image guidance is mandatory, and either the use of fluoroscopy or CT scan imaging is acceptable. Biplanar fluoroscopy has been advocated for use by some, but the author typically relies upon standard fluoroscopy in his practice.
- Patient positioning and assessment of all vulnerable nerves and bony prominences are assured.
- Full surgical sterile preparation is essential, as for any operative procedure.
- Appropriate bone biopsy needles with opacified polymethyl methacrylate are used exclusively.
- The author uses a bi-pedicular approach for both vertebroplasty and for balloon kyphoplasty, as shown in Figs. 35.2, 35.3, 35.4, and 35.5 wherein a vertebroplasty procedure was performed.
- It is critical to competently identify the targeted vertebra(ae) in conjunction with a complete and thorough review of the pre-procedure MRI or CT scan which identified the fracture originally.
- The medial cortex of the pedicle(s) must be visualized during the performance of the procedure.
- A gun barrel or tunnel view using the C-arm is recommended, although some select a direct anterior-posterior view, with both medial and lateral cortices being viewed continually.
- The vertebral end plates are aligned as closely as possible, taking into consideration the effects that the VCF deformity might have on assuring this contingency.
- Using an oblique fluoroscopic view, the pedicle of the level of interest is brought into the center of the vertebral body seen under fluoroscopy.
- The needle target is approximately at the 10 o'clock position of the pedicle (for left-sided approaches) and 2 o'clock for right-sided approaches.
- The skin and subcutaneous tissues are infiltrated using local anesthesia through a small-gauge hypodermic needle.
- A small skin incision is made using a #15 blade scalpel or equivalent.
- The vertebroplasty needle is advanced until it contacts the bony periosteum. The needle is advanced into the pedicle under fluoroscopy using either a twisting motion or else using an orthopedic type of hammer with gentle and rhythmic tapping. The medial cortex of the

pedicle remains in view under fluoroscopy at all times.

- Lateral fluoroscopic imaging is essential to assure that the needle is indeed in the vertebra and is not in the intervertebral disc or encroaching upon a neural foramen. Vertebroplasty requires that the needle be advanced into the anterior one third of the vertebra, whereas kyphoplasty advancement is into the posterior one third.
- Once proper needle placement has been assured, for vertebroplasty the cement is mixed and is injected slowly, under continuous live fluoroscopy in the lateral orientation, until the fracture channel is seen to fill without any posterior extravasation toward the spinal canal and without extravasation into the vertebral end plates into the intervertebral discs.
- For kyphoplasty, a hand-operated drill is used to create a space from the posterior third of the vertebral body to the anterior one third. A deflated balloon is advanced through the cannula into the cavity and is attached to a locking syringe with a digital manometer attached.
- Slow inflation of the balloon with iodinated contrast is now undertaken. The balloon is then deflated and is removed.
- The polymethyl methacrylate is prepared (PMMA). The PMMA contains sterile barium sulfate powder for radiographic opacity. Working time from initiation of the mixture varies between about 10–20 min.
- The volume of cement injected does not correlate with success of the procedure.
- To complete the injection for vertebroplasty, the stylet of the needle must be placed into the needle to avoid tracking of cement from the lumen of the needle backward, which could cause cement leakage into the neural foramen, spinal canal, or paraspinal muscles. For kyphoplasty, PMMA is injected using a blunt cannula during live fluoroscopy. The injection is terminated when the cavities are filled, along with any potential fracture lines outside the cavity. The needle stylet is replaced under live fluoroscopy.
- Sterile Band-Aids are applied over the cannula insertion sites.
- The patient is assessed for any neurological defects or deficiencies.

Summary

The care and management of the geriatric patient in pain is often a daunting challenge. Numerous physiologic changes occur with aging, which often precludes the safe use of pharmacotherapy and which argues in favor of using longer term, interventional pain-relieving modalities. Among the more commonly encountered pain entities seen with advanced age, we have highlighted the conditions of osteoporotic compression fractures, which may be amenable to advanced interventional approaches. In the present venue, it is impossible to review every disease entity associated with aging, as the task is monumental. As the population ages and as the relative percentage of elderly patients begins to increasingly assume a greater amount of care, health-care providers will be compelled to confront the inevitable consequences of being called upon with greater frequency to provide services to this special needs group. Being armed with a thorough knowledge of the physiological trespasses of aging, the pharmacological constraints imposed by those physiological processes, and the alternative interventional therapies that exist will assuredly help improve care to this distinct patient population.

Suggested Reading

1. United Nations, Department of Economic and Social Affairs, Population Division. *World population prospects: the 2012 revision, key findings and advance tables*. Working paper no. ESA/P/WP.227; 2013.
2. Jakobsson U, Klevsgard R, Westergren A, Hallberg I. Old people in pain: a comparative study. J Pain Symptom Manag. 2003;26:625–36.
3. Weiner D, Hanlon J. Pain in nursing home residents: management strategies. Drugs Aging. 2001;18:13–29.
4. Fine P. Chronic pain management in older adults: special considerations. J Pain Symptom Manag. 2009;38:S4–14.

5. Onder G, Landi F, Fusco D, Corsonello A, Tosato M, Battaglia M, Mastropaolo S, Settanni S, Antocicco M, Lattanzio F. Recommendations to prescribe in complex older adults: results of the CRIteria to assess appropriate medication use among elderly complex patients (CRIME) project. Drugs Aging. 2014;31:33–45.
6. Bjoro K, Herr K. Assessment of pain in the nonverbal or cognitively impaired older adult. Iin Geriatr Med. 2008;24:237–62.
7. Taylor R, Pergolizzi J, Raffa R, Nalamachu S, Balestrieri P. Pain and obesity in the older adult. Curr Pharm Des. 2014;20(38):6037–41.
8. Fine P. Treatment guidelines for the pharmacological management of pain in older persons. Pain Med. 2012;13:S57–66.
9. Tucker M, Andrew M, Ogle S, Davison J. Age-associated change in pain threshold measured by transcutaneous neuronal electrical stimulation. Age Ageing. 1989;18:241–6.
10. Guyton AC, Hall JE. Textbook of medical physiology. 11th ed: Elsevier Saunders, Philadelphia; 2006.
11. Weiner D, Rudy T, Kim Y, Golla S. Do medical factors predict disability in older adults with persistent low back pain? Pain. 2004;112:214–20.
12. Weiner D, Rudy T, Morrow L, Slaboda J, Lieber S. The relationship between pain, neuropsychological performance, and physical function in community-dwelling older adults with chronic low back pain. Pain Med. 2006;7:60–70.
13. Hadjistavropoulos T, Herr K, Turk DC, Fine PG, Dworkin RH, Helme R, Jackson K, Parmelee PA, Rudy TE, Lynn Beattie B, Chibnall JT, Craig KD, Ferrell B, Ferrell B, Fillingim RB, Gagliese L, Gallagher R, Gibson SJ, Harrison EL, Katz B, Keefe FJ, Lieber SJ, Lussier D, Schmader KE, Tait RC, Weiner DK, Williams J. An interdisciplinary expert consensus statement on assessment of pain in older persons. Clin J Pain. 2007;23:S1–43.
14. Karp J, Rudy T, Weiner D. Persistent pain biases item response on the geriatric depression scale (GDS): preliminary evidence for validity of the GDS PAIN. Pain Med. 2008;9:33–43.
15. Karp J, Shega J, Morone N, Weiner D. Advances in understanding the mechanisms and management of persistent pain in older adults. Br J Anaesth. 2008;101:111–20.
16. Shega J, Weiner D, Paice J, Bilir S, Rockwood K, Herr K, Ersek M, Emanuel L, Dale W. The association between noncancer pain, cognitive impairment, and functional disability: an analysis of the Canadian study of health and aging. J Gerontol A Biol Sci Med Sci. 2010;65:880–6.
17. Morone N, Abebe K, Morrow L, Weiner D. Pain and decrease cognitive function negatively impact physical functioning in older adults with knee osteoarthritis. Pain Med. 2014;15:1481–7.
18. Karp J, Rollman B, Reynolds C 3rd, Morse J, Lotrich F, Mazumdar S, Morone N, Weiner D. Addressing both depression and pain in late life: the methodology of the ADAPT study. Pain Med. 2012;13:405–18.
19. Stein W. Pain in the nursing home. Clin Geriatr Med. 2001;17:575–94.
20. Stewart K, Challis D, Carpenter I, Dickinson E. Assessment approaches for older people receiving social care. Int J Geriatr Psychiatry. 1999;14:147–56.
21. Horgas A, Dunn K. Pain in nursing home residents. Comparison of residents' self-report and nursing assistants' perceptions. Incongruencies exist in resident and caregiver reports of pain; therefore, pain management education is needed to prevent suffering. J Gerontol Nurs. 2001;27:44–53.
22. Wandner L, Heft M, Lok B, Hirsh A, George S, Horgas A, Atchison J, Torres C, Robinson M. The impact of patients' gender, race, and age on health care professionals' pain management decisions: an online survey using virtual human technology. Int J Nurs Stud. 2014;51:726–33.
23. Horgas A, Elliott A, Marsiske M. Pain assessment in persons with dementia: relationship between self-report and behavioral observation. J Am Geriatr Soc. 2009;57:126–32.
24. Weiner D, Peterson B, Keefe F. Chronic pain-associated behaviors in the nursing home: resident versus caregiver perceptions. Pain. 1999;80:577–88.
25. Deane G, Smith H. Overview of pain management in older persons. Clin Geriatr Med. 2008;24:185–201.
26. Bruckenthal P. Assessment of pain in the elderly adult. Clin Geriatr Med. 2008;24:213–36.
27. Reyes-Gibby C, Aday L, Cleeland C. Impact of pain on self-rated health in the community-dwelling older adults. Pain. 2002;95:75–82.
28. Weiner D, Rudy T. Attitudinal barriers to effective treatment of persistent pain in nursing home residents. J Am Geriatr Soc. 2002;50:2035–40.
29. Silverman S. The clinical consequences of vertebral compression fracture. Bone. 1992;13:S27–31.
30. Ruiz Santiago F, Santiago Chinchilla A, Guzmán Álvarez L, Pérez Abela AL, Castellano García Mdel M, Pajares López M. Comparative review of vertebroplasty and kyphoplasty. World J Radiol. 2014;6:329–43.
31. Xiao H, Yang J, Feng X, Chen P, Li Y, Huang C, Liang Y, Chen H. Comparing complications of vertebroplasty and kyphoplasty for treating osteoporotic vertebral compression fractures: a meta-analysis of the randomized and non-randomized controlled studies. Eur J Orthop Surg Traumatol. 2015;25 Suppl 1:S77–85.
32. Zhang L, Gu X, Zhang H, Zhang Q, Cai X, Tao K. Unilateral or bilateral percutaneous vertebroplasty for acute osteoporotic vertebral fracture: a prospective study. J Spinal Disord Tech. 2015;28(2):E85–8.

Pain in the Critically Ill Patient

36

Chiedozie Udeh

Key Concepts

- Critically ill patients commonly experience pain. More than 70% of patients report experiencing moderate to severe pain while in the intensive care unit (ICU). Causes include preexisting chronic pain and acute postsurgical pain plus pain due to multiple ICU procedures and monitoring equipment. Anxiety will exacerbate pain in these patients.
- Pain in critically ill patients is often underappreciated and undertreated. This is due to several factors: knowledge deficits on the part of the health-care team, erroneous belief that untreated pain has insignificant consequences, and lack of a systematic multidisciplinary approach to assessment and treatment of pain in critically ill patients.
- Untreated, undertreated, or overtreated pain can have adverse consequences, including delirium, respiratory depression, somnolence, withdrawal, delayed extubation, prolonged length of stay, depression, chronic pain, and post-traumatic stress disorder.
- Patient self-reports are the most reliable and recommended approach for assessment of pain in ICU patients. The 0–10 visual support numeric rating scale (NRS-V) is the most feasible and discriminative tool for assessment of pain in cognitively intact ICU patients. Physiologic parameters are unreliable as indicators of pain in the critically ill patient and should not be used to assess presence or severity of pain.
- Critically ill patients are frequently nonverbal/noncommunicative. Therefore observational tools are needed. The critical-care pain observation tool (CPOT) is superior to other psychometric tools for the assessment of pain in nonverbal patients.
- Given the complexity of the context of care in the ICU, the goal of pain management in critically ill patients is to decrease the severity of the pain as much as is safely possible. Pain levels should be decreased to a level that is tolerable and reduces the risk of long-term consequences, but also that in the short term, pain would not preclude patients from participating in necessary activities, such as early mobilization.
- A multimodal approach to pain management is recommended. Analgesia should be provided using an integrated protocol which prioritizes analgesia over sedation. Avoid unnecessary polypharmacy so as to limit adverse effects and interactions. Monitor frequently for effectiveness and for side effects. Adjust therapy as needed based on these assessments.

C. Udeh, MBBS, MHEcon (✉)
Center for Critical Care Medicine, Anesthesiology Institute, Cleveland Clinic, Cleveland, Ohio, USA
e-mail: udehc@ccf.org

J. Cheng, R.W. Rosenquist (eds.), *Fundamentals of Pain Medicine*,
https://doi.org/10.1007/978-3-319-64922-1_36

- Pharmacological options still largely revolve around opioids because of their potency, multiple routes of administration, low cost, and relative freedom from adverse hemodynamic effects. Whenever possible, opioids should be supplemented with appropriate adjuvants such as acetaminophen, nonsteroidal anti-inflammatory drugs (NSAIDs), and neuraxial or regional nerve blocks. These are opioid sparing and help to limit side effects overall.

Epidemiology of Pain in the Critically Ill Patient

More than 70% of critically ill patients will recall experiencing pain of moderate to severe intensity during hospitalization in the intensive care unit (ICU). With approximately five million admissions to the ICU annually, this represents a very large number of patients who have been subjected to, at the very least, significant unpleasantness. Although the problem is widespread, it has been demonstrated that minorities, females, and the elderly are less likely to receive adequate pain management. Historically, pain in critically ill patients had been poorly recognized and inadequately treated for several reasons:

- Deficits of knowledge and awareness on the part of the health-care team, regarding the extent, severity, and significance of pain in the ICU
- Pervasive personal, cultural, and institutional biases
- Erroneous beliefs including the presumption that sedation can substitute for analgesia, that untreated pain is of no consequences or worse, and that pain is a necessary stimulus to maintain alertness and encourage adequate breathing in critically ill patients
- Perception that pain cannot be reliably evaluated in critically ill patients
- Lack of a systematic approach to the assessment and treatment of pain in the ICU

Recent decades have seen expanded pain research. Much of the work has not been specific to the ICU setting. Nonetheless, issues pertaining to the assessment, treatment, and consequences of pain in critically ill patients have gained more attention. Professional societies have published guidelines for the management of pain in ICU patients. Indeed some regulatory agencies consider adequacy of pain management to be one indicator of the quality of care of hospitalized patients.

Despite improvements in knowledge and awareness, significant gaps still exist in implementing best practices. In many ICUs, objective psychometric tools are still not routinely used to assess pain in noncommunicative critically ill patients. Yet recent evolution in the management of the critically ill patient calls for increased emphasis on avoidance of deep sedation, and implementation of early mobilization. This underscores the need for adequate analgesia in these patients.

Sources of Pain in the ICU

The three main sources of pain in critically ill patients are:

- Acute pain from surgery or trauma
- Pain from ICU procedures and devices
- Pre-existing chronic pain

Among surgical patients, acute postsurgical pain is a major source of pain. However even nonsurgical patients are often subjected to multiple care-related procedures including placement of vascular access catheters, drains, and monitoring devices. There is also significant pain and discomfort from being confined to bed with restricted ability to change positions and tethered to multiple devices and monitors such as endotracheal tubes, intravenous lines, suction devices, compression devices, tubes, etc.

In the older age groups that comprise a majority of critically ill patients, pre-existing chronic pain is an important but commonly overlooked source of pain. Examples include chronic back pain, degenerative arthritis pain, gout, and neuropathic pain. Affected patients have usually been on maintenance analgesics prior to their hospitalization. Consequently they often require higher-than-usual doses of medications to achieve satisfactory analgesia when they encounter additional sources of pain. Moreover, if their routine medications are not resumed, they may be at risk of withdrawal symptoms thus compounding their condition.

Consequences of Pain and Its Management in the ICU

When pain is unrecognized, untreated, or inadequately treated in critically ill patients, the immediate consequence, of course, is profound patient distress. This could manifest as:

- Sobbing, moaning, or crying out vocally, if able
- Facial expressions and movements indicating discomfort such as tears, wincing, guarding, grimacing, furrowed brows, or muscle rigidity
- Signs of restlessness, agitation, or even violent behavior such as thrashing, pulling at catheters and tubes, or even hitting caregivers
- Patient–ventilator dyssynchrony

These are some of the signs used in psychometric scales to assess pain in the ICU. In the near term, patients with inadequate analgesia could develop paranoid delusions, anxiety, and delirium. They may become uncooperative or unable to participate in their care. These result in delayed extubation, prolonged ICU length of stay (LOS), and even increased mortality.

Research has shown that when a structured approach is used to proactively assess and direct pain management in critically ill patients, there are overall reductions, and more appropriate utilization of sedatives and analgesics. The avoidance of prolonged sedation may explain the decrease in LOS and mortality. Over the long term, suboptimal treatment of pain in critically ill patients is associated with increased risk of chronic pain syndromes, anxiety episodes, depression, and even post-traumatic stress disorder.

On the other hand, treatment of pain in the critically ill could also have serious adverse consequences. Opioids in particular may cause excessive somnolence and dangerous respiratory depression. Nausea, vomiting, ileus, and constipation are also common, leading to delayed recovery of bowel function after surgery, and interference with enteral nutrition. These could be exacerbated by critical illness-associated organ dysfunction. There may also be adverse synergistic interactions with other medications. In any case, the result could also be delayed extubation, prolonged LOS, and even mortality.

Barriers to Effective Pain Management in the ICU

Barriers still exist in ensuring that critically ill patients receive adequate analgesia. Gaps in knowledge and awareness as well as myths about the consequences of inadequately treated pain still persist. These require sustained effort at education and quality improvement for the current ICU workforce. Appropriate modification of the educational curriculum will prepare future generations of health-care team to properly address this issue. Beyond these, there are additional clinical, process, and technical barriers to adequate pain management in critically ill patients. These include:

- A complex clinical context of critical illness often marked by life-threatening physiological instability that drives attention to other priorities
- Difficulty with reliable assessment of pain because these patients are often unable to communicate due to their illness, sedation, restraints, or endotracheal tubes
- Paucity of treatment options specifically suitable for critically ill patients
- Increased risk of drug interactions due to concurrent use of multiple medications
- Difficulty with analgesic dosing due to organ system dysfunction:

  - Delirium and encephalopathy may limit use of opioids.
  - Hepatic and renal dysfunction will necessitate frequent dose adjustments or even exclude use of adjuncts such as acetaminophen or NSAIDs.
  - Sepsis and coagulopathy may preclude the use of neuraxial techniques such as epidural catheters or regional nerve blocks.
- Limited access to, or impaired function of, the enteral route of administration, effectively excluding several analgesic options

Assessment of Pain in the ICU

A proactive, frequent, and regular approach is crucial in assessing pain in critically ill patients. Additionally, there should be regular reassessment for efficacy after any therapy is administered for pain. It is pertinent to note that physiologic parameters such as vital signs are unreliable as indicators of pain, especially in critically ill patients. In these patients, hemodynamic derangements are common and neutralize what little value vital signs may otherwise have as indicators of the presence and severity of pain.

Pain is a subjective experience. In conscious patients, who are able to interact with caregivers, a patient self-report is thus the preferred method of assessing pain. Even delirious patients may be able to give a useful assessment of their pain level. A number of psychometric scales have been developed to facilitate this process including:

- The visual analogue scale (horizontal or vertical orientation)
- The verbal descriptor scale
- The verbal 0–10 numeric rating scale (NRS-O)
- The 0–10 numeric rating scale with visual support (NRS-V)

Most were adapted from scales developed and validated for the non-ICU setting. When these were compared in the ICU setting, the NRS-V was the most feasible and reliable scale. Whereas the NRS-O requires the patient to verbalize the number that best characterizes the severity of their pain, the NRS-V uses a card on which the numbers 0–10 are printed in enlarged bold fonts to facilitate the use in even intubated critically ill patients.

However many critically ill patients are nonverbal and unable to meaningfully interact with caregivers. Several behavioral pain scales have been developed for use in these noncommunicative critically ill patients:

- The pain assessment and intervention notation (PAIN)
- The nonverbal pain assessment tool (NPAT)
- The adult nonverbal pain scale (NVPS)
- The behavioral pain scale (BPS)
- The critical-care pain observation tool (CPOT)

These tools require some training but are not particularly difficult to use. They involve observation of the patient by the caregiver for specific pain-induced behaviors. Consequently they do have some limitations:

- They cannot be used in patients incapable of spontaneous neuromuscular activity.
- In general, there is some ambiguity in their item descriptors.
- They lack specificity for pain – observed behaviors may indicate other than pain.

A comparison of the scales in terms of their reported reliability and validity found that the CPOT appears superior to the other scales. The CPOT assesses pain behavior in four domains: facial expressions, body movements, muscle tension in upper limbs, and patient–ventilator synchrony or vocalizations in extubated patients.

Principles of Pain Management in the ICU

1. Multidisciplinary effort of doctors, nurses and pharmacists. The team should utilize a protocolized framework for pain assessment, drug selection, and monitoring.

Analgesia should be prioritized over sedation, and active patient participation is encouraged.
2. Goals should be to reduce pain to a tolerable level, minimize side effects and drug interactions, and facilitate patient participation in their care.
3. Proactive frequent assessment for the presence, source, and severity of pain.
4. A multimodal approach is recommended: Use pharmacological and non-pharmacological therapies (when appropriate). Employ regional analgesia techniques, if feasible.
5. Consider coexistence of chronic pain and account for its effect on analgesic requirement for superimposed acute pain.
6. Confirm dosages and resume chronic pain medications and anxiolytics; select appropriate substitutes if necessary.
7. Optimize analgesia by scheduled dosing of analgesics and setting appropriate safety "hold" parameters to reduce risk of excessive sedation or respiratory depression.
8. Allow supplemental doses of analgesics for breakthrough pain and before procedures; ensure dosing instructions and parameters are clear and unambiguous.
9. Reassess frequently for positive response. Proactive monitoring for side effects and adjust pain therapies as needed.
10. Proactive prophylaxis and management of side effects; for instance, the use of laxatives for opioid-induced constipation.

Therapies for Pain in the ICU

- Pharmacological options (opioids and non-opioid medications): Cognitively intact patients should have the option of using appropriately programmed patient-controlled analgesia (PCA) pumps for medication delivery. This provides additional autonomy and is especially helpful for those who cannot vocalize because of endotracheal intubation.
- Interventional regional analgesia techniques – for instance, intrathecal, epidural, and peripheral nerve blocks.
- Non-pharmacological options – for instance, music therapy, massage, and warm or cold compresses.

Opioids These potent analgesics act on *mu* receptors in the brain and spinal cord. They are the cornerstone of analgesic therapy in critically ill patients, in part because they are inexpensive and potent, with rapid onset and multiple routes of administration. Additionally opioids have minimal adverse hemodynamic effects and neither cause nor contribute to the development of hepatic or renal dysfunction. This makes them quite useful in ICU patients who often have hemodynamic instability and are at high risk of progressive organ dysfunction. Most opioids undergo hepatic metabolism and renal excretion. Dosage adjustments are thus necessary in patients with hepatic and renal dysfunction to reduce the risk of accumulation and side effects.

Common side effects include respiratory depression, somnolence, potentiation of sedatives, nausea, vomiting, ileus, and constipation. Tolerance to the analgesic and some side effects of opioids may manifest even with short-term use; such acute tolerance seems independent of opioid potency but rather is seen more with shorter acting opioids. Dose escalation or switch to different opioid (because cross-tolerance is incomplete) can help affected patients. Opioid-induced hyperalgesia (OIH) is also a concern; unlike with tolerance, dose escalation only exacerbates the pain. There may be a role for NMDA receptor blockers in preventing or mitigating OIH. With prolonged use, physical dependence may occur, and patients could experience symptoms of withdrawal if opioids are abruptly discontinued. Characteristics of some commonly used opioids are shown in Table 36.1.

Non-opioid Analgesics These are mostly utilized as dose-sparing adjuncts to opioids, but some possess sufficient potency to be the sole analgesic for mild to moderate pain. Commonly used non-opioid analgesics are shown in Table 36.2.

Table 36.1 Commonly used opioid analgesics

Agent	Onset	$T_{1/2}$	Intermittent dosing	Infusion dose range	Side effects/ comments
Morphine (iv, infusion)	5–10 min	3–4 h	2–4 mg IV q1–2 h	0.04–0.2 mg/kg/h	Prototypical opioid. Active metabolites
Fentanyl (iv, infusion)	1–2 min	2–4 h	0.25–0.5 mcg/kg/ q0.5–1 h	0.7–10 mcg/kg/h	50–100 times as potent as morphine. Minimal hemodynamic effects. Sympatholytic at high doses. Highly lipid soluble. Context-sensitive half-time increases with prolonged infusions
Fentanyl (transdermal patch)	4–8 h	17 h	25–100 μg/h change patch q72 h	N/A	Effects may persist >24 h after patch removal due to continued absorption from drug depot in skin
Hydromorphone (iv, infusion)	5–10 min	2–3 h	0.2–0.6 mg IV q2–3 h	5–50 mcg/kg/h	5–7 times as potent as morphine
Hydromorphone (oral. rectal)	20–30 min		2–8 mg q4–6 h	N/A	
Tramadol (oral)	20	6–8	25–100 mg Q4–6 h (max 400 mg/day)	N/A	Weak mu-opioid agonist. Metabolite has more potent opioid agonist activity
Methadone (oral)	10–20 min	8–59 h	10–40 mg q 6–12 h	N/A	Used for chronic pain and opioid dependence. Risk of serotonin syndrome and neuroleptic malignant syndrome with MAOIs and SSRIs. Monitor QTc interval
Remifentanil	1 min	3–10 min	N/A	0.5–1.5 mcg/kg loading dose, then 0.03–0.2 mcg/kg/ min	Metabolized by plasma esterases. Very short $T_{1/2.}$ Risk of acute withdrawal symptoms. Relatively expensive

- Nonsteroidal anti-inflammatory drugs (NSAIDs) achieve analgesia by inhibiting peripheral synthesis of prostaglandins. Their use in critically ill patients is limited by side effects – gastric mucosal ulceration, renal dysfunction, and possibly platelet dysfunction. Ketorolac is one of the most commonly used NSAIDs for analgesia in the ICU patient because it is available in parenteral form.
- Acetaminophen is thought to inhibit prostaglandins synthesis in the central nervous system. Until the year 2000, only enteral

Table 36.2 Commonly used non-opioid analgesics

Agent	Onset	$T_{1/2}$ (h)	Dose	Side effects/comments
Acetaminophen (oral/rectal)	15–30 min	2	325–650 mg q4–6 h (max dose 4 g/day)	Few side effects; hepatotoxic if daily limit exceeded; IV acetaminophen is relatively expensive
Acetaminophen (IV)	5–10 min	2–4	650 mg q4 h 1000 mg q6 h (max dose 4 g/day)	
Ketorolac (IV/IM)	20–30 min	2.4–8.6	15–30 mg q 6 h (max duration – 5 days)	Caution in ischemic heart disease; 90% renal excretion; lower doses in older patients and renal disease
Ketamine (IV infusion)	1–2 min	2–3	0.1–0.5 mg/kg (optional loading dose), then 0.05–0.4 mg/kg/h	Counteracts opioid-induced hyperalgesia. Dysphoria with higher doses
Dexmedetomidine (IV infusion)	5–10 min	2	1 mcg/kg (optional loading dose), then 0.2–0.7 mcg/kg/h	FDA-approved use – max 24 h; severe bradycardia and hypotension may occur; relatively expensive
Gabapentin (oral)	2–3 h	5–7	Starting dose –100 mg q8 h (max dose 5 mg/kg q8 h)	Indicated for neuropathic pain may cause drowsiness. Abrupt discontinuation may precipitate seizures. 100% renal excretion (unchanged)
Lidocaine (transdermal patch)	2–3 h	6–8	5% lidocaine patches apply 1–2 patches to painful site (max 3 patches simultaneously)	Change patches every 8–12 h; less than 5% systemic absorption; FDA approved for post-herpetic neuralgia
Lidocaine (IV infusion)	10–15 min	1.5–3.0	1.5 mg/kg (optional loading dose), then 1–2 mg/kg/h	Useful in neuropathic pain; use only in monitored settings; high levels may induce seizures or cardiac arrest – check serum levels daily

formulations were available. Given variable absorption and extensive first-pass hepatic metabolism, its analgesic effects are mild. Intravenous acetaminophen rapidly achieves higher plasma concentrations and provides modest analgesic effects. Due to the risk of hepatic injury, the maximum daily dose of acetaminophen is 4 g/day (less or even none, if hepatic dysfunction already exists). Oral acetaminophen is widely used in fixed dose combination pills with various opioids. This must be accounted for, so as not to exceed the daily limit.

- Gabapentin is a structural analogue of gamma-aminobutyric acid (GABA) but does not appear to mediate its analgesic effects via GABA receptors. It is an antiepileptic with modest analgesic benefit particularly in neuropathic pain. It is administered orally and dosage adjustments have to be done slowly to limit sedation.
- Ketamine is a phencyclidine derivative and acts centrally on the N-methyl-D-aspartate (NMDA) receptor. It is a potent anesthetic, but in lower doses, it provides superior analgesia without respiratory or hemodynamic depression. It is very useful in patients undergoing periodic painful procedures in the ICU such as painful dressing changes. Ketamine prevents and can reverse opioid-induced hyperalgesia

and tolerance; it is thus also useful in patients who chronically use or abuse opioids, for whom achieving adequate analgesia after surgery can be difficult.

- Dexmedetomidine is a central α2 adrenoceptor agonist used primarily for sedation. It has modest analgesic effect without respiratory depression. This makes it a useful adjunct for procedures in the ICU. Severe bradycardia and hypotension may occur so it is currently only FDA approved for maximum 24 h duration.
- Lidocaine is an amide local anesthetic with hepatic metabolism. It is often used as an antiarrhythmic agent in the ICU. Lidocaine infusions can provide modest systemic analgesia, but the need for continuous hemodynamic monitoring and checking of serum levels of lidocaine are important limitations. Transdermal lidocaine patches are available and can be useful for focal sources of pain, such as incision sites or around chest tubes insertion sites.

Interventional Regional Analgesia Techniques These include the use of intrathecal, epidural, peripheral nerve, and peri-incisional nerve blocks with local anesthetics either as a single injection or continuously via a catheter. Patient controlled pumps can be used with these catheters to provide supplemental boluses of local anesthetics for breakthrough pain. The quality of analgesia is generally superior to intravenous analgesics particularly in high-risk patients undergoing major thoracic, abdominal, or extremity surgeries.

Systemic effects of regional analgesia are minimized because the agents are delivered directly in the vicinity of the nerves. Central neuraxial blocks (intrathecal and more commonly epidural catheters) typically utilize a mixture of a low-dose opioid (e.g., fentanyl) plus a low concentration of local anesthetic (e.g., 0.0625–0.1% bupivacaine). This helps minimize the occurrence of hypotension from the sympatholytic effect of the local anesthetics. Coagulopathy, local or systemic infection, and the need for block placement by anesthesiologists are the common obstacles to wider use of these techniques.

Non-pharmacological Therapies There is a wide variety of non-pharmacological interventions for pain that have been described. The more common ones include the use of music therapy, focal massage, and hot or cold compresses. Their precise role in pain management in the ICU remains undefined, and supportive evidence for their efficacy is sparse. Some, like music therapy, seems to help distract patients and help them cope with their pain. In general, they are relatively inexpensive, and their use is acceptable if the patient finds it beneficial.

Patient Monitoring

Careful monitoring is required for safety and to ensure adequacy of analgesia. Caregivers should look for side effects, toxicity, and drug interactions. Focused clinical examination, sedation, and delirium scales should be used to assess level of sedation and mental status. There should be routine monitoring of respiratory rate, peripheral oxygen saturation and blood pressure, and end-tidal carbon dioxide (in intubated patients). It has been proposed that capnography should also be used in non-intubated patients receiving opioids; however, this is not yet widely accepted partly because of reliability concerns with the devices currently available.

Suggested Reading

1. Barr J, Fraser GL, Puntillo K, Ely EW, Gelinas C, Dasta JF, et al. Clinical practice guidelines for the management of pain, agitation, and delirium in adult patients in the intensive care unit. Crit Care Med. 2013;41(1):263–306.
2. Chanques G, Jaber S, Barbotte E, Violet S, Sebbane M, Perrigault PF, et al. Impact of systematic evaluation of pain and agitation in an intensive care unit. Crit Care Med. 2006;34(6):1691–9.
3. Chanques G, Viel E, Constantin JM, Jung B, de Lattre S, Carr J, et al. The measurement of pain in intensive care unit: comparison of 5 self-report intensity scales. Pain. 2010;151(3):711–21.

4. Erstad BL, Puntillo K, Gilbert HC, Grap MJ, Li D, Medina J, et al. Pain management principles in the critically ill. Chest. 2009;135(4):1075–86.
5. Gelinas C, Fillion L, Puntillo KA, Viens C, Fortier M. Validation of the critical-care pain observation tool in adult patients. Am J Crit Care. 2006;15(4):420–7.
6. Haslam L, Dale C, Knechtel L, Rose L. Pain descriptors for critically ill patients unable to self-report. J Adv Nurs. 2012;68(5):1082–9.
7. Lee M, Silverman S, Hansen H, et al. A comprehensive review of opioid induced hyperalgesia. Pain Physician. 2011;14:145–61.
8. Pasero C, Puntillo K, Li D, Mularski RA, Grap MJ, Erstad BL, et al. Structured approaches to pain management in the ICU. Chest. 2009;135(6):1665–72.
9. Puntillo K, Pasero C, Li D, Mularski RA, Grap MJ, Erstad BL, et al. Evaluation of pain in ICU patients. Chest. 2009;135(4):1069–74.
10. Rose L, Smith O, Gelinas C, Haslam L, Dale C, Luk E, et al. Critical care nurses' pain assessment and management practices: a survey in Canada. Am J Crit Care. 2012;21(4):251–9.
11. Sessler CN, Varney K. Patient-focused sedation and analgesia in the ICU. Chest. 2008;133(2):552–65.
12. Skrobik Y, Ahern S, Leblanc M, et al. Protocolized intensive care unit management of analgesia, sedation, and delirium improves analgesia and subsyndromal delirium rates. Anesth Analg. 2010;111(2):451–63.
13. Stites M. Observational pain scales in critically ill adults. Crit Care Nurse. 2013;33(3):68–78.

Index

J. Cheng, R.W. Rosenquist (eds.), *Fundamentals of Pain Medicine*,
https://doi.org/10.1007/978-3-319-64922-1

I

J

K

L